Research Methods
in
Clinical Oncology

Research Methods in Clinical Oncology

Brigid G. Leventhal, M.D.
Associate Professor
Oncology and Pediatrics
Johns Hopkins Hospital
Baltimore, Maryland

Robert E. Wittes, M.D.
Associate Director for Cancer Therapy Evaluation
Division of Cancer Treatment
National Cancer Institute
Bethesda, Maryland

Raven Press New York

Raven Press, 1185 Avenue of the Americas, New York, New York 10036

Made in the United States of America

Library of Congress Cataloging-in-Publication Data

Leventhal, Brigid G.
  Research methods in clinical oncology.

  Includes bibliographies and index.
  1. Cancer—Chemotherapy—Evaluation.   2. Antineoplastic agents—
Testing.   3. Clinical trials.
I. Wittes, Robert E.   II. Title.   [DNLM: 1. Clinical
Trials.   2. Neoplasms—drug therapy.   3. Neoplasms—
therapy.   4. Research Design. QZ 267 L657r]

RC271.C5L465   1988   616.99'4061'0724   85-43225
ISBN 0-88167-382-X

The material contained in this volume was submitted as previously unpublished material, except in the instances in which credit has been given to the source from which some of the illustrative material was derived.

Great care has been taken to maintain the accuracy of the information contained in the volume. However, neither Raven Press nor the authors can be held responsible for errors or for any consequences arising from the use of the information contained herein.

Materials appearing in this book prepared by individuals as part of their official duties as U.S. Government employees are not covered by the above-mentioned copyright.

9 8 7 6 5 4 3 2 1

Preface

This volume is intended as a short introductory textbook in clinical investigation in cancer treatment for those who are beginning their training in clinical oncology. We expect that even seasoned cancer clinicians may also find in it something of value.

The first few chapters of this book discuss how to make measurements. We then describe Phase I, II, and III trials. In Phase I, the nature of the agent's toxicity in man is established and a dose selected for future efficacy trials. The agent might be a drug, a biologic, or a new energy source for radiation therapy. During Phase II, the agent is tested against a spectrum of tumors in patients to determine whether it has clinical activity. A relatively small number of patients may be accrued in the initial stages of Phase II to give an estimate of activity, but if some activity is seen a larger number of patients will have to be studied to estimate response rates with reasonable precision. Phase III trials are comparative and assess the potential role of the new agent in the management of the disease. This question obviously must be answered about all treatments before they are accepted as standard.

We have attempted to make the discussion of the phases of development of a new agent relevant to modalities other than just chemotherapy, although the bulk of the discussion is most directly applicable to drugs. Chapters dealing with special problems of combination therapy, combined modality therapy, and biologic response modifiers are included. Next we describe how to plan a formal experiment (i.e., write a protocol). Because our experimentation involves human beings, certain issues of informed consent and regulatory requirements must be considered, in addition to scientific and medical ones. A concluding chapter describes what should be included in a report of a clinical trial. Even if the reader does not plan a clinical experiment, a more critical approach to the literature will allow him or her to face individual decision making in clinical medicine with greater confidence.

This book, then, is addressed to the clinician who is hoping to carry out clinical cancer trials or at least to understand the principal issues involved therein. While a few of the simpler techniques are described in detail, it is not intended as a statistical treatise. We hope to help the investigator steer a path between overenthusiastic adoption of an insufficiently tested new therapy and the overly pessimistic rejection of an approach that might, in fact, make a significant impact on survival even without curing the majority of patients.

Brigid G. Leventhal
Robert E. Wittes

Acknowledgments

The authors are grateful to Michael Kastan, M.D., Roy Beveridge, M.D., and Carl Leventhal, M.D., for their review of the manuscript. They also appreciate the suggestions of Larry Rubinstein, Ph.D., Stuart Grossman, M .D., Albert H. Owens, Jr., M.D., and Martin Abeloff, M.D. Secretarial assistance by Ms. Joan Bennett and Ms. Michele Heffler is also gratefully acknowledged.

Contents

CHAPTER 1

Introduction

At around the time of Sir William Osler there began a long period of therapeutic nihilism, and it came to a close with the introduction of penicillin. Since the 1940s medicine has been undergoing transformation from an art, as it was earlier termed, to a mixture of science and technology (1).

Lewis Thomas
1977

Over the past 50 years the practice of medicine has changed dramatically. Some new treatments, such as penicillin, have had such a convincing therapeutic impact that physicians could easily see their beneficial effect. But many useful advances in medicine may not produce similarly dramatic clinical results at first, and not all results that initially seem to be dramatic are sustained and reproducible. It therefore behooves all physicians to have some understanding of how advances in therapy are assessed. This book will discuss how to evaluate reliably the effects of treatment.

For many years surgery and radiotherapy were the only available treatments for cancer. Since few therapeutic options existed for a given clinical circumstance, there was little need to compare therapies. Twenty to thirty years ago, however, reports of potentially curative chemotherapy for disseminated cancer began to appear. Tumors such as choriocarcinoma, acute lymphatic leukemia, and Hodgkin's disease were all found to respond to more than one chemotherapeutic agent and it suddenly became necessary to ask comparative questions: Is agent A better than B for a particular tumor? Is a combination of A + B better than either agent alone? The evolution of new treatments required the development of techniques for measurement and for data analysis as well. The same methodology used to evaluate new drugs can be used, for example, to ask whether radiotherapy can replace radical surgery for the control of local breast cancer. Many of the statistical methods described in this book were developed only after 1960 in response to the need to establish ways of demonstrating that modest differences in response are, in fact, real. Such a demonstration may indicate productive new paths toward major advances in cancer treatment. Most treatments are not universally effective in reversing the course of disease but nonetheless may represent a significant step in the development of highly effective therapy, as was true with single drugs in the treatment of Hodgkin's disease and acute leukemia before the development of combinations. New single agents will have their toxicity evaluated in Phase I (see Chapter 4) and be studied for activity Phase II (see Chapter 5), but the real estimation of efficacy comes during controlled trials in Phase III (Table 1.1).

Controlled clinical trials are necessary to detect small advances in treatment, but even with dramatic advances a controlled clinical trial is usually the best way to prove definitively that a particular treatment represents improvement. The prolonged 10-year debate about the potential effect of postoperative adjuvant chemotherapy in osteosarcoma (2), which was finally answered in a controlled trial with 18 patients in each arm (3) after hundreds had been treated in an uncontrolled fashion, is an example. Thomas (1) asserts the value of such trials in his statement that ''Hunches and intuitive impressions are essential for getting the work started, but it is only through the quality of the numbers at the end that the truth can be told.''

Medical school curricula give little emphasis to the teaching of clinical trials methodology. Bernard Fisher (4) has asserted that the philosophy behind the clinical training of medical students is antithetical to the process, since training emphasizes individual decision making in each clinical situation. In advocating that the advancement of the science of medicine requires properly conducted clinical trials, Fisher goes on to say that ''just as sterile technique becomes a way of life for surgeons, so must all physicians be indoctrinated with the clinical trial mechanism so that it too becomes an integral part of their professional activities.''

All physicians should understand the nature of the clinical trial, not only those who participate in them but also those who must interpret the work of others and make decisions about current best therapy for their patient. If one does not understand how a clinical trial should be conducted, then one cannot really evaluate the results of a trial conducted by someone else. Roy (5) points out that the concept of ''physician versus clinical investigator'' as a polarized relationship is antithetical to the conduct of reasonable ethical discourse on the subject of clinical trials:

> A physician's moral obligation to offer each patient the best available treatment cannot be separated from the twin clinical and ethical imperatives to base that choice of treatment on the best available and obtainable evidence. The tension between the interdependent responsibilities of giving personal and compassionate care, as well as scientifically sound and validated treatment, is intrinsic to the practice of medicine

TABLE 1.1. *Phases of development of a new treatment*

Phase I: Agents selected for evaluation in man on the basis of broad activity in preclinical screens are tested in humans so that the toxicity in man can be established and the MTD[a] can be established. The procedures are described in Chapter 4.
Phase II: Drugs are tested in the appropriate number of patients with measurable disease and with specific diagnoses to determine whether or not a drug has activity against a particular tumor type. Generally, the tests are performed at doses that are about 80% of the MTD. The specific methodology is described in Chapter 5.
Phase III: The therapy is tested in a way that provides a quantitative estimate of the contribution it might make to the treatment of a particular disease. In general, this will involve comparative trials of the agent, described in Chapters 6 and 7.

---

[a]MTD, maximum tolerated dose.

today. . . . Controlled clinical trials—randomized when randomization is feasible, ethically achievable, and scientifically appropriate—are an integral part of the ethical imperative that physicians should know what they are doing when they intervene into the bodies, psyches, and biographies of vulnerable, suffering human beings.

A different description of the importance of good clinical research from the point of view of the medical oncologist was given by Yarbro (6), who laments the decrease in research emphasis in the training of medical oncology fellows:

There is so little that we have to offer so many of our patients that we tend to develop a sense of helplessness unless we are regularly involved in research projects that at least seem to offer hope for the future. . . . Research is not just a luxury for (oncologists), it may be a necessity to preserve our mental health.

If indeed research is necessary to our mental health, then it will only benefit us if it is properly done, because only under these circumstances does it provide new knowledge. Improperly conducted and/or interpreted trials produce confusion about what the physician should do for his patient and in that sense are part of the problem, not part of the solution.

REFERENCES

1. Thomas, L. (1977): Editorial. *Science*, 198.
2. Carter, S. K. (1984): Adjuvant chemotherapy in osteogenic sarcoma: The triumph that isn't? *J. Clin. Oncol.*, 2:147–148.
3. Link, M. P., Goorin, A. M., Miser, A. W., et al. (1986): The effect of adjuvant chemotherapy on relapse-free survival in patients with osteosarcoma of the extremity. *N. Engl. J. Med.*, 314:1600–1606.
4. Fisher, B. (1984): Clinical trials for the evaluation of cancer therapy. *Cancer, 54(Suppl.)*:2609–2617.
5. Roy, D. J. (1986): Controlled clinical trials: An ethical imperative. *J. Chronic. Dis.*, 39:159–162.
6. Yarbro, J. (1985): Quo vadis? *Semin. Oncol.*, 12:199–200.

CHAPTER 2

Quantitation

In any experiment accurate measurements are a necessity. In the laboratory the need for meticulous technique, pure reagents, accurate measurement, and sufficiently sensitive instrumentation has long been appreciated. In the same way, clinical endpoints must be accurately and reproducibly assessed. Precise and reproducible measurement is always to be preferred; in order to make some measurements maximally informative, it may be necessary to develop sensible semiquantitative scales to evaluate certain variables. This chapter considers some of the aims and pitfalls in making some common measurements in cancer therapy trials.

GENERAL PRINCIPLES

As in laboratory work, the key endpoints should be decided on before the study begins and should be specified in the protocol document, along with a clear description of how the endpoints are to be assessed and with what frequency. The endpoints that are appropriate for a specific clinical trial depend on the nature of the experiment. Dose-finding studies (Phase I) emphasize the determination of a maximally tolerated dose of an agent. Studies that seek to determine activity against particular tumor types (Phase II) require the measurement of tumor regression rates and durations. Comparative trials of different therapies (Phase III) generally focus on survival or progression-free interval, or various measures of symptom reduction and quality of life. Whatever one measures, however, certain general characteristics of the data-gathering process are particularly important. Standard techniques for staging, scales for response, and toxicity assessment should be employed and clearly described or referenced in the publication. Utilization of common criteria greatly facilitates comparison of results across studies and this makes the results easier to interpret. The research record, which includes flow sheets and on-study and off-study forms, must contain unambiguous and accurate measurements or description of all endpoints of interest at each designated time point. Whenever possible, measurements that are inherently rather imprecise or may involve a subjective component (e.g., tumor regression or assessment of performance status) should be performed by more than one observer. Radiographs and computerized tomography (CT) scans should, ideally, be submitted to a central panel for review. It should be stressed that the new imaging technology, involving digitized images from CT, magnetic resonance imaging (MRI) and radionuclide scans, will soon make possible much more satisfactory quantitative volumetric measures of tumor mass. Many of the problems discussed later in this chapter will then become as irrelevant to clinical research as a new design for a covered wagon would be to current transcontinental travel. Measurement techniques should not be changed in midstudy, however, no matter how much technology has improved. Certainly, the best diagnostic techniques should be used for optimal patient management, but the tests considered standard at the beginning of treatment should also be continued so that all patients in a trial are assessed in comparable fashion. In addition, in a comparative study, the intervals at which measurements are performed must be the same for both groups of patients. All actual measurements must be recorded so that, for example, if staging classifications change, it will be possible to reclassify patients retrospectively.

ASSESSMENT OF TUMOR SHRINKAGE

Since the aim of anticancer therapy is elimination of malignant cells from the host, reduction in a patient's tumor burden as a result of therapy would seem to be an obvious and sensible measure of treatment effect. Observable tumors are heterogeneous collections of cells, and successful antitumor therapy aims to destroy the stem cells that are capable of dividing and producing more malignant cells. Unhappily, we have no way of measuring this effect directly. We can, however, attempt to assess treatment activity by observing the relative extent of disease before and after institution of treatment.

MEASURABLE VERSUS EVALUABLE DISEASE

For most solid tumors, response assessment relies chiefly on some estimation of the extent to which therapy has reduced the patient's disease. In the context of experimental drug trials, one wishes to be as precise as possible about the nature of the treatment effect. For this reason it is often useful to distinguish between measurable and evaluable disease. As most investigators use these terms, ''measurable'' disease refers to tumors whose dimensions can be defined with reasonable accuracy in at least two dimensions. This usually requires that the disease be present as a mass that can be palpated or visualized either directly or by radiologic techniques. In contrast, ''evaluable'' disease has dimensions that cannot be precisely determined. Lymphangitic pulmonary metastases, multiple metastases to bone, miliary disease on serosal surfaces with or without effusions, and meningeal carcinomatosis are all examples of involvement that is evaluable rather than measurable. Figure 2.1 is an example of dramatic regression of a pleural effusion on radiograph, but the effusion is not the tumor, and so this change cannot be considered a measurable response. If a different technique had been used (e.g., CT scan) the mediastinal disease in this patient might have been measurable.

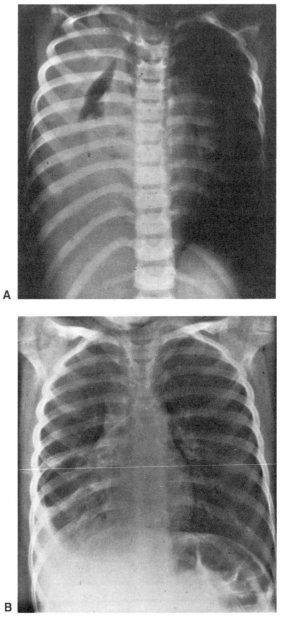

FIG. 2.1.   Chest radiographs before (**A**) and after (**B**) chemotherapy in a patient with me-diastinal and pleural disease. This patient had dramatic shrinkage in the size of her large pleural effusion, but this does not represent a measurable reduction in disease.

Laboratory studies of organ function do not measure the extent of tumor in that particular organ. In addition, although certain tumor markers such as carcinoembryonic antigen or alpha fetoprotein may be useful as general indicators of tumor status, they are not generally considered evidence of measurable disease. The heterogeneity within a tumor is such that one cannot be sure that all tumor cells are in fact making the marker, so even a negative result in a patient who was previously positive may not be strong evidence of the absence of tumor. There are certainly exceptions to this generalization with regard to particular tumors, such as gestational choriocarcinoma (1).

Certain tumors may be measured with relative precision both at the time of diagnosis and subsequent to it. Others, however, which are measured relatively easily at the time of presentation, may be difficult to measure when one is trying to determine response. It bears repeating that a partial response cannot be defined unless disease is both initially and subsequently measurable.

MEASUREMENT OF MEASURABLE DISEASE

Although they are easier to quantify than "evaluable" disease, measurable tumors still present certain problems in evaluation. Many currently available techniques give only a two-dimensional representation of a three-dimensional object. The limits of a lesion are often difficult to define, particularly when they overlie normal structures. Moreover, many techniques measure something quite different from tumor size. A CT scan of the brain with contrast will measure vascularity in the tumor and the surrounding peritumoral edema, which may vary independently of tumor size from patient to patient. Assays that depend on a metabolic function of the tumor, such as the ability of a labeled antibody to adhere to a cell making a tumor marker, or the uptake of a scanning isotope by a cell, may not be absolutely tumor specific. In addition, tumor cells may be extremely heterogeneous in their expression of the marker.

Problems that apply to the assessment of a change in the extent of a tumor include the fact that current diagnostic studies are not performed in a precisely reproducible fashion. For example, the interval between sections on a CT scan may be 10 mm in one study and 8 mm in another, and so a small lesion that appears on a follow-up study may merely have been missed initially. Certain studies may never return to a normal baseline, as in the case of a collapsed vertebra that does not remodel itself. In addition, certain studies may be more sensitive than others to a particular change in clinical status. Bone scans, for example, are more sensitive than plain films for the detection of new skeletal lesions, while radiographs may give a more complete picture of large bony lesions, at least in some cancers. Treatment and other factors may affect the appearance of repeat diagnostic studies; radiotherapy to an intrathoracic tumor mass may have a profound effect on the radiological appearance of the surrounding normal lung. Finally, although response assessment should involve repetition of all initial baseline studies, certain procedures, particularly invasive ones, cannot always be repeated to assess disease response.

PHYSICAL EXAMINATION OF PALPABLE MASSES

Several studies using simulated tumors have assessed the variation in the repeated measurement of a single object by one observer and the variation of measurement from one experienced observer to another. One such study is summarized in Table 2.1. The investigators used solid spheres of known dimensions and of various materials, placed under cover of foam rubber or a blanket in a random fashion. In general, the variation in size with repeated measurements by the same investigator is about 15% of the size of the object, and the interobserver variation is 20–30% (2–4). Despite this inaccuracy, however, it is still a good idea to attempt to measure palpable lesions in their maximal diameter with a calipers or a ruler and then measure the perpendicular diameter to get an estimate of tumor size. Since the error rate in assessing response decreases as the size or number of the assessed lesions increases (2), one should pick more than one signal lesion in a patient who has many (e.g., multiple enlarged lymph nodes in a patient with lymphoma). It also seems obvious that one should not define response as a change in size that appears to be within the error of the measurement.

Warr et al. (2) (Table 2.1) also assessed the reproducibility of the measurement of the extension of the liver edge below the costal margin at the midclavicular line. They studied 15 patients whose liver edges were palpated by several investigators at least 5 cm below the costal margin. A 30% decrease in liver size was felt to be the smallest shrinkage that could be reliably detected.

TABLE 2.1. *Range of measurements of standard masses*

Measurement	Percent false categorization		
	PR	PR + MR	Progression
Simulated nodules (1.0–2.6 cm)	12.6	31.0	34.3
Simulated nodules (3.2–6.5 cm)	1.3	19.7	24.0
Neck nodes	13.1	32.1	33.4
Lung metastases (CXR)	0.8	11.2	15.9
Liver size	(A) 8.5		28.7
	(B) 18.4		

NOTE. PR was a > 50% decrease in area, PR + MR was a > 25% decrease in area, and progression was > 25% increase in area except for the liver size. For liver size, PR was defined as > 50% decrease (A), or > 30% decrease (B), in the sum of the linear measurements of the liver edge below the costal margin in the midline and MCL; progression was defined as > 25% increase in the same measurement.
Reproduced from Ref. 2.

RADIOGRAPHIC METHODS OF MEASURING DISEASE

These techniques illustrate most clearly the problems involved in two-dimensional measurement of a three-dimensional lesion, in distinguishing tumor from normal structures, and in diagnostic sensitivity with improving technology. Warr et al. (2) assessed the ability of physicians to measure the same pulmonary nodules reproducibly on chest X-ray. Only discrete lesions were measured; nodules were excluded if there was adjacent pneumonitis or if they overlapped the hilum, cardiac silhouette, diaphragm, chest wall, or other lesions. A total of 37 lesions were chosen for assessment on 17 films. Each of eight physicians measured the maximum and greatest perpendicular diameter of marked lesions on three occasions at least 1 week apart. There was a false categorization of partial response 0.8% of the time on duplicate measures, and a false assessment of progression 16% of the time.

Despite the problems cited above, parenchymal lesions are easier to measure than lesions that abut on normal structures. In patients with small cell lung cancer, Chak et al. (5) compared the accuracy of the chest X-ray taken no more than 30 days before death with autopsy findings, and demonstrated the frequency of unsuspected involvement of hilar nodes (Table 2.2).

The accuracy of detecting both the nature and number of sites of involvement in the chest is greatly enhanced by CT scanning. Rostock et al. (6) studied thoracic CT scans on 42 newly diagnosed patients with Hodgkin's disease and found that 5 of 10 patients with negative chest X-rays had CT scans showing anterior mediastinal disease. Of the remaining 32 patients, 17 demonstrated extensive pericardial or chest wall invasion which led to alteration of their therapy; 2 additional patients had a retrocardiac mass (1) and pulmonary parenchymal involvement (1) not detected on chest X-ray. In all, more than half of the patients had their treatment changed because of the CT scan findings. Thus, CT scan does increase the sensitivity of detection of thoracic disease.

The obvious consequence of this increased sensitivity is an increase in false positives with the use of CT. In looking at the lungs to detect small metastases of

TABLE 2.2. *Comparison of chest X-ray and postmortem findings in small cell lung cancer*

Site	Radiographic findings	Autopsy[a]	
		Abnormal	Normal
Lung parenchyma	Abnormal	24	2
	Normal	5	7
Hilar nodes	Abnormal	3	2
	Normal	19	14

[a]Abnormal, small cell carcinoma; Normal, no small cell carcinoma.
From Ref. 5.

osteogenic sarcoma in newly diagnosed patients at the National Cancer Institute, the results shown in Table 2.3 were obtained (7). CT defined almost three times as many nodules as conventional radiographs. These additional nodules were usually pleural or subpleural and 3–6 mm in diameter, but 60% of the additional nodules defined by CT and resected proved to be benign granulomas or pleural-based nodes at thoracotomy. It is not surprising that with an increase in sensitivity there was a decrease in specificity, particularly during the early evolution of expertise with a new technique. As experience with CT scanning increases, these false-positive calls should decrease. It is important to remember how large the subjective component is in the interpretation of many of these studies, particularly in borderline cases.

CT scans, if properly analyzed, can in fact produce a three-dimensional assessment of organ or tumor size. In measuring total organ volume of liver, spleen, and kidneys with CT scans at postmortem, Heymsfeld et al. (8) reported the accuracy to be ± 5%. Significant quantitative improvement in the measurement techniques for repeat studies will require increased standardization of the way in which the technique is applied. For example, to measure changes in the size of a brain tumor from one scan to the next, all procedural variables must be held constant, i.e., the same amount of contrast must be given during each procedure, the same distance maintained between cuts, the patient's head held at the same angle, and the steroid dose remain unchanged.

In a study of 33 patients with hepatoma, Ettinger et al. (9) performed a volumetric analysis of tumor size. Examinations were performed on a whole-body scanner at contiguous 8-mm intervals, using a standard slice thickness and scan time. Normal and tumor-bearing regions of interest were contoured manually in each CT slice. Then the entire sequence of each patient's CT slices were digitized on a minicomputer. The tumor volume determinations made by these methods were reproducible to ± 10%. Such techniques allow one to measure both the size of the liver and the amount of tumor within it to a degree of accuracy not possible with physical examination alone.

MRI has the advantages of not requiring contrast and not exposing the patient to radiation, and is replacing CT scanning in the evaluation of some anatomic sites. The same considerations concerning the importance of standardizing the measurements apply.

TABLE 2.3. *Comparison of conventional and computed tomographs in detecting pulmonary metastases*

	No. nodules		Metastases	
	Seen	Resected	No.	%
Chest X-ray	21	21	19	90
Computed tomography	69	47	31	66

From Ref. 7.

RADIOISOTOPIC SCANNING

These studies are not as easily quantified as the physical or radiographic measurements, since most of them depend on a metabolic function of the tumor cell or the reactive tissue around it. In addition, clinically useful techniques for quantitating the extent of involvement have not been available. Still, for diseases that consistently provoke a blastic reaction in surrounding bone, the ^{99}Te diphosphonate bone scan is the best way to screen for metastatic disease. In a study of 34 women with osseous metastases from breast cancer, the bone scan was found to be a more accurate and sensitive indicator of the status of bone metastases than the radiograph (10). With the use of a digital model, the investigators were able to measure accurately the area of skeletal involvement with serial bone scans, and they considered this the optimal technique to assess the response of bone metastases in this disease. The findings in the radiographs generally appeared later than those in the bone scan.

In multiple myeloma, however, a disease with a largely osteolytic pattern of bony involvement, radionuclide imaging appears to underestimate the extent of radiographically evident disease about one-third of the time (11). On the basis of a limited number of serial images, Woolfenden et al. (11) have postulated a transition with increasing lesion size from (a) abnormal scintigram + normal radiograph to (b) abnormal scintigram + abnormal radiograph, and finally to (c) normal scintigram + abnormal radiograph, implying that the more extensive the bony destruction the *less* likely the lesion was to be detected on bone scan.

One must always keep in mind the possible effect of prior therapy on the diagnostic technique itself. In the case of bone scans, radiotherapy often results in localized and permanent depression in the uptake of bone-seeking radionuclide because of localized decrease of blood flow and degeneration of the microvasculature (12). Thus, if disease spreads to a previously irradiated area, it may not be detected.

The performance of one diagnostic test may interfere with another. Gallium scan detects leukocytes in inflammatory sites as well as those activated as part of a malignant lymphoma. If a normal cell has been exposed to an inflammatory stimulus, such as the dye used in lymphangiograms, then it will be rendered gallium-avid. Thus, there is little utility to a gallium scan in screening for lymphoma in a patient who has recently had a lymphangiogram.

DEFINITION OF RESPONSE

Response is assessed by comparing the extent of a patient's disease after a certain amount of therapy with the baseline pretreatment status. For this comparison to reflect the effect of treatment accurately, the baseline measurements should have been taken just before the start of therapy. Utilizing baseline measurements that reflect tumor status weeks prior to treatment may well result in an underestimation of therapeutic effect.

To measure masses one takes the greatest diameter and then the largest diameter perpendicular to the first. The response criteria currently in common use depend on a comparison of the sum of the products of the two perpendicular diameters of all, or a representative selection of, measured lesions before and after treatment. The sum of the products can be denoted by S. Complete response represents a fall of S to 0, while partial response represents a fall in S to less than 50% of pretreatment baseline (Table 2.4).

Note that this response scale considers only objective shrinkage of tumor masses; subjective improvement, relief of troublesome symptoms, and increase in performance status do not count in evaluation of response status. Note also that the calculation of tumor burden, involving as it does the sum of the product of two rather than three diameters, yields a figure that bears no necessary direct relation to tumor volume as such. For example when a 3×3-cm object shrinks to 2×2 cm, the tumor "size" calculated as above, has shrunk 56%. It is likely, however, that the third dimension of that tumor has not remained constant during this time. If shrinkage affects all three dimensions equally, then the actual decrease in volume is about 70% [$\Delta V = \frac{4}{3} (r_1^3 - r_2^3)$]. Thus, if three-dimensional measurements become the basis for response assessment, the definition of partial response may have to change if it is to retain an equivalent clinical significance.

GENERAL FEATURES OF RESPONSE EVALUATION

Certain general features of the evaluation of responses that relate to the limits of error in the method of measurement noted above bear particular emphasis:

1. Since the purpose of these measurements is to get an estimate of overall reduction in tumor burden, the investigator should endeavor to include a truly representative sample of marker lesions in the evaluation. If the patient has only a few measurable lesions, all should be followed. If the number of lesions is too large to make this feasible, a representative sample should be selected. If multiple

TABLE 2.4. *Definition of response*

Complete response: Complete disappearance of all measurable disease for some minimum time period, usually 1 month.
Partial response: Shrinkage of tumor such that S posttreatment is < 50% of S pretreatment for some minimum time period (usually 1 month), in the absence of growth of any lesion or the appearance of new lesions.
Minor response: Shrinkage of tumor insufficient to meet the criterion of partial response.
Stable disease: No significant change in tumor size or extent during the observation period.
Progression: Increase in tumor size such that S posttreatment exceeds S pretreatment by some fixed amount, usually 25 or 50%, *or* the appearance of any new lesions during the observation period.

S, sum of the products of two major perpendicular diameters of all measured lesions.

anatomic sites are involved, marker lesions should be selected from a variety of sites.

2. Since the variability of measurements of the same tumor on physical examination of palpable masses or organs is generally in the range of 20–30%, it would not be useful to attempt to measure accurately any response smaller than this. Even if new imaging technologies allow reliable detection of smaller volume changes and permit us to quantify accurately shrinkage of 25% in measurable disease, such a small change in tumor size would generally not have any great significance for the patient. It might, however, give a hint of drug activity from which one might predict more productive uses for the new agent. In addition, a sustained but small increase in tumor size might well be an early warning that a particular therapy is not working and should not be pursued, thereby sparing the patient needless toxicity.

3. In any trial the complete response rate will depend on how diligently one searches for evidence of residual tumor. Two trials of the same therapy may yield widely discrepant complete response rates if they employ different methods of posttreatment restaging. For example, a trial using noninvasive clinical staging to define complete response in ovarian cancer could never be compared with one where second-look laparotomy was used as the ultimate measurement. Different investigators who have studied patients with ovarian cancer judged clinically free of disease after therapy have found rather consistent results at second-look laparotomy with only 35–40% of patients found to be truly disease free (see Table 2.5).

4. Because of the problems with measurement error outlined above, it is advisable, whenever possible, to have measurements confirmed independently by a second observer and to have tumor shrinkage sustained over more than one observation period, before the patient is termed a responder.

PROBLEMS WITH MEASUREMENT IN SPECIAL SITUATIONS

Some tumors are not measurable at both the beginning and end of therapy. A particularly difficult anatomic area to evaluate is the brain. In this setting, although disease may be measurable at the onset of therapy, it may no longer be so later in the disease. Brain tissue which has been resected along with tumor will not remodel itself and brain function that has been ablated may not be restored despite successful antitumor therapy. Areas of intracranial tumor that have shown speckled calcification may coalesce to large calcified masses easily visible on CT scan; these

TABLE 2.5. *Second-look surgery in ovarian cancer patients clinically free of disease*

Ref.	No. pts.	No residual disease	Microscopic residual only
Smirz et al. (13)	88	35 (40%)	16 (18%)
Miller et al. (14)	88	38 (43%)	16 (18%)
Gershenson et al. (15)	246	85 (35%)	50 (20%)

masses may or may not contain viable tumor cells. For these patients, second-look surgery is often difficult or impossible and it may be reasonable to consider ''stable disease'' or even improvement in specific aspects of the neurologic examination as part of the report of treatment effect.

Some normal structures infiltrated by tumor never return to a normal anatomic baseline. Assessing complete or partial response may be extremely difficult under these circumstances. Perhaps the best known example is that of the mediastinal abnormalities in patients with nodular sclerosing Hodgkin's disease, which return slowly, if at all, towards normal even after successful therapy in patients who remain in remission for many years. Jochelson et al. (16) reported the analysis of chest roentgenograms from 65 patients with mediastinal adenopathy as part of Hodgkin's disease. On completion of treatment with radiotherapy, and in some cases chemotherapy, 57 (88%) had some residual mediastinal abnormality. Long-term follow-up (median 48 months) revealed continued abnormalities in 24 (40%) of these 57 patients and there was no higher incidence of recurrence in those with than those without persistent mediastinal abnormalities.

Certain tumors require return of normal organ function as part of the definition of response. The most notable example of this is acute leukemia. Normally, for other tumor types, infiltration of the bone marrow is considered evaluable rather than measurable disease. Certain techniques have been proposed as quantitative measures of the replacement of bone marrow with leukemia cells, since this is assumed to be a relatively homogeneous infiltration of marrow (17). However, most definitions of complete remission in leukemia include not only the elimination of leukemia cells from the marrow but also the return of normal function. Although the degree of tumor lysis is of interest, an aplastic marrow, free of leukemia cells, is not a complete response.

MEANING OF RESPONSE CATEGORIES

Which of these response categories represent real clinical benefit to the patient? Responses of major magnitude (complete or partial response) are the endpoints of greatest interest in Phase II drug testing. Treatments yielding a high complete response rate are often associated with a significant number of long-term survivors; thus complete response is the most highly-prized, short-term therapeutic endpoint, since it points to the possibility of long survival in at least a fraction of the patient population. Complete response should not, however, be confused with cure or long-term survival; it simply denotes the disappearance of all evidence of cancer for some minimum time period. Generally, of course, treatments that are curative are associated with a high rate of complete response, but it is also unfortunately the case that patients in complete response, even that which is surgically confirmed, can suffer relapse. When Young et al. (18) reviewed the prognosis after restaging laparotomy in ovarian carcinoma, they found that patients with initial Stage III and IV disease still had a relatively high percentage of tumor recurrence within 2–5 years, even when the second-look laparotomies had been negative.

The partial response is an important signal of drug activity against individual tumor types and may also be associated with substantial relief of symptoms for the duration of the response. Minor responses are generally quite short and most often are of little clinical value. When minor responses occur in a Phase I study, however, they may help point to tumors for priority assessment in Phase II. The "stable disease" category is very difficult to assess since the rate of measurement of tumor progression prior to entry on study is usually undefined, and since tumors progress at different rates during different time periods in the same patient.

As noted before, certain diseases, such as prostate cancer, which metastasize primarily to nonmeasurable sites such as bone, may require trials in which all patients have only evaluable disease. Under such circumstances it is impossible to rely on conventional response endpoints, and initial studies of drug effectiveness may have to be done in a controlled Phase III setting (19) with survival as the endpoint.

DISEASE PROGRESSION

Disease progression is usually defined as either the appearance of new lesions or an increase in the size of a measurable lesion by 25–50%. If 25% were taken as the criterion, this would mean that a nodule on chest X-ray which initially measured 1 cm in diameter would be considered as "progressive disease" if the next diameter measured 1.25 cm. It would therefore seem more prudent to use the 50% criterion over at least two measurements for disease progression as well. The appearance of new lesions, which are unfortunately often multiple, is easier to evaluate. It is important to remember, however, that if a lesion is said to be "new," that organ system must have been shown to be free of disease before the study began.

LOCAL VERSUS SYSTEMIC RECURRENCE

It is most important to record carefully the sites of progression of the disease, particularly in trials that include modalities other than chemotherapy. Both surgery and radiotherapy aim primarily for local control of disease, and in evaluating their effectiveness we must know whether local control was, in fact, achieved. If a patient with osteosarcoma relapses in the lung and not at the primary surgical site, then the relapse was probably secondary to micrometastases already present at the time of the initial surgery. If the relapse is local, then it may be secondary to an inadequate resection. The approach to solving these two problems may be quite different. Evaluation of disease status at the site of primary treatment is also subject to certain methodologic difficulties; the site may be distorted or scarred after primary therapy and may never return to normal. In addition, although local disease control may be improved with a particular treatment, overall survival may be unaffected. An example is the evaluation by the European Organization on Research and Treatment of Cancer (EORTC) of radiation therapy given preoperatively to half a group of patients with resectable rectal carcinoma. The 5-year survival rate was 65% and showed no difference between the two groups, but the time to local recurrence was highly significantly different between the two treatment groups ($p = 0.001$) (20). Under these circumstances it is likely that an impact on survival will occur only with the addition of more effective systemic therapy for disease.

MEASURING DURATION OF OBJECTIVE BENEFIT

Having discussed the measurement of response, we now turn to standard ways of expressing the duration of benefit from therapy. Table 2.6 summarizes the definitions of the various intervals that are most commonly used to do this. Response duration only refers to patients who have an initial response to therapy, while progression-free interval refers to all patients. The start time for measuring response duration is somewhat arbitrary. Many investigators prefer to start the clock from the beginning of therapy, since this date is accurately known and not dependent on the schedule of response assessment. Others prefer to measure the interval from the time at which response was first documented. There is no very strong reason to prefer one convention over the other; clinical trials reports should simply make clear how the interval is calculated. The time at which progression is documented clearly depends on the frequency and completeness with which the tests are performed; as noted elsewhere, these should be decided upon before start of the study. The diagnostic tests and follow-up interval for assessing response duration or survival must be performed according to a stipulated schedule that is identical for all treatments being compared. Disease-free survival and overall survival are very important measures of therapeutic benefit for patients with fatal disease. Except in circumstances where improvement in survival with a new therapy is very dramatic, survival benefit can be assessed reliably only in formal comparative trials. We shall, therefore, defer a full discussion of this endpoint to Chapter 6.

A few comments concerning the measurement of survival are in order. If one wishes to measure survival from the time of diagnosis, the same techniques should be used for diagnosis in the entire cohort of patients. Feinstein et al. (21) found that a cohort of patients with lung cancer first treated in 1977 had a higher 6-month survival rate than a cohort treated between 1953 and 1964 at the same institutions. The more recent cohort, however, had undergone many new diagnostic imaging procedures. He attributed this apparent survival improvement to a phenomenon that epidemiologists have called "zero-time shift" or "lead-time bias." This occurs when a screening test or other appropriate diagnostic procedure leads to earlier detection of disease, so the patient does not live longer, but is simply known to have the disease longer before he dies.

In 1974, at the time of public disclosure that the wives of the U.S. President and Vice President had breast cancer, there was a major public effort to promote screening for the disease by mammography. Disease was detected in so many

TABLE 2.6. *Endpoints in measuring disease response*

Endpoint	Patient category to which endpoint applies		How endpoint interval is measured	
	Gross disease present[a]	Gross disease absent	From	To
Response duration	CR, PR, MR	(Not used)	Start of therapy or first documentation of response	Documented progression
Progression-free interval	CR, PR, MR, SD	(Rarely used)	Start of therapy	Documented progression
Disease-free survival (or relapse-free survival)	CR	All	Time rendered disease free	Disease recurrence
Survival	All	All	Time rendered disease free or start of therapy	Death

[a]CR, complete response; PR, partial response; MR, minor response; SD, stable disease.

patients that there was an apparent peak in incidence of the disease well beyond the limits of random variation. This peak may well reflect the inclusion of very small invasive lesions, as well as a proportion of benign and borderline lesions that in other years would not have been detected and reported (22). A clinical study mounted in this year would be likely to show improved survival if comparisons were made with historical controls rather than concurrent randomized controls; many patients were diagnosed with nonpalpable lesions, and some patients may have been included whose lesions might have been considered benign in other years.

Paradoxically, because survival rates are necessarily based only on patients with invasive cancer, diagnosis and treatment of tumor in a preinvasive phase can create an appearance of decreased survival. Cases diagnosed at the *in situ* stage (prior to local invasion) are not included in survival calculations for cancer patients, and yet these cases have the best prognosis. Patients cured of *in situ* carcinoma do not go on to develop invasive disease. This has the effect in subsequent years of shifting the stage distribution of invasive cancer away from the more favorable early stages and toward advanced stages with a poor prognosis. This has been given as an explanation for the lack of improvement in the 5-year survival rate over a 20-year period for women with invasive cervical cancer, in spite of a dramatic decrease in the mortality rate of that disease (23).

For overall survival, the time of death is the endpoint. It is worth repeating that the cause of death, be it disease, toxicity, or other, must be carefully determined. Sometimes, as is discussed elsewhere in this book, a treatment might increase death from other causes while decreasing cancer deaths (24), or one more toxic treatment might result in an increase in early deaths but an eventual improvement in the percentage of patients with long-term survival (25). These endpoints are summarized in Table 2.6.

STAGING

The systematic assessment of the size and extent of the primary tumor as well as the degree of locoregional extension and distant spread at the time of presentation is called staging. Once the patient's initial workup and evaluation of extent of disease has been completed, the patients can be assigned a stage appropriate for the particular tumor. Over the years many staging systems for cancer have evolved. For many types of carcinomas and sarcomas, the so-called TNM system for classification of primary tumor size and extent (T), nodal involvement (N), and other metastatic disease (M), is the most appropriate staging scheme to use; the definitions of the various T, N, and M categories for particular primary sites have been established by expert committees and are described in detail in most oncology textbooks.

Staging systems are subject to periodic revision, as knowledge accumulates of disease behavior and prognostic factors. For example, at the present time an international commission is proposing to change some of the definitions of T, N, and

M in relation to lung cancer (26) as shown in Table 2.7. The changes are proposed because those patients with ipsilateral nodes, but not contralateral nodes, are likely to have disease resected and thereby have a better prognosis, while patients with positive supraclavicular nodes do not represent "distant" disease, since they are likely to have their disease included in the radiation field. This type of change in staging designation occurs with some regularity, particularly as more is known about the response to treatment of certain classes of patients. If one has recorded only the global classification and not one's original measurements, it will not be possible to reclassify one's patients retrospectively by the new system.

Though widely employed, the TNM system is not used universally for all tumor types. Lymphomas, testis cancer, colorectal cancer, and many pediatric neoplasms use staging systems that have been constructed for these particular settings.

The tests that should be a part of the staging of each cancer patient in a clinical trial are determined by the known patterns of spread for the particular tumor type. A bone marrow examination, for example, is a reasonable staging procedure in all patients with non-Hodgkin's lymphoma, but unnecessary for patients with primary colon cancer. A detailed discussion of the proper techniques for staging individual tumors is beyond the scope of this volume. We do emphasize, however, that the staging studies required for each patient must be clearly specified in the protocol.

If the initial assessment of tumor size is a surgical one, then the initial operation may be important for staging as well as therapy. Many staging systems have as an initial descriptor whether or not tumor was completely resected. Since surgical technique varies from one individual to another, a patient who presented with the same amount of tumor might be completely resected (Stage I) in one institution or left with at least microscopic residual disease (Stage II) in another. In addition, surgeons who are more experienced in managing a particular disease may do a more complete exploration for disease at the time of the initial surgery. A significant proportion of patients referred to the National Cancer Institute and initially classified as having Stage I and II ovarian carcinoma were found to have more extensive disease at pretreatment laparoscopy or second-look surgery (18). Sites of disease that had been commonly overlooked were the diaphragm and aortic lymph nodes. In large multiinstitutional studies it is often a good idea to stratify patients by institution so that differences in response to therapy are not attributed to the biology of the disease or to the adjuvant therapy when they reflect instead differences in institutional approach to the patient.

TABLE 2.7. *Proposed changes in lung cancer staging*

Current classification	New classification
N2—Metastases to ipsilateral mediastinal nodes	N2
N2—Metastases to contralateral mediastinal nodes	N3
M1—Metases to supraclavicular nodes	N3

From Ref. 26.

Sometimes patients on clinical trials must undergo a more extensive staging evaluation than those treated conventionally. For example, a study of chemotherapy ± radiation in Hodgkin's disease might require all patients to have a laparotomy to define radiotherapy fields, while similar patients treated off study with chemotherapy only might not require this evaluation. On the other hand, the number of staging procedures required of all patients should be minimized, so that costs and risks can be kept as low as possible and protocol compliance maximized.

WILL ROGERS PHENOMENON

Feinstein et al. (21) found that the more recent cohort of patients with lung cancer who had undergone new diagnostic imaging procedures, in addition to having higher overall survival, had higher survival rates for subgroups in each of the three main TNM stages than the cohort treated earlier at the same institutions.

A change with time in the diagnostic techniques employed can change the prognosis of patients within each stage in a surprising way. This effect has been dubbed "The Will Rogers phenomenon" (21). To Will Rogers is attributed the quip that when the Okies left Oklahoma and moved to California they raised the average intelligence level in both states. In clinical terms this has been reinterpreted as follows. If one takes a group of patients with osteosarcoma, for example, who were originally considered free of pulmonary metastases on the basis of chest X-ray alone, and reclassifies them on the basis of pulmonary metastatic disease seen only on CT scan and not seen on chest X-ray, then the survival of the "localized disease" patients will go up because those patients with the greater amount of disease will be removed from that group, but the survival of the "disseminated disease" patients will also go up since a group with a smaller amount of disease has been added in. Thus, with no basic advances in therapy at all, an improvement of survival in both groups of patients will be seen. This phenomenon occurred in the patients analyzed by Feinstein et al. (21). The 1953–1964 cohort had not undergone the new forms of imaging (radionuclide scanning, CT, and ultrasonography) that had been developed and extensively used since 1964. Therefore, many of the more recently diagnosed patients who previously would have been classified in a "good" stage were assigned to a "bad" stage. Because the prognosis of those who migrated, although worse than that for other members of the good-stage group, was better than that for other members of the bad-stage group, survival rates rose in each group without any change in individual outcomes (Table 2.8). When classified according to symptom stages that would be unaltered by changes in diagnostic techniques, the two cohorts had similar survival rates (21).

CONCLUSIONS

Clinical experiments require good measurement technique just as any other experiment does. Endpoints must be defined prior to beginning the study, disease

TABLE 2.8. *Will Rogers phenomenon (the effects of restaging on the survival of cohorts with no change in therapy)*

Effects of stage migration on six-month survival rates in the 1977 cohort[a]

Old-data TNM stage[a]		Stage migration six-month survival		New data TNM stage[a]
I: 32/42 (76)	→	I: 22/24	(92)	I: 22/24 (92)
	↘	II: 1/1	(100)	
	↘	III: 9/17	(53)	
II: 17/25 (68)	→	II: 12/17	(71)	II: 13–18 (72)
	↘	III: 5/8	(63)	
III: 23/64 (36)	→	III: 23/64	(36)	III: 37/89 (42)
		Total 72/131 (55)		

[a]TNM denotes tumor, nodes, and metastases. Values are number of patients, with percentages in parenthesis.
Reproduced from Ref. 21.

must be measurable if responses are to be assessed, and the techniques used must be performed as accurately and reproducibly as possible. If the techniques are less than perfect, the investigator should be aware of their limitations so as not to make claims that are outside the limits of the method. Accurate and, whenever possible, duplicated recordings should be made of original data so that if classification schemes change patients will remain evaluable.

REFERENCES

1. Hertz, R., Lewis, J., and Lipsett, M. B. (1956): Five years experience with the chemotherapy of metastatic trophoblastic diseases in women. *Am. J. Obstet. Gynecol.*, 86:808–814.
2. Warr, D., McKinney, S., and Tannock, I. (1984): Influence of measurement error on assessment of response in anticancer chemotherapy: proposal for new criteria of tumor response. *J. Clin. Oncol.*, 2:1040–1049.
3. Moertel, C. G., and Hanley, J. A. (1976): The effect of measuring error on the results of therapeutic trials in advanced cancer. *Cancer*, 38:388–394.
4. Lavin, P. T., and Flowerdew, G. (1980): Studies in variation associated with the measurement of solid tumors. *Cancer*, 46:1286–1290.
5. Chak, Y., Paryami, S. B., Sikic, B. I., et al. (1983): Diagnostic accuracies of clinical studies in patients with small cell carcinoma of the lung. *J. Clin. Oncol.*, 1:290–294.
6. Rostock, R. A., Siegelman, S. S., Lenhard, R. E., et al. (1983): Thoracic CT scanning for mediastinal Hodgkin's disease: Results and thereapeutic implications. *Int. J. Radiat. Oncol. Biol. Phys.*, 9:1451–1457.
7. Schaner, E. G., Change, A. E., Doppman, J. L., et al. (1978): Comparison of computed and conventional whole lung tomography in detecting pulmonary nodules: A prospective radiologic pathologic study. *Am. J. Roentgenol.*, 131:51–54.

8. Heymsfeld, S. B., Fulenwider, T., Nordlinger, B., et al. (1979): Accurate measurement of liver, kidney, and spleen volume and mass by computerized axial tomography. *Ann. Intern. Med.*, 90:185–187.

9. Ettinger, D. S., Leichner, P. K., Siegelman, S. S., et al. (1985): Computed tomography assisted volumetric analysis of primary liver tumor as a measure of response to therapy. *Am. J. Clin. Oncol.*, 8:413–418.

10. Citrin, D. L., Hougen, C., Zweibel, W., et al. (1981): The use of serial bone scans in assessing response of bone metastases to systemic treatment. *Cancer*, 47:680–685.

11. Woolfenden, J. M., Pitt, M. J., Durie, B. G., and Moon, T. E. (1980): Comparison of bone scintigraphy and radiography in multiple myeloma. *Radiology*, 134:723–728.

12. O'Mara, R. E. (1976): Skeletal scanning in neoplastic disease. *Cancer*, 37:480–486.

13. Smirz, L. R., Stehman, F. B., Ulbright, T. M., et al. (1985): Second-look laparotomy after chemotherapy in the management of ovarian malignancy. *Am. J. Obstet. Gynecol.*, 152:661–668.

14. Miller, D. S., Ballon, S. C., Teng, N. N. H., et al. (1986): A critical reassessment of second-look laparotomy in epithelial ovarian carcinoma. *Cancer*, 57:530–535.

15. Gershenson, D. M., Copeland, L. J., Wharton, J. T., et al. (1985): Prognosis of surgically determined complete responders in advanced ovarian cancer. *Cancer*, 55:1129–1135.

16. Jochelson, M., Mauch, P., Balikian, J., et al. (1985): The significance of the residual mediastinal mass in treated Hodgkin's disease. *J. Clin. Oncol.*, 3:637–640.

17. Blumenreich, M. S., Strife, A., and Clarkson, B. D. (1983): A new technique to quantify cytoreduction in the bone marrow induced by cytotoxic chemotherapy. *J. Clin. Oncol.*, 1:552–558.

18. Young, R. C., Knapp, R. C., Fuks, Z., and DiSaia, P. J. (1985): Cancer of the ovary. In: *Cancer: Principles and Practice of Oncology*, edited by V. T. DeVita, Jr., S. Hellman, and S. A. Rosenberg, pp. 1083–1117, 2nd ed. Lippincott, Philadelphia.

19. Eisenberger, M. A., Simon, R., O'Dwyer, P. J., et al. (1985): A reevaluation of nonhormal cytotoxic chemotherapy in the treatment of prostatic carcinoma. *J. Clin. Oncol.*, 3:827–841.

20. Gerard, A., Berrod, J.-L., Pene, F., et al. (1985): Interim analysis of a phase III study on preoperative radiation therapy in resectable rectal carcinoma: Trial of the Gastrointestinal Tract Cancer Cooperative Group of the European Organization for Research on Treatment of Cancer (EORTC). *Cancer*, 55:2373–2379.

21. Feinstein, A. R., Sosin, D. M., and Wells, C. K. (1985): The Will Rogers phenomenon: Stage migration and new diagnostic techniques as a source of misleading statistics for survival in cancer. *N. Engl. J. Med.*, 312:1604–1608.

22. Bailar, J. C., III, and Smith, E. M. (1986): Progress against cancer? *N. Engl. J. Med.*, 314:1226–1232.

23. Enstrom, J. E., and Austin, D. F. (1977): Interpreting cancer survival rates. *Science*, 195:847–851.

24. Blackard, C. E., Doe, R. P., Mellinger, G. T., and Byar, D. P. (1970): Incidence of cardiovascular disease and death in patients receiving diethylstilbestrol for carcinoma of the prostate. *Cancer*, 26:249–256.

25. Schein, P. S. (for the Gastrointestinal Tumor Study Group) (1982): A comparison of combination chemotherapy and combined modality therapy for locally advanced gastric carcinoma. *Cancer*, 49:1771–1777.

26. Mountain, C. F. (1986): A new international staging system for lung cancer. *Chest*, 89(*Suppl. 4*):225–233.

CHAPTER 3

Treatment Toxicity and Quality of Life

The key to the evaluation of any new treatment is a weighing of benefits and costs. We have chosen to discuss toxicity and quality of life in a single chapter for several reasons. First, toxicity has an obvious impact on quality of life. In addition, measurements of toxicity and quality of life must both be tailored to the particular treatment and/or disease. One needs to assess the effect of amputation, both medically and psychosocially, in deciding on the proper treatment for a patient with osteosarcoma, but not for most other tumors we treat. And finally, although toxicity is more often objectively measurable than quality of life, the measurement of some of the features of both represent an attempt to quantify elements of the patients' experience that are subjective rather than quantitatively "measurable." In his classic discussion of the analysis of survival statistics, Mantel (1) notes:

> It is assumed here that improved survival is not accompanied by deleterious aspects such as blindness. If they were present, any appropriate comparison would have to take this into account. What is required is a value or utility function defining the value of living to a certain age or for a certain period of time beyond therapy. One could then weigh the statistical comparisons with such a value function before assessing them for statistical significance. The difficulty with this approach lies in the lack of any general agreement on the value function to use. The economist, the theologian and the philosopher would probably provide quite different value functions. In the absence of an agreed on value function, such a concept for comparing survival patterns cannot be implemented.

Even in the absence of such a "value function" the physician must still attempt a description of the adverse impact of treatment and the effects of both treatment and disease on quality of life. This chapter describes attempts to do this.

TOXICITY

The essential requirements for studying toxicity are (a) to decide in advance what toxicities are likely to be important, what measurements or observations will be made to identify them, and how often the measurements will be made; (b) to make the measurements as quantitative as possible, using standard scales whenever available, so that studies can be compared; (c) to make a reasonable initial screen of the patients' status to assist eventually in separating disease-related signs and symptoms from those due to the treatment; (d) to make sure that anticipated toxicities are sufficiently well recorded; and (e) to appreciate that certain unanticipated events may represent previously undescribed toxicity.

Most trials are designed to assess acute toxicity, i.e., that which occurs during or within a few weeks of treatment. Chronic and late toxicities also occur and become particularly important in situations where treatment is curative; thus, careful long-term follow-up is essential. The risk of oxygen toxicity, for example, in a patient who has received bleomycin and later requires surgery is currently unknown, but is of potential importance to those individuals cured of their primary tumor with bleomycin-containing combinations.

ANTICIPATING IMPORTANT TOXICITIES

In Phase I trials, toxicities are anticipated on the basis of preclinical screens. These screens are known not to predict well for effects on certain organ systems such as the central nervous system. In the later stages of drug development, information gained from the early trials allows relatively detailed planning about what toxicities to look for and how often. Although assessment of hematopoietic, renal, and hepatic function is appropriate in virtually every study, the particular selection of tests should be tailored to the clinical setting. Serum amylase, total protein, albumin, and clotting protein studies should be measured from time to time when asparaginase is being given, but are not required routinely in a study of vinca alkaloids.

When toxicity has been reported in a particular organ system, it behooves the investigator to identify the assays that predict or define the toxicity most efficiently, i.e., with the fewest and simplest tests per patient. It may well be that a single CO diffusion study will be a sufficient screen for pulmonary function if one is concerned about the development of pulmonary fibrosis. However, in certain situations, tests should be done before and after exercise to detect minimal changes in pulmonary or cardiac function. As knowledge in other areas of medicine advances, the studies that should be used to assess toxicity in any particular organ system will change. State of the art medicine should be used to provide the appropriate degree of sensitivity in the assessment of toxicity during clinical oncology trials.

QUANTITATION OF TOXICITY

Measurements should be quantitative wherever possible, even if the toxicity is not an expression of a quantitative variable such as white blood cell count. Assigning a numerical degree of severity to a toxicity will make it much easier to summarize data and compare patient groups. One should make the criteria as objective as possible for symptoms that are difficult to measure. Nausea may be arbitrarily quantitated, for example, as with or without vomiting, responsive to antiemetics or not. In fact, the severity of a number of the more subjective symptoms may be quantitated as to whether or not they are severe enough to require intervention;

diarrhea with dehydration requiring fluid replacement, or constipation requiring nasogastric tube for decompression are examples of severe gastrointestinal dysfunction. Such criteria do not avoid some inconsistency stemming from different thresholds for intervention among different physicians, but these would still result in a depiction of symptoms that is more reproducible and clinically relevant than terms such as "mild," "moderate," or "severe" used without more specific qualifiers.

Obviously, all investigators performing a trial must agree on toxicity grading criteria before starting the study. The use of standard criteria allows comparison from one trial to the next. One set of such standard toxicity criteria, those used by the Eastern Cooperative Oncology Group (ECOG), are given in Table 3.1 (2). A general standardized system of assessing toxicity would certainly be desirable. Some years ago the World Health Organization (WHO) proposed such a scheme (3), but it was not rapidly accepted in the clinical oncology community. There are as yet no uniform criteria for toxicity reporting among the U.S. clinical trials groups. In comparing the toxicity scales from three cooperative groups, Vietti (4) found variations in the definitions of grades for several important toxicities. This was particularly true where the toxicity was reflected in less easily quantified signs or symptoms (e.g., severity of diarrhea), rather than in laboratory numbers. Bloody diarrhea requiring fluids or transfusions represented Grade 3 toxicity for two of the groups and Grade 4 for the third, but even degrees of laboratory abnormalities may be given different weights in different groups; a BUN level three times normal is Grade 3 for one group and Grade 2 for another.

The standard listing of toxicity criteria usually groups measurable laboratory parameters into grades as well. This allows one to give a succinct and reproducible definition of the toxicity that would lead to altered dosing in a clinical trial, for example, "drug will be held for any toxicity more severe than ECOG Grade 2." This practice tends to standardize protocol writing and investigator behavior.

Duration of toxicity should be reported as well as severity. While most patients might tolerate well a white count that stays below 500 for 3 days, one that stays at that level for 30 days is likely to be associated with severe complications. Mucositis preventing a patient from eating is bothersome if it lasts a day or two, but could be life-threatening if it interferes with overall nutritional status for weeks. The duration of any toxic sign or symptom will only be known if the protocol explicitly requires that the observations be made at fixed intervals, which will vary according to the type of trial. Detailed observations may be required once or twice weekly or even daily during a Phase I study, and only every few weeks during a Phase II or III study. If the trial is comparative, however, observations should be made at comparable intervals in all groups of patients.

INITIAL SCREENING

Initial screening studies are critical in order to distinguish preexisting conditions from treatment-related toxicity and will vary according to the nature of the patient

TABLE 3.1. ECOG toxicity criteria

Symptom		Toxicity grade[a]				
		0	1	2	3	4
Leukopenia	WBC × 10³	≥ 4.5	3.0–< 4.5	2.0–< 3.0	1.0–< 2.0	< 1.0
	Neut × 10³	≥ 1.9	1.5–< 1.9	1.0–< 1.5	0.5–< 1.0	< 0.5
Thrombocytopenia	Plt × 10³	≥ 130	90–< 130	50–< 90	25–< 50	< 25
Anemia	Hgb g%	≥ 11	9.5–10.9	< 9.5	—	—
	Hct %	≥ 32	28–31.9	< 28	—	—
	Clinical	—		Sx of anemia	Req. transfusions	
Hemorrhage		None	Minimal	Mod (not debilitating)	Debilitating	Life threatening
Infection		None	No active Rx	Requires active Rx	Debilitating	Life threatening
GU[b]	BUN mg%	≤ 20	21–40	41–60	> 60	Symptomatic uremia
	Creatinine	≤ 1.2	1.3–2.0	2.1–4.0	> 4.0	
	Proteinuria	Neg.	1+	2 + –3 +	4 +	
	Hematuria	Neg.	Micro-cult-positive	Gross-cult-positive	Gross + clots	c̄ Obst. uropathy
Hepatic[c]	SGOT	< 1.5 × nl	1.5–2 × Normal	2.1–5 × Normal	> 5 × Normal	—
	Alk. phos.	< 1.5 × nl	1.5–2 × Normal	2.1–5 × Normal	> 5 × Normal	—
	Bilirubin	< 1.5 × nl	1.5–2 × Normal	2.1–5 × Normal	> 5 × Normal	—
	Clinical				Precoma	Hepatic coma
N & V		None	Nausea	N & V controllable	Vomiting intractable	—
Diarrhea		None	No dehydration	Dehydration	Grossly bloody	—
Pulm[d]	PFT	Nl	25–50% Decrease in Dco or VC	> 50% decrease in Dco or VC	—	—
	Clinical	—	Mild Sx	Moderate Sx	Severe Sx-intermittent O₂	Assisted vent or continuous O₂
Cardiac	Clinical	Nl	ST-T changes	Atrial arrhythmias	Mild CHF	Severe or refract. CHF
		Nl	Sinus tachy. > 110 at rest	Unifocal PVCs	Multifocal PVCs	Ventric tachy
		—	—	—	Pericarditis	Tamponade

	None	Decr. DTRs	Absent DTRs	Disabling sens. loss	Resp dysfunction 2° to weakness
Neuro PN	None	Mild paresthesias Mild constipation —	Severe paresthesias Severe constipation Mild weakness —	Severe PN pain Obstipation Severe weakness Bladder dysfunct.	Obstipation req. surg. Paralysis (confining pt. to bed/wheelchair)
CNS	None	Mild anxiety Mild depression Mild headache Lethargy — —	Severe anxiety Mod. depression Mod. headache Somnolence Tremor Mild hyperactivity	Confused or manic Severe depression Severe headache Cord dysfunction Confined to bed due to CNS dysfunct	Seizures Suicidal Coma — —
Skin and mucosa	Nl —	Transient erythema Pigmentation, atrophy	Vesiculation Subepidermal fibrosis	Ulceration Necrosis	— —
Stomatitis	None	Soreness	Ulcers—can eat	Ulcers—cannot eat	—
Alopecia	None	Alopecia—mild	Alopecia—severe		—
Allergy	None	Transient rash Drug fever ≤ 38°C (≤ 100.4°F)	Urticaria Drug fever > 38°C (> 100.4°F) Mild brochospasm	Serum sickness Bronchospasm—req. parenteral meds.	Anaphylaxis
Fever[e]	≤ 37.5°C	≤ 38°C (≤ 100.4°F)	> 38°C (> 100.4°F)	Severe c̄ chills (> 40°C)	Fever c̄ hypotension
Local Tox.	None	Pain	Pain + phlebitis	Ulceration	—

[a] The toxicity grade should reflect the most severe degree occurring during the evaluated period, not an average. When two criteria are available for similar toxicities, e.g., leukopenia, neutropenia, the one resulting in the more severe toxicity grade should be used. Toxicity grade = 5 if that toxicity caused the death of the patient. Refer to detailed toxicity guidelines or to study chairman for toxicity not covered on this table.
[b] Urinary tract infection should be graded under infection, not GU. Hematuria resulting from thrombocytopenia is graded under hemorrhage.
[c] Viral hepatitis should be recorded as infection rather than liver toxicity.
[d] Pneumonia is considered infection and not graded as pulmonary toxicity unless felt to be resultant from pulmonary changes directly induced by treatment.
[e] Fever felt to be caused by drug allergy should be graded as allergy. Fever due to infection is graded under infection only.
From Ref. 2.

and of the treatment. Important aspects of the patients' normal status must be recorded in appropriate detail. In a pediatric study of leukemia patients, initial growth status relative to standard growth curves as well as school performance may be extremely important baseline parameters for assessment of the eventual toxic effect of prophylactic therapy to the central nervous system. In any group of patients receiving anthracyclines, some baseline assessment of cardiac function is important. However, in patients who are either quite young or in whom large doses are not contemplated, an echocardiographic assessment of ejection fraction might be considered an adequate screen, while in older patients or those in whom larger total doses were to be given, a more detailed evaluation including exercise tolerance might be desirable.

When possible, the severity of preexisting disease should be quantitated when considering what degrees of toxicity will be tolerated or how the toxicity will be defined. It is possible, of course, to exclude patients with certain preexisting conditions from study. A patient with a history of pancreatitis might be excluded from a study of asparaginase without jeopardizing patient accrual in any significant fashion. However, certain preexisting conditions are common enough in the target population that it makes more sense to describe these conditions than to exclude patients who have them. For example, in a study of diethylstilbesterol (DES) for its clinical effect in prostatic cancer, where the average age of patients studied was about 70, a scale was developed to grade the cardiovascular status of the patients during the study as well as at the time of entry (5) (Table 3.2). In addition, all patients going on study should have an assessment of the function of the organ systems important in the metabolism of the drug in question, to assure that the drug will be handled in as predictable a fashion as possible.

RECORDING ANTICIPATED EVENTS

Once a toxicity has become established as a side effect of a particular agent, its occurrence often goes unrecorded, particularly if this side effect is not dangerous

TABLE 3.2. *Example of pretherapy patient stratification criteria: Clinical cardiovascular status of study patients*[a]

0: No history of cardiovascular disease; normal EKG.
1: History of cardiovascular disease; not incapacitated; normal EKG.
2: Either no history or history of cardiovascular disease; not incapacitated; abnormal EKG.
3: Definite history of cardiovascular disease; mildly to moderately incapacitated; abnormal EKG.
4: Definite history of cardiovascular disease; severely incapacitated; abnormal EKG.
5: Death due to cardiovascular disease.

---

[a]For this study the degree to which the patients were overweight, their blood pressure, and the presence or absence of diabetes were also considered as potentially important determinants of the risk of significant toxicity.
From Ref. 5.

to the patient. Alopecia, for example, although extremely bothersome to the patient, may be recorded so infrequently that one cannot determine in a retrospective chart review how many patients in a particular study lost some, all, or none of their hair. Neuropathic effects of vincristine such as loss of reflexes, foot drop, and even cranial nerve signs such as ptosis may not appear in the record. If these items, which are associated with obvious physical signs, are poorly recorded, then symptoms experienced only by the patient and not externally visible will be even less often noted in the record. If one wishes to know the true incidence of a symptom such as nausea or fatigue, then it must be actively elicited and recorded with the same regularity in all patient groups in a particular study. For some key symptoms, a check sheet filled out by the nurse and/or patient may help to assure that such data are routinely collected.

UNANTICIPATED EVENTS AND TOXICITY

Any adverse event that occurs during the course of a patient's treatment must be explained rationally. In the early studies of ifosfamide, emphasis in reporting was on the dramatic toxicities expected from a cyclophosphamide analog, namely myelosuppression and hematuria. However, more recent studies have demonstrated the occurrence of central nervous system changes including moderate to marked mental confusion (6). The symptoms generally appeared some days after the start of treatment with the agent and disappeared once the agent was discontinued. This latter observation, particularly, allowed investigators to attribute the symptoms to the agent in question. The patients under study in these reports often had disseminated disease and were sometimes infected. The likelihood is high that, at least in some patients, these symptoms might have been attributed to other causes such as intracranial metastases or fever. It is important to consider that the drug may be the cause of a problem unless another cause can be proven.

ACCURATE ATTRIBUTION OF ADVERSE EVENTS

Although adverse events should be attributed to a drug unless there is another rational explanation, the attribution of particular signs or symptoms to treatment is often uncertain. Disease-related signs and symptoms may resemble treatment-related effects. Schein et al. (7) had difficulty distinguishing the anorexia, weight loss, and malabsorption associated with adenocarcinoma of the pancreas from the similar problems a patient might encounter undergoing combined modality therapy including irradiation of the epigastrium. This distinction might be impossible, even in a controlled trial, if the patients receiving no treatment were being assessed only for survival and not having their symptoms as carefully recorded as those in the treatment group.

Possible explanations other than antineoplastic therapy for abnormal laboratory values should also be recorded. A patient receiving aminoglycoside antibiotics or amphotericin may have a creatinine elevation because of nephrotoxic anticancer therapy, the antibiotic, the combination of the two, or disease progression. Investigators should decide in advance which "complications" such as infections or antibiotic therapy should be recorded and how.

In any trial where toxicity information is available, the anticipated toxicities will have been discussed with the patient prior to the administration of the drug. This prior discussion, or previous courses of treatment itself, might make the occurrence of subjective symptoms more likely. The frequency of this sort of "anticipatory" symptom can be appreciated when one realizes how common nausea and vomiting prior to the administration of medication, or even prior to a visit to the clinic, can be in patients on chemotherapy (8).

The frequency and importance of placebo effects, i.e., side effects that are not attributable to the biological properties of the treatment, are rarely studied in cancer therapy. One early report with a small number of patients looking at 5-fluorouracil versus placebo in bladder cancer showed a surprisingly similar distribution of signs and symptoms in both groups of patients (9). Table 3.3 gives an indication of how common such effects can be in other medical contexts (10).

Since the most severe potential toxicity is death, all deaths on study must be reported and the causes of death carefully analyzed. Often by the time a patient dies there are multiple contributing causes including both treatment and disease. All causes should be noted, and death should not be attributed to progressive disease if indeed the treatment may be at fault. A patient with widespread metastatic cancer dying of sepsis that occurred after induction of treatment-related marrow hypoplasia is, from the point of view of the study, a patient who died of treatment-related effects, even though it is perfectly proper to list the disseminated cancer as a contributing cause. This is a difficult area requiring expert judgment.

Blackard et al. (5), in the previously cited study of Stage III and IV prostate carcinoma, analyzed the causes of death in patients who were randomized to receive

TABLE 3.3. *Toxicity during placebo controlled trial of procardia*

Adverse effect	Procardia (%) (N = 226)	Placebo (%) (N = 235)
Dizziness, lightheadedness, giddiness	27	15
Flushing, heat sensation	25	8
Headache	23	20
Weakness	12	10
Nausea, heartburn	11	8
Muscle cramps, tremor	8	3
Peripheral edema	7	1
Nervousness, mood changes	7	4
Palpitation	7	5
Dyspnea, cough, wheezing	6	3
Nasal congestion, sore throat	6	8

Reprinted from Ref. 10.

either placebo or 5 mg of DES daily. Though the overall mortality in both groups was the same, an examination of the causes of death revealed the pattern shown in Table 3.4. DES had significantly decreased the number of deaths from prostate cancer but had significantly increased the number of patients with clinically evident cardiovascular disease, if both those who died and those who remained alive with newly diagnosed disease were included. The cardiovascular disease included arteriosclerotic heart disease with congestive heart failure and/or myocardial infarction, cerebrovascular accident, pulmonary embolus, and hypertensive cardiovascular disease. The pretreatment cardiovascular status of estrogen-treated patients was generally better than those treated with placebo, so that one could not ascribe the increase in cardiovascular disease to the patients' pretreatment status. Overall survival analysis alone would have missed this important toxicity, which was reduced in subsequent studies with lower doses of DES.

ANALYSIS OF DRUG TOXICITY DATA

The true incidence of any particular toxicity is likely to be very difficult to establish. Single agents are rarely studied alone in any large number of patients. Since asparaginase is a foreign protein, one might expect anaphylaxis to occur more frequently on an intermittent than on a daily or continuous schedule. In early studies of L-asparaginase, anaphylaxis was reported with the incidence varying by study as shown in Table 3.5 (11–17). It can be seen that even in these trials, where an effort was made to define the least toxic schedule, the efforts were unsuccessful. In the first three trials where daily treatment is compared with intermittent dosing, the incidence of anaphylaxis is slightly higher on the intermittent schedule. However, the range is very wide, the numbers small, and the assessment of the higher incidence in the later trials of daily administration of drug alone is confounded by the longer duration of treatment in this group. A more precise estimate of the relative incidence of anaphylaxis as a function of schedule would require a controlled comparative trial in larger numbers of patients.

Controlled studies of toxicity alone are rare. Currently, the greatest need in the therapy of most cancers is to improve complete response rate and survival; so long as toxicity is tolerable, it is unlikely that a more active schedule or dose would be

TABLE 3.4. *Analysis of causes of death*

		Dead		Alive with new CV disease	Mean age (yr.)
	N	CA prostate	CV disease		
Placebo	114	28	32	7	70.3
DES (5 mg q.d.)	119	15	44	14	70.7

CA, cancer; CV, cardiovascular.
From Ref. 5.

TABLE 3.5. *Incidence of anaphylaxis in studies of asparaginase as a single agent*

Schedule	No. pts.	No. with anaphylaxis	Fraction with anaphylaxis	Ref.
Daily	9	0	0	
b.i.w.	7	1	0.14	11
Daily	17	0	0	
b.i.w.	18	6	0.33	12
Daily	16	3	0.19	
b.i.w.	16	4	0.25	13
b.i.w.	11	1	0.09	
Weekly	10	1	0.10	14
Daily	40	6	0.15	15
Daily (b.i.w.)	29	13	0.45	16
Daily	120	42	0.35 (children)	
	127	33	0.26 (adults)	17
Total	420	111	0.24	

abandoned in favor of a less active one just because the latter is less toxic. In a few situations where therapy has been highly successful but toxic, randomized studies have been done to attempt to determine whether less intensive therapy would be as effective. Patients with nonseminomatous testicular cancer historically had experienced a 5% death rate due to toxicity with agranulocytic septicemia as the leading cause of death. Stoter et al. (18), therefore, looked at high-dose versus low-dose vinblastine in cisplatin–vinblastine–bleomycin combination chemotherapy of nonseminomatous testicular cancer. They found that vinblastine at 0.3 mg/kg/cycle was as effective and caused less leukopenia than vinblastine at 0.4 mg/kg/cycle. Several pediatric trials have been designed with toxicity reduction in mind (19). Most often, however, the comparative toxicity of two or more regimens must be extracted from analysis of trials designed to demonstrate efficacy.

Simply reporting the severity and duration of toxicities observed in a clinical trial is an inadequate use of potentially valuable data (3). The most critical additional question is whether the induction of toxic effects was required to produce a favorable antineoplastic response. Post hoc subset analysis cannot be used to prove this point, but if it appears that patients who received full dose did better than those who did not, a randomized trial of dose and schedule might be useful to see if this is important. A special part of the analysis of toxicity data requires sequential examination of observations made in each patient to determine whether a toxicity recurs with repetitive dosing and whether or not it is cumulative in nature. In order to conclude that toxicity is cumulative, a progressive worsening of toxicity with repeated treatment without dose escalation must be demonstrated. If an unusual feature of toxicity is to be studied, appropriate measurements must be made. If one wishes to decrease the number of inpatient hospital days (20), for example, as part of the plan of study, it is important to provide a place where this information can be recorded and retrieved. In this particular example, it might also be important to establish that this is not achieved at the price of a great increase in the number of outpatient visits.

In order to avoid bias in the performance of toxicity analyses, every patient receiving therapy should be included, though not all may be available for analysis of response or survival. A patient who is lost to follow-up because he refuses to take any further therapy should be included in the discussion of toxicity. Then, in analyzing the relative toxicities of two regimens in a comparative study, one should consider the number of courses that were given at full dose, how often the dose had to be cut, and how many courses were included on each arm. It would be foolish to say that arm A is less toxic, if no patients still had low white counts after two courses when they had all had their doses decreased for leukopenia after the first course, while treatment had been continued at full dose on arm B because it was tolerated. Subset analysis should be done to see whether certain types of patients experience specific toxicities. Some drugs, for example, might cause impotence or loss of libido in males but have no equivalent effect in females.

If the study involved a combination, the contribution of each agent to the overall toxicity should be assessed and a decision made as to whether the toxicity of one agent inhibited the ability to give the maximum dose of the other. A new drug added to a combination may enhance previously known toxicities of the other agents. The toxicity of methotrexate might be significantly increased by the simultaneous administration of cisplatin, for example, if the nephrotoxicity of the latter delayed excretion of the former. These sorts of interactions may be obvious or they may be more subtle; in the latter case they may only be proved by analysis of toxicity in comparative randomized trials.

CHRONIC AND LATE TOXICITIES

The first concern in a clinical trial is acute toxicity, but as more and more patients are cured, chronic and late toxicities of therapy become increasingly important. In the early days of radiotherapy the size of a single dose was decreased with protraction of overall treatment duration until acute toxic responses (e.g., of skin and mucosa) no longer limited the total dose that could be delivered to a tumor. However, when protraction was sufficient to minimize acute reactions, the total dose became limited by the development of late complications (e.g., dermal necrosis and bone fracture). Tissues are now divided by radiotherapists into early and late responding. Repair of sublethal damage occurs in both, but regeneration of surviving target cells during the course of fractionated radiotherapy is less in the late-responding tissues; in some, regeneration may not occur at all (21). This has been an important factor in limiting the dose of radiation that can be administered to the brain for treatment of clinically inapparent disease in leukemia. Although the children show no acute evidence of brain damage, their overall mental function as studied on IQ tests and reflected in school performance, shows a marked deterioration relative to sibling or nonirradiated patient controls (22,23).

Some very important toxicities may not be detected in the initial trials of a drug. Phase I trials by their nature are usually short-term studies and the effects of chronic drug administration will not be appreciated. Chronic or cumulative toxicities will generally become evident only if the drug has some activity, since otherwise treatment courses are short. Thus, the most useful agents have the most surprises to spring on us. The cardiotoxicity of anthracyclines is now well known, but when daunorubicin, the first compound in this class, first went into clinical trial in this country, the only anticipated toxicity was myelosuppression. This had been so dramatic in the acute trials that no observations of cardiotoxicity had been made either in animals or in the initial cohort of patients receiving the drug. In early preclinical studies in Italy (24), and in clinical studies of children with acute leukemia treated in France (25), there was no mention of cardiotoxicity.

The earliest clinical experience with daunorubicin in the U.S. was reported in 1967 (26). This series included 68 children, 19 of whom had received a total of 25 mg/kg or more of daunomycin. At the time of the report 5 were alive. Of the 14 that had died, 7 had developed cardiopulmonary symptoms characterized by tachycardia with or without arrhythmia, gallop rhythm, and in some cases overt congestive heart failure. The publication assessed these findings as follows:

> These patients had evidence of widespread cancer and in most cases there were adequate explanations for their clinical difficulties. Because these findings occurred, however, in patients who received more than 25 mg/kg of daunomycin, it was necessary to consider the possibility that death was due to a late toxic effect of daunomycin.

A group-wide study in CALGB (Cancer and Leukemia Group B) was started in 1966 (27) and reached similar conclusions. This study included 96 evaluable patients with acute leukemia treated at three different dosage levels. The investigators suspected the presence of cardiac toxicity as follows:

> Cardiac toxicity possibly occurred 9 times, 6 times among responders and 3 times in nonresponders. . . . With cardiac findings at cumulative doses of 300–1050 mg/m^2 and questionable cardiac involvement at 90–850 mg/m^2 a definite relationship between total dose and cardiac toxicity cannot be established. However, no patient in the series received over 600 mg/m^2 without developing evidence suggestive of cardiac toxicity.

Thus, two large studies involving a total of 164 children served only to suggest cardiac toxicity rather than establish its definite existence. The papers documenting cardiac toxicity in animal model systems and working out the quantitative toxic doses in man did not appear until the 1970s. It might have taken an even larger number of patients to discover the cardiotoxicity of daunorubicin if the initial trials had been performed in adults, in whom alternative causes of cardiac dysfunction are common. This example is a reminder that late toxicity, even when it is common, may be missed in a Phase I trial, particularly because it is often qualitatively different from early toxicity.

Some treatment-related toxicities may not occur for many years after cure has been effected. It would be ideal if a tumor registry could obtain yearly follow-up on all patients treated for cancer so that some estimate of the incidence of other disease could be obtained for comparison with the general statistics. Pediatric oncologists have speculated, for example, that children who have been treated with anthracyclines, because of loss of myocardial cells, may have an earlier incidence of adult cardiovascular disease than would otherwise occur, but this will require decades of follow-up.

A particularly serious late effect is the occurrence of second malignancies. In patients where cure has been possible for many years such as those with Hodgkin's disease, these occur at a rate which appears to be above that expected in the general population (28). This result was not appreciated until 5 or more years after the initial beneficial therapeutic result of chemotherapy in this disease was known. The attempt to reduce the incidence of these devastating late toxicities has been a significant factor in the design of current trials for treatment of Hodgkin's disease.

QUALITY OF LIFE

An overall assessment of the impact of disease and treatment on the life of the patient is usually subsumed under the rubric of quality of life. It seems obvious that developing measures of quality of life is more difficult than measuring survival and response rate. It is difficult to decide what to measure and it is unlikely that any particular test for quality of life can be measured against a single external standard in the way, for example, that achievement test scores might be compared against grades in an academic subject.

Any test should be both valid and reliable. Validity refers to the ability of the test to measure what we want it to measure. This is assessed by (a) looking at the test to see whether the questions asked are appropriate and comprehensive, (b) seeing whether the test items are answered in an internally consistent fashion, and (c) determining comparability of this test with other available measures of the question under consideration, such as other tests, psychological/psychiatric evaluation, and other methods that can assess behavior such as compliance with treatment regimens and successful resumption of normal activity. One must establish the validity of a new measure before it is generally adopted.

If a test is to be of value, it must also be reliable. It must consistently score the same value when measuring what is thought to be the same value of the process. For example, a reliable blood sugar measure should provide very similar results when tested on multiple occasions against a fixed solution of known glucose concentration.

A familiar functional outcome measure employed in oncology is the Karnofsky performance status scale which will be discussed in Chapter 6. This scale is a valid predictor of outcome, but it is obvious that the indices used on this scale are incomplete measures of overall quality of life and seem to reflect physical function better than psychological well-being. A number of questionnaires to assess the latter have been developed.

SELF-REPORT QUESTIONNAIRES

In general, well-designed self-administered questionnaires that do not require the intervention of health professionals have been most satisfactory for evaluating patient adjustment to treatment and disease. Involving a health professional is expensive and also may bias the results since the questions may be ''interpreted'' for the patient.

A widely used instrument is the SCL-90 (29). It has been applied in an adjuvant chemotherapy trial of ECOG. The instrument consists of 90 questions, each having 5 possible answers, ranging from ''not at all distressed by the complaint'' to ''extremely distressed by the complaint.'' Subscores may be derived, for example, for general neurotic feelings, somatic symptoms, fear, depression, and problems in functioning. The reliability and validity of the SCL-90 have been quite high (30) and its use has been associated with high compliance despite repeated administration. The patient's score can therefore be followed over a period of time to elicit and evaluate trends.

Schipper and Levitt (31) have developed the Functional Living Index: Cancer (FLIC), a 22-item, self-administered questionnaire to measure what they call the four central aspects of quality of life: physical/occupational function, psychological state, sociability, and somatic discomfort. The FLIC is also currently in use in several clinical trials.

At the Dutch Cancer Institute a so-called ''complaint questionnaire'' has been in use for several years (30). Participating investigators considered this questionnaire a valid measurement of the discomfort of chemotherapy. Patients who reported many complaints on this questionnaire also indicated that they felt more ill, needed more rest during the day, were hindered more in their daily activities, and used more kinds of medicine than those reporting fewer complaints. The list has been shown to differentiate well between patients receiving chemotherapy and controls. It also distinguishes periods of rest from periods of treatment.

Many instruments that may have been validated on a general population, or even a population in which psychological disturbance is suspected, may not have been properly validated for a cancer population. Using standard indices for depression, Plumb and Holland (32) discovered that the somatic symptoms of anorexia and fatigue, which were often attributable to therapy, led to a misleadingly high score on the depression index and could not be used for scoring cancer patients on treatment. When patients were scored on the nonsomatic or psychological items only, they were no more depressed than next-of-kin controls, and significantly less depressed than people with a history of suicide attempt. Specific scales must be developed to measure anxiety in cancer patients. Even if a problem with anxiety or depression is discovered, these are common conditions and may have predated the diagnosis of cancer. In fact, Plumb and Holland (33) noted that those cancer patients who were most depressed were those who had a prior history of depression and a "tendency to brood." They found no correlation between the severity of depression and the nearness of death.

It is also important to know that an instrument does not correlate with variables it is not supposed to measure. The Dutch complaint questionnaire was used in a study of 20 patients with advanced testicular cancer (30) treated with combination chemotherapy and their partners. Only a very slight correlation was found between the number of complaints and a neuroticism score. This may be regarded as an indication that the questionnaire measures something other than neuroticism. The study also emphasizes another important point. A common pitfall in quality-of-life studies is to consider only physician- or patient-perceived factors. The concerns of primary family members are also likely to have a significant impact on a patient's adjustment to the stresses of diagnosis and treatment. A study of the effect of corticosteroids on mental and emotional state in pediatric patients with leukemia and lymphoma employed both parent and child evaluations (34). Certain behaviors, such as difficulty in controlling temper, were more worrisome for the parent than for the young child.

SPECIALIZED INSTRUMENTS

Global scales that might assess the functional capacity of an adult are not applicable to children. A scale that scores play activities as to whether or not they are age appropriate can be used for children from age 6 months through 16 years. This contains a combination of observed and reported behavior (35).

A number of more specialized scales for measurement of specific problems may assist in developing risk–benefit ratios (30). Many of these specialized tests involve the evaluation of local therapy and therefore look at comparisons of surgical or radiotherapeutic procedures. Harwood and Rawlinson (36) assessed vocal function in 129 patients following treatment for laryngeal cancer. The patients were randomly selected from a group who had already had either surgery or radiation. Not surprisingly, they found that the quality of vocalization was much more satisfactory in the irradiated group: 44% of the surgical patients and only 2.5% of those successfully irradiated were unable to use the telephone. The answers to other questions relating to use of voice for socializing were similar. In another study (37) when healthy volunteers were offered a theoretical choice of laryngectomy with a 60% 5-year survival and loss of normal speech versus radiotherapy with a 30–40% 5-year survival but preservation of nearly normal speech, 20% said they would choose radiation instead of surgery. For this 20% then, what they perceived as enhanced quality of life may be more important than quantity of life. It remains to be seen what these individuals whould choose if faced with a real decision. The authors of both reports conclude that in view of the superior quality of voice and life in the successfully irradiated patients, irradiation with surgery in reserve is the optimal treatment for patients with laryngeal cancer.

Assessment of functional results of local treatment may serve to allay previous fears and prejudices of the physicians in terms of what represents acceptable therapy. Until recently, patients with carcinoma of the lower two-thirds of the rectum had been treated by abdominoperineal resection. This leaves the patient with a colostomy and possible neurological damage to bladder and sexual apparatus inflicted by the pelvic dissection. With the development of new surgical techniques, many low rectal carcinomas are now being treated by sphincter-saving resection. Initially, surgeons feared that these new procedures would invariably result in incontinence and that the extensive pelvic dissection would still leave the patient with other neurologic problems. Williams and Johnston (38) studied patients after each surgical procedure with the use of a self-administered questionnaire. With the sphincter-saving procedure 30 patients (75%) were entirely continent; 13/18 (83%) who were employed had returned to work and 6/20 men (30%) had impaired sexual function. Each patient with a colostomy was incontinent and 25 (66%) had leaks from their appliance; only 6/15 (40%) returned to work and in 12/18 men (67%) sexual function was impaired. The apparent superior quality of life after sphincter-saving resection justified the continued development of this technique. If the data from the control group had not been available it would have been difficult to decide whether 83% returning to work or 30% having impaired sexual function after the new operation was a positive or negative result.

A study of amputation in osteosarcoma was performed by another group of surgeons (39) who stated: ''At the beginning of this project we had a definite bias. We were convinced that sparing a limb as opposed to amputating it offered a quality of life advantage (that is, less extensive loss of function).'' After eligibility was determined, patients were randomized in a 2:1 ratio to limb-sparing surgery + radiation therapy + chemotherapy versus amputation + chemotherapy. After studying the patients with several scales they found either no difference for some functions such as emotional behavior, or a better score for the amputees than for the patients who had had the limb-sparing surgery. In this admittedly very small study the Katz activities of Daily Living Scale recorded complete functioning in all amputees but only in 7/12 limb-spared patients. Thus, the investigators could not substantiate their initial bias that a limb-sparing operation would have a better functional result. They point out that the results of this small study may not be representative, and that only patients who may have been prepared to lose a limb would have agreed to randomization. These results emphasize the importance of actually collecting the data from the patients rather than simply assigning them to the procedure that one feels will be the most emotionally and/or physically acceptable. The proper assessment of the impact of therapy on the lives of patients should be attempted both for the global and the more disease-related aspects of quality of life. Patients may be willing to substitute even some quantity of life for a better functional outcome, and this decision should not be made for them in advance. Data should be collected in such a way that the choice a patient is making is as clear and logical as it can possibly be.

REFERENCES

1. Mantel, N. (1966): Evaluation of survival data and two new rank order statistics arising in its consideration. *Cancer Chemother. Rep.,* 50:163–170.
2. Oken, M. M., Creech, R. H., Tormey, D. C., et al. (1982): Toxicity and response criteria of the Eastern Cooperative Oncology Group. *Am. J. Clin. Oncol.,* 5:649–655.
3. Kisner, D. L. (1984): Reporting treatment toxicities. In: *Cancer Clinical Trials: Methods and Practice,* edited by M. E. Buyse, M. J. Staquet, and R. J. Sylvester, pp. 178–190. Oxford University Press, Oxford.
4. Vietti, T. J. (1980): Evaluation of toxicity: Clinical issues. *Cancer Treat. Rep.,* 64:457–461.
5. Blackard, C. E., Doe, R. P., Mellinger, G. T., and Byar, D. P. (1970): Incidence of cardiovascular disease and death in patients receiving diethylstilbestrol for carcinoma of the prostate. *Cancer,* 26:249–256.
6. Klegar, K., Ryan, L., Elias, A. D., et al. (1986): Ifosfamide (IFF) for advanced previously treated sarcomas: Phase II. *Proc. A.S.C.O.* 5:514.
7. Schein, P. S. (for the Gastrointestinal Tumor Study Group) (1982): A comparison of combination chemotherapy and combined modality therapy for locally advanced gastric carcinoma. *Cancer,* 49:1771–1777.
8. Nerenz, D. R., Leventhal, H., Easterling, D. V., and Love, R. R. (1986): Anxiety and drug taste as predictors of anticipatory nausea in cancer chemotherapy. *J. Clin. Oncol.,* 4:224–233.
9. Prout, G. R., Bross, I. D. J., Slack, N. H., and Ausman, R. K. (1968): Carcinoma of the bladder. 5-Fluorouracil and the critical role of the placebo. A cooperative group report. I. *Cancer,* 22:926–931.
10. Physicians' Desk Reference (1987): 41st ed., Edward R. Barnhart, publisher. Medical Economics Co., Oradell, New Jersey.
11. Pratt, C. B., Simone, J. V., Zee, P., et al. (1970): Comparison of daily versus weekly L-asparaginase for the treatment of childhood acute leukemia. *J. Pediatr.,* 77:474–483.
12. Jaffe, N., Traggis, D., Das, L., et al. (1972): Comparison of daily and twice-weekly schedule of L-asparaginase in childhood leukemia. *Pediatrics,* 49:590–595.
13. Jaffe, N., Traggis, D., Das, L., et al. (1973): Favorable remission induction rate with twice weekly doses of L-asparaginase. *Cancer Res.,* 33:1–4.
14. Pratt, C. B, Choi, S., and Holton, C. P. (1971): Low-dosage asparaginase treatment of childhood acute lymphocytic leukemia. *Am. J. Dis. Child.,* 121:406–409.
15. Capizzi, R. L., Bertino, J. R., Skeel, R. T., et al. (1971): L-Asparaginase: Clinical, biochemical, pharmacological, and immunological studies. *Ann. Intern. Med.,* 74:893–901.
16. Jaffe, N., Traggis, D., Das, L., et al. (1971): L-Asparaginase in the treatment of neoplastic diseases in children. *Cancer Res.,* 31:942–949.
17. Oettgen, H. F., Stephenson, P. A., Schwartz, M. K., et al. (1970): Toxicity of E. coli L-asparaginase in man. *Cancer,* 25:253–278.
18. Stoter, G., Sleyfer, D. T., ten Bokkel Huinink, W., et al. (1986): High-dose versus low-dose vinblastine in cisplatin–vinblastine–bleomycin combination chemotherapy of non-seminomatous testicular cancer: A randomized study of the EORTC genitourinary tract cancer cooperative group. *J. Clin. Oncol.,* 4:1199–1206.
19. D'Angio, G. J., Evans, A. E., Breslow, N., et al. (1976): The treatment of Wilms' tumor: Result of the National Wilms' Tumor Study. *Cancer,* 38:633–646.
20. National Wilms' Tumor Study 4, protocol.
21. Withers, H. R., Thames, H. D., and Peters, L. J. (1984): Dose-fractionation and volume effects in normal tissues and tumors. *Cancer Treat. Symp.,* 1:75–83.
22. Pfefferbaum-Levine, B., Copeland, D. R., Fletcher, J. M., et al. (1984): Neuropsychologic assessment of long-term survivors of childhood leukemia. *Am. J. Pediatr. Hematol. Oncol.,* 6:123–128.
23. Robison, L. L., Nesbit, M. E., Jr., Sather, H. N., et al. (1984): Factors associated with IQ scores in long-term survivors of childhood acute lymphoblastic leukemia. *Am. J. Pediatr. Hematol. Oncol.,* 6:115–122.
24. DiMarco, A., Gaetani, M., Dorigotti, L., et al. (1963): Studi sperimentali sull'attivita' antineoplastica del nuovo antibiotico daunomicina. *Tumori,* 49:203–217.
25. Jacquillat, C., Tanzer, J., Boiron, M., et al. (1966): Rubidomycin. A new agent active in the treatment of acute lymphoblastic leukemia. *Lancet,* ii:27–28.
26. Tan, C., Tasaka, H., Yu, K., et al. (1967): Daunomycin, an antitumor antibiotic, in the treatment

of neoplastic disease. Clinical evaluation with special reference to childhood leukemia. *Cancer*, 20:333–353.

27. Jones, B., Holland, J. F., Morrison, A. R., et al. (1971): Daunorubicin (NSC 82151) in the treatment of advanced childhood lymphoblastic leukemia. *Cancer Res.*, 31:84–90.

28. Coleman, N. (1986): Secondary malignancy after treatment of Hodgkin's disease: An evolving picture. *J. Clin. Oncol.*, 4:821–824.

29. DeRogatis, L. R. (1977): *The SCL-90 Manual*. Johns Hopkins University Press, Baltimore.

30. Van Dam, F. S. A. M., Linssen, C. A. G., and Couzijn, A. L. (1984): Evaluating "quality of life" in cancer clinical trials. In: *Cancer Clinical Trials: Methods and Practice*, edited by M. E. Buyse, M. J. Staquet, and R. J. Sylvester. pp. 26–43. Oxford University Press, Oxford.

31. Schipper, H., and Levitt, M. (1985): Measuring quality of life: Risks and benefits. *Cancer Treat. Rep.*, 69:1115–1123.

32. Plumb, M. M., and Holland, J. (1977): Comparative studies of psychological function in patients with advanced cancer. I. Self reported expressive symptoms. *Psychosom. Med.*, 39:264–276.

33. Plumb, M. M., and Holland, J. (1981): Comparative studies of psychological function in patients with advanced cancer, II. Interviewer rated current and past psychological symptoms. *Psychosom. Med.*, 43:243–254.

34. Harris, J. C., Carel, C. A., Rosenberg, L. A., et al. (1986): Intermittent high dose corticosteroid treatment in childhood cancer: Behavioral and emotional consequences. *J. Am. Acad. Child Psychiatry*, 25:120–124.

35. Lansky, L. L., List, M. A., Lanksy, S. B., et al. (1985): Toward the development of a play performance scale for children (PPSC). *Cancer*, 56:1837–1840.

36. Harwood, A. R., and Rawlinson, E. (1983): The quality of life of patients following treatment for laryngeal cancer. *Int. J. Radiat. Oncol. Biol. Phys.*, 9:335–338.

37. McNeil, B. J., Weicheselbaum, R., and Pauker, S. J. (1981): Speech and survival: Trade offs between quality and quantity of life in laryngeal cancer. *N. Engl. J. Med.*, 305:982–987.

38. Williams, N. S., and Johnston, D. (1983): The quality of life after rectal excision for low rectal cancer. *Br. J. Surg.*, 70:219–225.

39. Sugarbaker, P. H., Barofsky, I., Rosenberg, S. A., and Gianola, F. J. (1982): Quality of life assessment of patients in extremity sarcoma clinical trials. *Surgery*, 91:17–23.

CHAPTER 4

Phase I Trials

The principal scientific goal of the Phase I trail of a new agent is to determine a dose suitable for later activity and efficacy testing. Drugs are generally selected for clinical testing because of preclinical activity against tumors of either animal or human origin. A Phase I study begins at a low dose that is very likely to be safe, based on information derived from prior experience in animals. Small cohorts of patients are then treated at progressively higher doses until reproducible biological effects are noted. Escalation generally continues until drug-related toxicity reaches some predetermined level at which it was agreed that the trial would stop, or until unexpected and unacceptable toxicity has been seen. We then say that the maximum tolerated dose (MTD) has been reached. The recommended dose for Phase II studies is usually 75–90% of the MTD. Since the MTD is generally determined on experience in a relatively small number of patients, it should be seen as a useful guide to the starting dose for Phase II trials but sometimes must be modified as experience with the drug increases.

Phase I is also the usual setting for studying the clinical pharmacology of a new agent. Appropriate pharmacokinetic studies characterize the behavior in body fluids of the parent drug and its metabolites and determine the drug's excretion patterns. This information may be very important in helping to decide the most appropriate schedule for wider study in Phase II and in estimating the likely impact of altered renal or hepatic function on the clinical behavior of the new drug.

The MTD is a relative concept and depends on the level of toxicity that physicians and patients are willing to tolerate. An impetus to reopen Phase I investigations and to explore the administration of doses higher than the originally defined MTD would be the discovery of antitumor efficacy during Phase II testing, particularly if the initial dose-limiting toxicity is hematologic. The drug may then be studied in this new cycle of Phase I trials in conjunction with intensive blood product or autologous bone marrow support until some other less correctable dose-limiting toxicity is encountered. In the same way, new radiation schedules such as multiple daily fractions, or new energy sources such as high linear energy transfer (LET) radiation require formal Phase I study.

Physicians should always remember that cancer patients agree to participate in Phase I trials because of the possibility of therapeutic benefit, even if they realize that the probability of benefit is small. Some patients may also be motivated by the altruistic desire to help others. The goal of the physician in Phase I trials is also to benefit the individual patient. At first glance this may seem incompatible with the format of the trial design. The dilemmas implicit in the conduct of early clinical trials in patients with far-advanced malignancy are discussed at the end of the chapter.

SELECTING DRUGS FOR CLINICAL TESTING

Several papers (1,2) have examined the evolution of screening programs used to predict which drugs deserve to be tested in the clinic. Compounds are selected for screening in preclinical systems for a variety of reasons. Some have a structure which, it is predicted, will be active in the killing of tumor cells; many of these may be chemical analogs of drugs already known to be active. Some have shown toxicity in animal systems, which suggests antiproliferative activity. Crude periwinkle extract first attracted attention as a possible antidiabetic agent, and was found to cause leukopenia in animals. Purification of the active principle yielded vinblastine (3). Other compounds such as 5-fluorouracil or the adenosine deaminase inhibitor deoxycoformycin, were rationally designed to interfere with a particular enzyme or biosynthetic pathway.

Other compounds may be tested for purely empirical reasons, perhaps because they have a novel structure unlike those that have previously been tested. In the past such drugs have been screened for activity in transplantable murine tumors. The National Cancer Institute (NCI) screening system has included L1210 and P388 leukemia as well as mouse colon, breast, lung carcinomas, and B16 melanoma. More recently, studies have also been done in human tumor xenografts in nude mice. In an effort in increase the yield of new agents active against the common adult solid tumors, the NCI is shifting its emphasis away from transplantable murine tumors and toward human tumor cell lines *in vitro*.

Currently, investigators attempt to test compounds in both fast- and slow-growing tumors since the earlier screens, which relied heavily on murine leukemia assays for initial detection of activity, favored detection only of compounds active against fast-growing tumors. There is not necessarily good agreement between these various assays nor does the result in any particular assay correlate well with clinical activity. On the other hand, broad spectrum activity in experimental tumors appears to correlate with at least minimal clinical activity (1).

SELECTING PATIENTS FOR TRIAL

Experimental anticancer agents usually have significant toxicities, whether or not they prove to be effective. Biologically inactive doses, biologically active doses, and highly toxic or lethal doses may be close to each other. For this reason it seems ethically justifiable to administer these drugs to human beings only if they are being given with some therapeutic intent. Thus, Phase I trials of anticancer drugs are always performed in patients with cancer who have active disease and not, as with many other drug classes, in normal volunteers.

The initial Phase I evaluations are always performed in adults; studies in children, which are discussed in more detail below, follow determination of the adult MTD. In addition, Phase I studies in solid tumor patients are usually separated from those performed in acute leukemia. For obvious reasons the evaluation of drug effects on normal bone marrow is impossible in relapsed leukemia patients. In addition, it has been generally accepted in the oncology community that, at least for myeloid leukemia, myelosuppressive activity and antileukemic activity are likely to go hand in hand and that "emptying out" the bone marrow may be necessary to achieve a complete remission. Drug dosing is thus generally more aggressive in leukemia trials, and the MTD in leukemia is often significantly higher than the conventionally accepted MTD for solid tumors. As techniques for supportive care improve, this distinction may become unnecessary.

The scientific objective of a Phase I study is determination of the MTD for a particular drug. Eligibility is not, therefore, generally restricted to patients with a particular disease type. If, however, preclinical information suggests strongly that the drug is likely to be active only in a particular tumor (e.g., a hormonal agent in breast cancer), Phase I studies might reasonably be restricted to patients in this group. Also, since the determination of response rates is not a primary goal of Phase I, the presence of measurable tumor masses (see Chapter 2) is not required, and patients who have only evaluable disease should not be excluded from Phase I trials. Good medical practice, of course, dictates that a patient's extent of disease be estimated as accurately as possible prior to therapy and, if possible, response should be carefully followed in the course of the trial. This practice permits intelligent decision making about the advisability of continuing therapy after each course and permits one to develop a preliminary sense of drug activity before the formal Phase II evaluation. However, responses in Phase I are not a substitute for a formal Phase II evaluation, and the absence of response in Phase I should not impede the progression of a drug into Phase II.

Several other requirements for patient entry are conventionally employed in most Phase I studies. Patients should have good performance status (ECOG 0–2) at the start of treatment and an estimated life expectancy of at least 8–12 weeks. Although patients entering Phase I studies commonly have had significant amounts of prior therapy, including chemotherapy, entry onto Phase I studies should be restricted to patients with the minimum amount of previous treatment that is feasible for the disease in question. The patient should have been off prior therapy for some minimal period of time (generally 2–6 weeks) to insure that the effects seen in the trial are those of the agent of interest and not residual toxicity from a prior course of treatment. Finally, the patient should have adequate major organ function, so that the metabolism of the new agent will be normal. All these criteria tend to minimize the chance that the patient will suffer unnecessary severe toxicity from the new agent and to maximize the chance that the agent will be adequately evaluated. By requiring that patients in Phase I trials, despite having advanced disease, have relatively normal major physiological parameters, the criteria also tend to insure that the scientific results of a Phase I study will be relevant to patients with less-advanced disease.

Prior to the start of treatment, patients should have a complete history and physical examination with determination of extent of disease and reasonable documentation of evaluable and measurable parameters. In addition, they should have a hemogram, hepatic and renal function tests, serum electrolytes, glucose, uric acid, urinalysis, chest roentgenogram, and electrocardiogram. Special baseline studies such as pulmonary function tests, ophthalmology exam, and audiometry may also be appropriate, depending on previous findings with the particular drug in preclinical toxicology.

It is not necessary that a patient have received prior conventional therapy before being entered on a Phase I trial if there is no effective chemotherapy for their disease. In fact, under such circumstances it may be preferable to have Phase I trials performed in previously untreated patients. Even if a reasonable time has elapsed since the last dose of chemotherapy, the toxicity observed in a Phase I trial may be affected by toxicity from prior therapy, such as might result from a diminished marrow reserve. A falsely low MTD may be arrived at if only pretreated patients are studied. In a Phase I study of difluoromethylornithine (DFMO) (4), 4 of the 22 patients studied had received no prior chemotherapy. Thrombocytopenia, which was dose-limiting, occurred in 11 of 16 patients who had received prior chemotherapy and in none of the four who had not. It is not unusual, in fact, for the recommended Phase II dose to be different for previously treated and untreated patients. In a study of 9-beta-D-arabinofuranosyl-2-fluoroadenine-5'-monophosphate (NSC 312887) Hutton et al. (5) recommended a starting dose of 18 mg/m^2/day for patients with prior chemotherapy or radiotherapy and 25 mg/m^2 for those without prior therapy, a difference of about 35%.

SAFE STARTING DOSE

Although the extrapolation of toxicity data from animal to man poses many difficulties, established guidelines can predict a safe starting dose in man with reasonable accuracy. Currently, all the comparisons from one species to another are based on the seminal analysis of Freireich et al.(6) and are expressed as doses in mg/m^2. Since the 1950s, data have been accumulating about the relative toxicity of drugs in man compared with the mouse, rat, dog, and monkey. Grieshaber and Marsoni (7) describe the process by which this large data base of human and animal toxicology was assembled and reviewed in the late 1970s, in order to determine whether it was possible to streamline the preclinical toxicity testing of antineoplastics without sacrificing safety. In 1979, the Food and Drug Administration Oncologic Drugs Advisory Committee concurred with the concept that preclinical studies in the mouse could predict a safe starting dose for the testing of antineoplastic drugs in man. They also recommended that one additional experimental species be tested to assess the safety of proposed human starting doses and to predict qualitative organ toxicity. The beagle dog was deemed the best choice because of the extensive background information already available.

In current murine toxicology studies, the dose of drug that is lethal to 10, 50, and 90% of nontumor-bearing animals is established (LD 10, LD 50, LD 90) by analysis of multiple doses given to several hundred animals. The murine LD 10 dose is converted to its equivalent dose in mg/m^2 (the so-called mouse equivalent LD 10 or MELD 10). The starting dose for trials in man has been established as $\frac{1}{10}$ the MELD 10 or less. The interested reader is referred to the work of Guarino et al. (8) for an appreciation of some of the problems of arriving at a precise number for the LD 10 or the LD 50. As the authors state: "[the LD 50] should not be considered the equivalent of a melting point on pure organic compounds." There are variations between strains of mice, route of administration, and vehicle. There are even variations when the same individual tries to reproduce the same experiment in the same laboratory. In addition, the toxicity curves can be relatively flat. For 8 of 16 compounds analyzed in the report by Guarino et al. (8), the LD 90 was less than twice the LD 10 in mg/kg.

Once the MELD 10 is known, the beagle dog is then used in studies done around the MELD 10 to determine its relative safety. If no severe toxicity is observed in dogs at $\frac{1}{10}$ the MELD 10, then this becomes the starting dose for man. If severe toxicity is observed in dogs at this dose, the dose is reduced until minimal or no toxicity is found. In such cases the initial human doses would be based on the human equivalent in mg/m^2 of ⅓ the dog dose experimentally determined to cause minimal reversible toxicity or to an equivalent fraction of the LD 10 in mice (7).

The rat is also being studied, once the MELD 10 is known, to see whether it can be used to predict specific organ toxicities in man. The rat is easier to work with than the mouse since the organs are larger and serial blood samples can be drawn for hematologic and chemical determinations. A summary of the kinds of information derived from studies in each species is shown in Table 4.1.

Despite the use of more than one species, certain toxicities cannot be assessed easily in animal model systems. Skin, cardiac, and peripheral nervous system toxicity are not well predicted, and the detection of central nervous system (CNS) toxicity is dependent on the care with which animals are assessed neurologically (9). Also, specific manifestations of toxicity are less well predicted than broad organ toxicities; for example, hematopoietic toxicity may be expressed as anemia in animals and leukopenia in man.

TABLE 4.1 *Preclinical Toxicology Studies*

Schedule	Mouse	Dog	Rat
Single dose	LD 10, LD 50, LD 90	Qualitative toxicity	Qualitative toxicity
Daily × 5	LD 10, LD 50, LD 90	Qualitative toxicity	Qualitative toxicity
Others as needed			

Grieshaber and Marsoni (7) have reviewed the relationship of preclinical toxicology to findings in early clinical trials to see how well the current toxicology protocol predicts safe starting doses and qualitative toxicities in man. They reviewed seven agents which had undergone preclinical toxicology studies as described above and which had completed Phase I studies in man. Five drugs on seven schedules were started at $\frac{1}{10}$ the MELD 10. The entry level dose was reduced for three drugs because serious toxicity was found in dogs for each drug at $\frac{1}{10}$ MELD 10. These serious toxic effects involved the alimentary tract, liver, kidney, prostate, and bone marrow. As a result of these preclinical findings, the starting doses in man were lowered to $\frac{1}{30}$ or $\frac{1}{60}$ MELD 10. It appeared that there was a tendency for the dog to overpredict toxicity, since humans tolerated these drugs at $\frac{1}{10}$ the MELD 10 with no adverse effects; however, once dose-limiting toxicities did appear in man, the nature of the toxicity was as predicted by the large animal model. In one of the seven drugs (fludarabine), myelosuppression was seen in man at a dose which both the mouse and the dog would have predicted to be tolerable. The authors conclude that the preclinical toxicity screen with two species is valuable in predicting the potential risk to humans even though the recommended safe starting doses are occasionally too low and a few extra dose escalations are required in man.

DRUG SCHEDULES

Not all drugs are going to be effective at the same dose and schedule. In designing the Phase I trial, one must give some thought not only to what will be tolerated but also to what drug administration schedule is logical. Ideally, before starting a Phase I trial one would like to have an idea of what level of drug in the blood one wishes to achieve and for how long. This is not an easy task, since for many drugs good pharmacologic measurement methods are not available at the time Phase I trials are instituted. However, when such methods become available, even if the mechanism of action of a drug is not understood, it will be possible to measure the drug concentration that is associated with antitumor effect and/or toxicity in *in vitro* or *in vivo* systems. If proper pharmacokinetic studies can be done, then the practical achievable level can be assessed and the level associated with therapeutic effect or toxicity can be noted, even if the schedules are determined empirically and the desirable drug level can be assessed and the level for efficacy is not known.

The concentration of drug that can be achieved depends on a number of factors such as absorption, distribution, metabolism, excretion, and normal tissue sensitivity, all of which may vary from one species to another. Pharmacologic ideas that seem sound during *in vitro* experiments may turn out to be inapplicable *in vivo* because the requisite concentrations of drug simply cannot be achieved in an animal. In some studies, the concentration of drug actually achieved in the tumor can be measured if the tumor cells are readily accessible. Repeated assays of drug levels in leukemia cells are quite feasible, for example.

Collins et al. (10) have reemphasized the importance not only of the peak drug concentration achieved after a single dose but also of the area under the concentration versus time curve (C × T). This concept began with the observation by German pharmacologists during World War I that mustard agents were equally toxic whether a high concentration was inhaled for a short time or a low concentration was inhaled for a long time. The essential feature is that C × T is the determinant of effect rather than C itself. Not all drugs, however, depend strictly on the absolute concentration achieved or on the C × T. Antimetabolites, for example, whose action depends on the inhibition of synthesis of macromolecular systems, may be more dependent on time of exposure above a certain threshold concentration. Lower doses, which may still be toxic, can be totally ineffective no matter how long they are maintained.

It may be possible to select a schedule with a specific biochemical rationale. For example, an enzyme inhibitor must attain drug concentrations that will inhibit the enzyme in tumor tissue *in vivo*. DFMO arrests growth in culture of a number of different experimental tumors. The mechanism of action is thought to be the inhibition of ornithine decarboxylase and, with it, blockage of the conversion of ornithine to putrescine, the first and rate-limiting step in the polyamine biosynthetic pathway. It makes sense then, that in order for the drug to be useful in clinical trials, a dose has to be achieved in which the concentration of DFMO in the steady state is within the range needed for inhibition of ornithine decarboxylase in cell culture systems as well as for inhibitory activity against various human tumors *in vitro*. In a recently completed Phase I trial (4), the highest dose achieved (3 gm/m^2 every 6 h by mouth for 28 days) did indeed achieve these concentrations, as did somewhat lower doses. The investigators recommended a Phase II dose of 2.25 gm/m^2 every 6 h. The pharmacokinetic analysis in this paper is so carefully done that it is possible to suggest that even an every-8-h schedule of administration would achieve the relevant concentrations of drug, and this might be a more practical schedule for administration. Obviously, because of the relatively short plasma half-life of this compound, determining the MTD of a single dose given every 3 weeks would have been a waste of both patient and investigator effort.

DOSE ESCALATION

After the schedule and starting dose have been decided on, subsequent doses must be escalated until the MTD is reached. The MTD may be defined in advance as a dose that produces an arbitrary level of a predicatable toxicity in a certain percentage of patients, or it may be determined when some unexpected and poorly reversible toxicity occurs.

As Collins et al. (10) have pointed out, the process of dose escalation is governed by a fundamental conflict. There is a need to go slowly to avoid the sudden appearance of very severe toxicity; on the other hand, if one goes too slowly, large numbers of patients are treated at submaximal doses. The dangers of escalation that is too rapid are easily understood. To guard against this, in most trials, at least 3 patients are placed on the initial dose and adequate time is allowed for follow-up of toxicity before entering patients on the next dose. In practice, this generally means that 3–6 weeks elapse after each course to allow the return of counts or chemistries to normal. As toxicity occurs, more patients are entered at each dose level until the MTD is reached. This may mean that 6–8 patients per dose level are entered on a few of the higher levels. This allows one to have a very rough estimate of the incidence of toxicity that can be expected at any dose level. It also guards against stopping a trial prematurely because one patient has an unusual reaction to the drug. It should be emphasized again here that this means the MTD is usually determined on the basis of observations in a rather small number of patients.

There are also dangers if escalation proceeds too slowly. Principally, there is the obligation to the individual patient to try to administer doses of the drug that are potentially therapeutic. A recent review of Phase I studies by the NCI (11) showed that about 40% of the patients on Phase I trials were treated at doses at or above that recommended as the eventual Phase II dose. Thus, current escalation schemes do permit a significant proportion of patients to receive adequate doses of the experimental agent.

As a result of consideration of these conflicting pressures, the escalation scheme that has been most widely adopted is the "modified Fibonacci" scheme (10) (Fig. 4.1). The starting dose is established as discussed above, and the second step is to double the starting dose; the third step is 67% greater than the second, the fourth is 50% greater than the third, and each subsequent step is 33% greater than that preceding it. Figure 4.1 demonstrates the relative number of steps required if one starts at $\frac{1}{10}$ or $\frac{1}{30}$ the MELD 10.

How efficient is this strategy in terms of the number of dose escalations required to reach the MTD? Collins et al. (10) have looked at the wide range in the eventual MTD in man relative to the mouse LD 10. For the 17 drugs they analyzed, the median MTD in humans was equal to the mouse LD 10 and the median number of steps to reach the MTD was five or six. For a number of the drugs, however, ten or more escalations were required (Fig. 4.2).

In practice, escalation is not always done strictly by the Fibonacci scheme. One specific example is shown in Table 4.2. The starting dose for this study was $\frac{1}{30}$ the MELD 10 because of findings in preclinical toxicology. A classic escalation was proposed but one level was skipped. In fact, no toxicity was seen at doses less than 1500 mg/m^2. At doses of 2000 and 2500 mg/m^2 Grade 2 hepatic and symptomatic toxicity occurred in about half the courses, although there was no obvious difference between the two doses. Because moderate toxicity was seen at this level, more patients were treated so that the investigators could assure themselves that these responses were relatively typical. At 3125 mg/m^2 Grade 3 hepatic and symptomatic toxicity occurred in two of two patients and the study was terminated. Based on this study, the investigators recommend that Phase II therapy should be initiated at the 2000-mg/m^2 dose level and escalated to 2500 mg/m^2 if the initial dose is well tolerated.

In the DFMO study previously cited (4), the investigators added steps rather than skip escalations as the predicted MTD was approached, because European studies

MODIFIED FIBONACCI SCHEME
OF DOSE ESCALATION

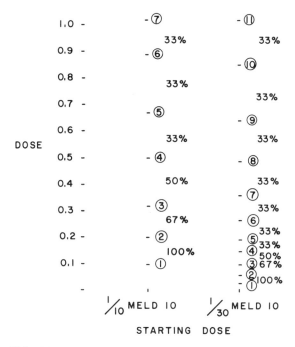

FIG. 4.1. Number of dose escalations that would be performed if a compound were started at $\frac{1}{10}$ or $\frac{1}{30}$ the MELD 10.

in man had revealed possible serious gastrointestinal toxicity. The escalation scheme that was used is shown in Table 4.3. Following completion of the 28-day course at any level, a further 2 weeks elapsed before new patients were entered on the study at the next higher dose level. There was no escalation of dose for any individual patient. Most current Phase I trials are done with *these sorts of* cautious modifications of the Fibonacci scheme, and so far this practice has proven to be relatively safe.

Other schedules based on pharmacologic rationales may prove to be more efficient. A focus of considerable current interest (10) is the possibility that toxicity may be equivalent between mouse and man at equivalent blood levels of drug. If so, then differences in MTD and MELD 10 may reflect differences in metabolism, excretion, or some other process which might be species related such as drug binding (10). For drugs where this turns out to be the case, escalation can perhaps be determined by the blood levels achieved in man compared with mouse, rather than by a completely empirical schedule. Doxorubicin, for example, has an MTD in man (90 mg/m²) fivefold greater than the MELD 10 (18 mg/m²) (13); however, this apparent tolerance is based on the fact that humans have a higher clearance

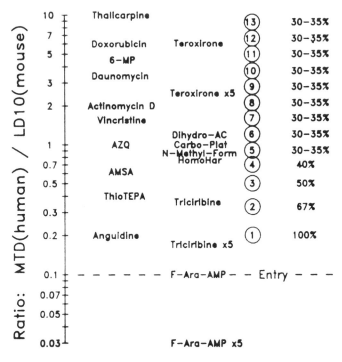

FIG. 4.2. Analysis of dosage escalations actually required for 17 drugs during Phase I trials when $\frac{1}{10}$ the MELD 10 is used and a modified Fibonacci escalation. The median number of escalation steps was 5–6. For 5 of the drugs more escalations were required. (Reprinted from Ref. 10.)

TABLE 4.2 *Dose Escalations in Phase I Trial of N-methylformamide*

Starting Weekly Dose (mg/m²)	No. patients (evaluable)	No. courses (evaluable)	% Dose increased
125	3(3)	3(3)	—
250	3(3)	3(3)	100
413	4(4)	4(4)	65
625	3(3)	3(3)	51
875	—	—	—
1125	4(3)	4(3)	80
1500	4(4)	5(5)	33
2000	11(9)	14(12)	33
2500	8(6)	9(7)	25
3125	2(2)	2(2)	25

From Ref. 12.

TABLE 4.3 *Dose Escalation in Phase I Trial of DFMO*

Oral dose every 6 hr. for 28 days (gm/mQ2w)	% Dose increased
0.75	—
1.50	100
2.25	50
3.00	33.3
3.75	25
4.50	20
5.25	16.7

From Ref. 4.

$(ml/min/m^2)$ for doxorubicin than mice, so that for any single dose administered the blood level in man will be lower than that in a mouse. When the drugs are compared at equal blood levels, there is considerable agreement in the organ toxicity between the two species. If these data had been known when the initial Phase I trials were being performed, rapid dose escalation past the early dose levels in man, based on plasma levels, could have been accomplished.

TERMINATING THE STUDY

The maximum toxicity to be tolerated and the interval at which tests should be performed to determine toxicity should be defined as precisely as possible before the study begins. Prior to the start of treatment in the DFMO study (4), it was agreed that the MTD would be defined as that dose of drug at which Grade 2 ECOG toxicity appeared. In order to make sure that this level of toxicity is seen consistently, as soon as one patient exhibits this phenomenon, then extra patients should be treated at this dose level before escalation proceeds.

During treatment, physical examinations, hemograms, and hepatic and renal function tests were repeated at a minimum of weekly intervals. If one uses one of these general toxicity scales to define an acceptable toxicity level, then reactions in most of the organ systems will be included. It is important to remember that unexpected toxicities can occur, even with the first dose of an agent. In general, patients should be admitted for the first courses of any drug at the starting dose in case of unexpected toxicity. Once it is clear that the patients will not sustain untoward events of major proportion, then they can be treated as outpatients.

Certain toxicities are extremely difficult to detect in rodents and even in dogs. These include neurologic side effects, visual or auditory effects, and effects on the skin. Patients must be examined and carefully questioned for the existence of such signs as mucositis or alopecia and symptoms such as dizziness, which might reflect orthostatic hypotension. A mental status examination should be given to detect mental confusion (14), since significant aberrations in mental status may occur before they are detected in casual conversation.

These issues are of significant practical importance. In a Phase I study of 1-(2'-deoxy-2'-fluoro-1-beta-D-arabinofuranosyl)-5-methyluracil (FMAU) (15), there were no CNS side effects at doses of 32 mg/m²/day or less, but in 6 evaluable patients treated with doses of 64 or 128 mg/m²/day, CNS dysfunction consisting of severe encephalopathy with extrapyramidal dysfunction occurred in 3 and contributed to 2 deaths. Two of these 3 patients, including one who died, had prior whole brain irradiation. This emphasizes the importance of the interactions with prior therapy in a Phase I setting.

In another Phase I trial with acivicin (16), 13 patients who received 17 courses at doses at or above 5.5 mg/m²/day developed neurotoxicity. This was characterized by reversible asthenia (11 courses), disorientation (6), lethargy (3), depression (2), paranoia (2), amnesia (1), hostility (1), and transient unconsciousness (1). The symptoms cleared spontaneously and no permanent neurologic dysfunction was noted. Neurotoxicity was more common in patients requiring opiates for analgesia where all of 17 evaluable courses showed neurotoxicity versus 5/12 courses in patients not on analgesics, and in those with increased third-space fluid (6/17 courses versus 1/12). This again emphasizes the interaction with other therapies and specifically with those therapies (analgesics) that are common in advanced cancer and are not given to animals in whom the drugs are tested.

The frequency with which tests are performed during the administration of the drug should be related to the likelihood and time course of a particular toxic side effect and the planned frequency of drug administration. In studying a myelosuppressive agent, one should obviously determine blood counts at the time of the expected nadir. For a potentially cardiotoxic agent, such as a new anthracycline analog, suitable tests of cardiac function must be performed periodically. Since the probability of drug-induced cardiac toxicity is generally a function of cumulative dose, it seems appropriate to increase the frequency of cardiac monitoring as the patient accumulates progressively larger amounts of drug.

One cannot predict exactly which toxicities are going to occur, particularly in the Phase I setting. In addition, certain side effects may greatly bother the patients even when they are not life threatening. In a Phase I investigation of Ametantrone (17), all patients with fair complexions receiving two or more courses of drug developed a cumulative blue-gray skin discoloration. Skin biopsies revealed no detectable drug. After the drug was stopped, a peeling of the epidermis occurred along with a gradual fading of the blue-gray skin tint over the ensuing months. However, even 5 months after discontinuation of the drug, 2 of these patients still had blue-gray discoloration of the skin. This is cited to serve as a dramatic reminder to insert a sentence in all consent forms that "unpredicted toxicities may occur."

Although most toxicities from chemotherapy are reversible, occasionally irreversible and even fatal side effects may occur. In early clinical trials of tricyclic nucleoside phosphate (18), 20 adults were treated with intravenous infusions given over 15 min once every 3 weeks, in doses ranging from 25 to 350 mg/m². Hyperglycemia and elevation of hepatocellular enzymes were observed beginning at a dose of 250 mg/m²; 5 patients received a dose of 350 mg/m², 2 of whom developed irreversible and fatal liver damage. Because preclinical studies had predicted that hepatotoxicity might be significant with this drug, the only surprise was the severity of the liver damage, but we should remember that an occasional lethal reaction may occur, particularly during a Phase I trial. It is only because the MTD has been established that such reactions are rarely seen in Phase III studies.

In evaluating toxicity in a Phase I trial, it is most important to separate the effects of a drug from those of a disease. As noted above, this is one important reason why patients should have relatively normal organ function at the beginning of the trial. Hematopoietic toxicity, for example, cannot be assessed reliably in a patient whose bone marrow is infiltrated with tumor or was hypocellular before starting the trial. In general, one tends to believe that an adverse event is drug related if there is a temporal relation between drug administration and the appearance of the reaction, or if there seems to be a definite dose–effect relationship with increasing incidence or severity of the putative toxicity at higher doses. With the small numbers of patients treated at any particular dose in a Phase I study, however, these correlations can be difficult to establish.

For these reasons, postmortem examinations are important in patients who have participated in Phase I trials, particularly in those who have done so shortly before death. Unsuspected new infiltration of tumor into the liver might explain abnormal liver function tests, and intracranial metastases could explain CNS symptoms that might have otherwise been ascribed to the drug. Conversely, pathologically documented absence of tumor involvement in a particular organ implicates the drug or its metabolites as possible causes of the observed abnormalities. Although the physician may think that the cause of death in a patient is known, and the family may feel that the patient "has suffered enough," the contribution the patient makes to our knowledge about the new agent and to the potential benefit of this treatment for other patients should not be overlooked or go undiscussed.

Some very important toxicities may not be detected in Phase I trials, which by their nature are usually short-term studies. Thus, the effects of chronic drug administration may not be appreciated. Chronic toxicities are an important issue medically only for relatively active drugs, simply because these are the only agents that are given on a chronic basis. Delineation of chronic toxicities generally occurs, therefore, in the later stages of drug development and continues well into the postmarketing period.

Late toxicity is a particular problem in the Phase I evaluation of new radiotherapy techniques and schedules. As dosing or fractionation is changed there may be a loss in the differential toxicity for normal and tumor tissue, but the effect may not be appreciated for several months after the dose is given. This means that Phase I studies in radiotherapy may require months rather than weeks of delay between entry of patients at each dose escalation (19).

MTD IS A RELATIVE CONCEPT

As previously mentioned, the Phase I study of DFMO was stopped at the point at which Grade 2 ECOG toxicity appeared. This means that doses of drug that suppressed the platelet count to below $50,000/mm^3$ would not be recommended for initial investigations of efficacy with this drug. Under other circumstances, however, such modest degrees of thrombocytopenia might not be considered dose limiting. Investigators are particularly likely to want to study very high doses of a drug with myelosuppressive dose-limiting toxicities at conventional doses if the initial studies have shown some activity in Phase II trials. Etoposide is active in a number of tumors including small cell carcinoma of the lung. Once this was established, investigators wished to explore the effects of higher doses to see whether remission rates would increase correspondingly. In a repeat Phase I study of high-dose etoposide (20), where the doses studied were 10 times or more as high as those studied in the initial trials, the number of days patients spent with platelet counts below $20,000/mm^3$ and the number of platelet transfusions required were recorded but were not regarded as limiting further escalation; the dose-limiting toxicity was considered to be mucositis. In other words, thrombocytopenia, as long as it could be controlled with transfusions, was not considered reason to stop the dose escalation.

As noted above, investigators are particularly likely to explore extremely high doses of a drug if the initial dose-limiting toxicity has been hematologic, since current techniques of blood component support and the widespread availability of broad-spectrum antibiotics can often reduce the probability of fatal complications to within acceptable limits. Duration of marrow hypoplasia may be significantly reduced by infusion of autologous bone marrow cells, which might be considered a form of ''biologic rescue'' with stem cells stored in a viable state before high-dose drug administration. Drugs may also be pushed well beyond the conventional MTD if a pharmacologic rescue technique becomes available, such as with methotrexate and leukovorin.

One must remember that these repeat trials at higher doses are true Phase I trials, and that the ''next dose-limiting toxicity'' of high-dose agents after myelotoxicity may occur in different organ systems from those affected at low doses. The potentially lethal pulmonary toxicity of the nitrosoureas was not appreciated until these drugs were used in high doses in the autologous marrow transplant setting (21).

PHASE I STUDIES IN CHILDREN

The low incidence and high responsiveness of childhood cancer relative to adult cancer greatly influence the way new drugs are evaluated in this population. Children are (a) more likely to have a tumor for which some initial potentially curative therapy is already available and should be given; (b) less able to give truly informed consent themselves for a study; and (c) less likely to be available in adequate numbers for a timely evaluation of any significant number of new agents. Phase I studies in children, therefore, are usually not performed until the MTD in adults is already known and are often restricted to agents that have shown some activity in adult tumors.

In a recent review of qualitative and quantitative toxic effects of antineoplastic agents in adults and children, Marsoni et al. (22) discovered some difference in the thresholds for developing toxicity in the two populations. Children with solid tumors appear to have a greater dose tolerance than adults, while children with leukemia appear to have a tolerance equivalent to adults. However, the authors remind us that from a physiological point of view, children are not "little adults," but rather immature individuals subject to a continuous state of development. Marked variations exist in drug distribution and elimination via renal excretion or hepatic metabolism according to age; the relative volumes of the body water compartment, total body water, and extracellular water decrease progressively from infancy to adulthood. This might lead one to predict a greater tolerance in children for some agents, and in fact, a larger volume of distribution in children was documented for ICRF 187, a compound that children tolerated in doses almost three times those of adults (23). Greater rates of plasma elimination in children than adults have been reported for cyclophosphamide, methotrexate, and etoposide. The overall rate of hepatic metabolism also decreases from late infancy through childhood to adolescence and adulthood. This factor may have played a role in the increased toxicity observed with indicine-*N*-oxide in younger children where hepatic metabolism is thought to be responsible for the production of the toxic metabolite dehydroindicine. Thus, although the overall trend is for children to show the same or better tolerance for drugs than adults, an occasional agent is more toxic in children than adults and separate Phase I studies should certainly be performed. The NCI is currently recommending (22) that Phase I trials in children (a) begin in patients with solid tumors and leukemia at 80% of the MTD in adults with solid tumors; (b) be designed so that separate groups of patients with leukemia and solid tumors are entered at each level; and (c) be escalated at fixed 20% increments, i.e., at a more conservative rate than the modified Fibonacci scheme. The toxic effects observed in patients with leukemias (for whom myelosuppression is a sought after effect) should be distinguished from those observed in patients with solid tumors. If myelosuppression is the dose-limiting toxicity in solid tumors, drug dose should be escalated beyond the MTD in patients with leukemia.

ANTITUMOR ACTIVITY

Estey et al. (11) analyzed the response rate seen in Phase I trials reported to the NCI and performed between 1974 and 1982. Of 1921 patients, 719 had measurable disease. Among these latter patients there were 5 complete remissions (0.7%) and 16 partial remissions (2.2%) for an objective response rate of 2.9%. Thus the probability of a clinically significant response in Phase I trials is low. These authors compared Phase I and Phase II data where both were available for the same drug. They found that the median overall Phase I response rate for drugs later found to be active in Phase II was 4.3% (range 1.5–11.8%) compared with a response rate of 2.7% (range 0–5.7%) for drugs later found to be inactive. The difference was not significant. They conclude that it would be inadvisable to establish a policy of discontinuing the development of drugs that show no responses in Phase I. Table 4.4 shows the five drugs that had the lowest response rate in their formal Phase I studies and their eventual fate in Phase II. This low level of therapeutic activity in Phase I trials, even in those agents which eventually prove active in Phase II, is in contrast to the activity seen in the Phase I trials performed before 1974 with those agents that now have established therapeutic activity. In Phase I trials of vincristine, for example, the response rate was 40%. These older drugs were more often tested in patients with responsive tumors and in previously untreated patients, while 94% of the patients going on Phase I trials more recently have received some prior therapy (11). The lesson is clearly that Phase I trials must be designed so that the maximum information is gained with the smallest possible number of patients being exposed to potentially ineffective doses of the drug.

DILEMMAS IN PHASE I

The scientific imperatives of the Phase I study are compelling ones, for it is clear that there can be no clinical development of new agents without a careful dose-finding phase. From a medical and ethical perspective, however, several features of the Phase I trial are disquieting to many physicians. How can one discuss the risks and benefits of a treatment with a patient if neither risk nor benefit is known? Since these dose-finding studies are the earliest clinical experience with new anti-cancer agents, there is no previous track record on which to make even a preliminary judgment about efficacy. The physician, therefore, can impart to his patient no particular confidence that Phase I drug treatment has any solid chance to success at all, since essentially nothing is known about the agent's behavior in human beings. Second, since the Phase I study has dose escalation built into the structure

TABLE 4.4 *Phase I versus Phase II Responses*

	Phase I			Phase II Best Response		
Drug	Response rate (CR + PR)	Studies (N)	Patients (N)	Tumor type	CR + PR	80% CI
Alanosine	0	3	116	Inactive		
Anguidine	0	4	122	Inactive		
PALA	1.3	6	237	Inactive		
Aclacinomycin (17–26)	1.5	6	134	Leukemia	21%	
Carboplatin (31–45)	1.9	5	155	Ovarian	38%	

CR, complete response; PR, partial response.

of the trial, the patient entering the study at a level less than the eventual MTD is being exposed to a less than full (and therefore presumably less than optimal) dose; in the early stages of the trial, the difference between the administered dose and any biologically effective dose may be very large indeed. Third, patients entering Phase I trials are those for whom effective conventional therapy either does not exist at all or has been exhausted. These patients, by definition, then, have drug-resistant disease and must have a very low probability of responding even to a Phase I drug that might subsequently prove active in a less-resistant patient population. These features of Phase I studies are difficult enough for many physicians to come to terms with, but in addition to the facts themselves the nature of the informed consent process requires that they all be discussed rather explicitly with the patient at the time a Phase I trial is proposed. Small wonder, then, that many physicians shy away from participation in Phase I studies and prefer to treat their patients with some conventional approach.

Nevertheless, for many patients interested in continuing efforts at active therapy, entry onto a Phase I study is the most promising approach that can be offered. New agents are brought to clinical trial because one or more desirable properties have been uncovered in preclinical testing. Although their credentials as clinically active antitumor agents have not yet been established, their spectrum of activity in preclinical models make the presumption of clinical activity at least reasonable. A demonstration in the laboratory of lack of cross-resistance with other available antitumor agents strengthens the attractiveness of new agents for testing in drug-resistant patient populations. The use of a Phase I agent, particularly one with a novel chemical structure or one known to be noncross-resistant with existing drugs, may realistically be a more hopeful therapeutic approach for the patient who is eligible for a Phase I trial than the use of a conventional cytotoxic agent that is already known to have a very low probability of success. The fact that many patients are treated in Phase I at less than the MTD is, in a sense, quite beside the point. Good Phase I trials are designed in such a way that *all* patients on the trial are treated at the maximal dose that is known to be safe for them at the time they are entered. The corollary here is that over-accrual of patients onto subtoxic and subtherapeutic levels in the course of dose escalation is bad clinical trials practice and bad medical practice, and the 3–6 patients per escalation dose recommended here should not be exceeded unless the toxicity data are unclear at any particular level.

Admittedly, patients entering Phase I studies over the past several years have had little probability of demonstrable benefit. However, patients selected for these studies are those for whom no better therapy is available, and therefore one might have expected a low rate of response from alternative conventional treatment of these very patients under the same circumstances. It is critical that the patients be provided with enough information to make an informed decision about their participation. But when presenting the patient with the information it is just as important to stress the positive reasons why the drug has been selected for clinical trial, as it is to emphasize the lack of knowledge about the potential efficacy and side effects in man. Many patients who come to centers offering experimental drug therapy do so with the intention of taking advantage of all opportunities for participating in the testing of promising new therapies. This group of patients is self-selected for an activist approach to treatment, and some are genuinely motivated by the knowledge that their participation in a clinical trial may help other patients, even if it does not benefit them directly. For such patients, participation in early new drug trials is important ethically as well as psychologically. The ethical imperative, then, is to be sure that the trials are designed sufficiently well so that useful information can be accrued about the drug as a result of the patient's participation.

REFERENCES

1. Goldin, A., Venditti, J. M., Macdonald, J. D., et al. (1981): Current results of the screening program of the Division of Cancer Treatment, National Cancer Institute. *Eur. J. Cancer*, 17:119–142.
2. Spreafico, F., Edelstein, M., and Lelieveld, P. (1984): Experimental bases for drug selection. In: *Cancer Clinical Trials: Methods and Practice*, edited by M. E. Buyse, M. J. Staquet, and R. J. Sylvester, pp. 193–209. Oxford University Press, Oxford.
3. Noble, R. L., Beer, C. T., and Cutts, J. H. (1958): Further biological activities of vincaleuko-blastine—An alkaloid isolated from *vinca rosea (L.) Biochem. Pharmacol.*, 1:347–348.
4. Abeloff, M. D., Slavik, M., Luk, G. D., et al. (1984): Phase I trial and pharmacokinetic studies of alpha difluoromethylornithine—An inhibitor of polyamine biosynthesis. *J. Clin. Oncol.*, 2:124–130.
5. Hutton , J. J., Von Hoff, D. D., Kuhn, J., et al. (1984): Phase I clinical investigation of 9-beta-D-arabinofuranosyl-2-fluoroadenine-5'-monophosphate (NSC 312887), a new purine antimetabolite. *Cancer Res.*, 44:4183–4186.
6. Freireich, E. J., Gehan, E. A., Rall, D. P., et al. (1966): Quantitative comparison of toxicity of anticancer agents in mouse, rat, hamster, dog, monkey and man. *Cancer Chemother. Rep.*, 50:219–244.
7. Grieshaber, C. K., and Marsoni, S. (1986): The relation of preclinical toxicology to findings in early clinical trials. *Cancer Treat. Rep.*, 70:65–72.
8. Guarino, A. M., Rozencweig, M., Kline, I., et al. (1979): Adequacies and inadequacies in assessing murine toxicity data with antineoplastic agents. *Cancer Res.*, 39:2204–2210.
9. Owens, A. H., Jr. (1962): Predicting anticancer drug effects in man from laboratory animal studies. *J. Chronic Dis.*, 15:223–228.
10. Collins, J. M., Zaharko, D. S., Dedrick, R. L., and Chabner, B. A. (1986): Potential roles for preclinical pharmacology in Phase I clinical trials. *Cancer Treat. Rep.*, 70:73–80.
11. Estey, E., Hoth, D., Simon, R., et al.: Therapeutic response in Phase I trials of anti-neoplastic agents. *Cancer Treat. Rep.*, 70:1105–1115.
12. Ettinger, D. S., Orr, D. W., Rice, A. P., and Donehower, R. C. (1985): Phase I study of N-methylformamide in patients with advanced cancer. *Cancer Treat. Rep.*, 69:489–493.
13. Greene, R. F., Collins, J. M., Jenkins, J. F., et al. (1983): Plasma pharmacokinetics of adriamycin and adrimycinol: Implications for the design of *in vitro* experiments and treatment protocols. *Cancer Res.*, 43:3417–3421.
14. Folstein, M. F., Fetting, J. H., Lobo, A., et al. (1984): Cognitive assessment of cancer patients. *Cancer*, 53:2250–2257.
15. Fanucchi, M. P., Leyland-Jones, B., Young, C. W., et al. (1985): Phase I trial of 1-(2'-deoxy-2'-fluoro-1-beta-D-arabinofuranosyl)-5methyluracil (FMAU). *Cancer Treat. Rep.*, 69:55–59.
16. Sridhar, K. S., Ohnuma, T., Chahinian, A. P., and Holland, J. F. (1983): Phase I study of Acivicin in patients with advanced cancer. *Cancer Treat. Rep.*, 67:987–991.
17. Loesch, D. M., von Hoff, D. D., Kuhn J., et al. (1983): Phase I investigation of Ametantrone. *Cancer Treat. Rep.*, 67:987–991.
18. Mittelman, A., Casper, E. S., Godwin, T. A., et al. (1983): Phase I study of tricyclic nucleoside phosphate. *Cancer Treat. Rep.*, 67:159–162.

19. Rubin, P., Keys, H., and Salazar, O. (1981): New designs for radiation oncology research in clinical trials. *Semin. Oncol.*, 8:453–472.
20. Postmus, P. E., Mulder, N. H., Sleijfer, D. T., et al. (1984): High-dose etoposide for refractory malignancies: A Phase I study. *Cancer Treat. Rep.*, 68:1471–1474.
21. Weiss, R. B., Poster, D. S., and Penta, J. S. (1985): The nitrosoureas and pulmonary toxicity. *Cancer Treat. Rev.*, 8:111–125.
22. Marsoni, E., Ungerleider, R. S., Hurson, S. B., et al. (1985): Tolerance to antineoplastic agents in children and adults. *Cancer Treat. Rep.*, 69:1263–1269.
23. Holcenberg, J. S., Tutsch, K. D., Earhart, R. H., et al. (1986): Phase I study of ICRF-187 in pediatric cancer patients and comparison of its pharmacokinetics in children and adults. *Cancer Treat. Rep.*, 70:703–709.

CHAPTER 5

Phase II Trials

Once the dose of an agent that can be administered safely to man has been determined in Phase I, the next step is to determine in which tumor types the drug has activity. The specific purpose of a Phase II trial is to develop estimates of the response rate of patients with specified tumor types to a particular drug. To do this, a population of patients is treated with a dose that is usually 75–90% of that previously determined to be maximally tolerable in Phase I. The underlying assumption for chemotherapeutic agents and radiotherapy is that the higher the dose, the more likely a response. This may not be true for biologic response modifiers (see Chapter 10).

As noted in the previous chapter, response rates in Phase I trials do not clearly predict eventual clinical activity (1). In the absence of limiting toxic effects that are not clearly dose dependent or very severe, there are currently no good medical or scientific grounds for terminating a drug's clinical development short of a Phase II evaluation (2). The preclinical screens do not predict which specific tumor types should be selected for study. Agents active in breast cancer models will not necessarily be active in clinical breast cancer. Phase I and II trials are performed independently of each other and involve different criteria of patient selection and different drug doses. Responses that may occur in a Phase 1 study may be useful in indicating high priority directions for Phase II study. They cannot, however, be used as part of the Phase II assessment and are therefore not employed in computing response rates in Phase II.

In order to use the response data from Phase II studies to plan future comparative trials in Phase III, 15–25 or more patients with each tumor type of interest are placed on study. If no responses are seen, then the drug is likely to be dropped from future development. If activity is seen, enough patients should be treated to develop a rough idea of the level of activity of the drug. These estimates will then be used in planning subsequent trials of efficacy.

Since tumor shrinkage is a major endpoint of interest in a Phase II study, the patients treated in Phase II must have tumors for which changes in size can be quantitatively assessed. The other important endpoints of interest are the duration of the responses and the toxic cost of achieving therapeutic effects. Although Phase II trials are usually not comparative in design, investigators consider their results in light of all available knowledge about the treatment of a cancer to decide whether further trials are justified.

Phase II, therefore, is intended to determine activity. It does not determine efficacy; the question of how useful a new treatment will be in controlling a disease is implicitly a comparative one and cannot be addressed without a carefully selected control population. Phase II results determine whether a new treatment should be pursued further, and with what level of priority relative to other agents. Thus the outcome of Phase II is a decisive point in a drug's development.

DETERMINING TUMOR TYPES FOR STUDY

Occasionally a drug will be designed with a particular tumor type in mind. Hormonal agents might be studied only in malignancies of the appropriate target organ. Certain lipid-soluble agents are tested with the hope that they may prove useful in brain tumors, although study need not be limited to this group. Streptozotocin was brought to clinical trial in the hope that the toxicity to pancreatic islet cells observed in animal experiments would predict activity against islet cell tumors in man.

Most drugs, however, are selected for cytotoxic activity that may not be disease specific. When a new drug shows broad activity in a preclinical screen, it is important to test it in as many tumor types as possible. Although past screening methods have detected drugs that are more active in the hematologic malignancies than in the common epithelial tumors, it would be self-defeating to exclude these common cancers from Phase II testing, since these are the ones for which effective systemic treatment is most desperately needed.

In the past, individual Phase II studies often included a broad range of different malignancies which resulted in an inadequate number of patients of any given type. Currently, the National Cancer Institute (NCI) attempts to sponsor at least one or two trials with an adequate number of patients in each major tumor type (e.g., breast, colon, lung) as well as hematologic malignancies. An adequate number of patients is defined below. As more is learned about the importance of subcategories within a single tumor, it becomes necessary to select certain subsets of patients for separate trials. In lung cancer studies, because small cell lung cancer is more readily responsive than non-small cell cancer to currently available agents, pooling patients with these two diagnoses in a Phase II study to detect response rate in lung cancer overall would not make sense. Responses in patients with small cell cancer do not necessarily indicate drug activity in non-small cell cancer. If it is desirable to conduct a simultaneous Phase II study in both of these types of patients, then they should be considered separate strata and the minimum number of patients needed with each diagnosis to assess response should be entered on study.

Before planning for a trial gets too far along, one must assess the patient resources for each proposed study to be sure that there are sufficient patients to complete the trial in a timely fashion. It would be unproductive to be putting one's third patient on a study of a drug at a time when another institution has already established that it is inactive after having treated 35 similar patients. In the course of Phase II evaluation of a particular agent, several trials in patients with a variety of different diagnoses will be going on simultaneously in different institutions. The drug sponsor will be aware of all trials underway with the agent and will not provide drug for a trial which is considered to represent unnecessary duplication.

SELECTING PATIENTS FOR TRIAL

In contrast to Phase I trials, all patients entered on Phase II studies must have *measurable* disease. The distinction between measurable and evaluable disease is discussed at length in Chapter 2. In short, measurable disease is that for which quantitative changes in size can be appreciated. Disease that can be graded as present or absent, such as marrow infiltration, bone scan lesions, or effusions, is considered evaluable but not measurable. Since there is no way to describe a partial response (more than 50% shrinkage of disease) in patients who have only evaluable disease, these patients should not be entered on early Phase II trials. The entry of poorly measurable cases early in Phase II will very likely yield an ambiguous answer about the drug's activity. Once a drug has been shown to be active, subsequent evaluation may assess its effecct in evaluable disease. For example, the initial evaluation of a new agent in breast cancer should involve patients with clearly defined and measurable lesions in soft-tissue or visceral sites; patients with disease only in bony sites should probably be treated at a later phase of the agent's development after the drug has been shown to be active.

In certain tumor types, such as prostate cancer, this can mean that Phase II trials are very difficult to do. A recent review of the efficacy of nonhormonal cytotoxic chemotherapy in the treatment of prostatic carcinoma (3) found that only approximately 5% of patients studied fulfilled the usual criteria for complete and/or partial responses (CR + PR), while the vast majority of patients reported as "responders" were actually in the "stable disease" category. Since the rate at which disease progresses in any individual patient is unpredictable, "stable disease" as an indicator of antitumor response is highly questionable. In this situation survival might be a preferable endpoint, and would have to be assessed in controlled trials.

PREVIOUSLY TREATED PATIENTS

When a drug enters Phase II trials in a particular tumor, it should be tested in the patient group which is most likely to show a favorable effect, provided that it is ethically permissible to do so; otherwise, the chances of missing the activity and potential usefulness of the drug are increased. This criterion is best fulfilled by patients with maximum performance status and the minimum amount of prior therapy, especially chemotherapy, that ethical medical practice permits.

Extent of prior therapy is an extremely important variable in Phase II trials. In general, patients who have been treated previously are likely to be less responsive to a new agent than those who have had no prior treatment. In some cases this effect is very striking. In previously treated small cell lung cancer, Antman et al. (4) recently reported no responses to etoposide in 23 evaluable patients (95% CI = 0–15%)[1]. A previous study of untreated patients on the same schedule (5) had produced 7 partial responders in 13 patients (95% CI = 25–80%). If the Antman study had been the first one published, then the drug might never have been tried further in this tumor. Antman and her colleagues attributed the poor response in their patients to the amount of prior therapy the patients had received, although none had received prior etoposide. Several other examples of this type of apparent clinical cross-resistance show that consistently lower response rates are achieved in previously treated than in previously untreated patients (2).

The effect of prior therapy may be less striking if the tumor is highly responsive or the agent extremely effective. In a study (6) of high-dose cytarabine and asparaginase in patients with acute nonlymphocytic leukemia, 7/18 patients showed a complete remission; they had received a median of 2 prior induction courses (range 1–5). The 11 who failed to respond had had a median of 3 prior induction courses (range 1–4). Although the overall median number of prior treatments is minimally higher in patients who have shown no response, there were still complete responses in patients who had up to 5 prior treatments. With a very active agent such as cisplatin, responses may also be seen in previously treated patients. In one study of osteogenic sarcoma, responses were seen in 5/31 previously treated as well as 2/6 previously untreated patients (7).

The reason for the rather consistent decrease in response potential in previously treated patients is not entirely clear. One possible explanation is that although the mechanism of action of the drug under study may be different from that of the drugs already administered, drugs with a different mechanism of action may share a common mechanism of resistance. For example, exposure to vincristine *in vitro* can induce resistance to anthracyclines as well as to a number of other natural products (8). The phenomenon of multidrug resistance is the subject of intensive investigation at present.

There may be one unusual exception to this rule of behavior in very responsive tumors. Certain studies show that in some cases patients who had an initial response to therapy and then relapsed may have a higher response rate to the new agent than a previously untreated group of patients with the same diagnosis. Patients with Hodgkin's disease who initially responded to radiotherapy and then relapsed are more likely to achieve remission with chemotherapy than a group of previously untreated patients (9). In at least one study, patients with acute nonlymphocytic leukemia who relapsed after successful POMP (prednisone, oncovin, methotrexate, and purinethol) induction had a higher response rate to cytarabine than previously untreated patients (10). In this situation, the patients who had a remission may be classified as "responders" to chemotherapy in general.

---

[1]95% CI = the 95% confidence interval of the response rate. See Appendix 3.

The importance of the effect of prior therapy may vary by tumor type, tumor size, and drug. Phase II studies in tumors for which no good standard therapy exists should therefore be done in previously untreated patients. For the less sensitive epithelial cancers (non-small cell lung cancer; epidermoid cancers of head and neck, cervix, and esophagus; and colorectal cancer) and most soft tissue sarcomas, a serious Phase II effort should emphasize entry of patients with no prior history of exposure to cytotoxic agents.

The issue of when to do Phase II studies in patients with responsive tumors is still a difficult and unresolved problem. Most investigators consider single-agent Phase II studies to be a justifiable form of treatment only after potentially curative therapy has been exhausted. This means that patients with testicular cancer or Hodgkin's disease will generally have failed a minimum of two treatment regimens employing as many as eight drugs before first exposure to a new agent. Under these circumstances the chance of detecting an effective new agent may be very low. Some investigators have suggested that in this situation, if patients have relapsed after initial curative therapy, then a short Phase II trial of a new drug in an ''experimental window'' may be justifiable before the next standard regimen is attempted. The assumption here is that one to two courses of a new agent will not decrease the effectiveness of subsequent standard treatment. Since this has not yet been clearly shown in any clinical context, many investigators are not comfortable with this approach and prefer to reserve Phase II agents until all standard curative approaches have failed.

DRUG SCHEDULES

Ideally, pharmacokinetic and pharmacologic data collected during Phase I studies should enable one to select the best schedule for Phase II studies. Drugs with very short plasma half-lives should probably be given by continuous infusion or in multiple daily doses per course; for agents with long half-lives, intermittent administration may be justifiable. In addition, studies of schedule dependency in animal tumor systems sometimes assist in choice of a schedule for clinical use. The finding of greatly increased efficacy in murine models with frequent (e.g., every 3 hr) as opposed to intermittent (every 3 days) administration would tend to motivate study of daily administration or continuous infusion in the clinic. In the past, the choice of which schedule to bring into Phase II was often made on the basis of convenience. Whenever possible, the parmacologic and biological properties of the agent should be the major determinant of schedule selection.

The clinical activity of some agents appears to be dependent on schedule. Etoposide, for example, given 5 days weekly seems to produce more responses than weekly administration of the same total dose in small cell lung cancer (1) (Table 5.1).

For some agents neither pharmacologic studies nor preclinical murine tumor experiments suggest the likelihood of strong schedule dependency. Under these

TABLE 5.1. *Schedule-dependent responses of etoposide in small cell lung cancer*

Schedule (i.v.)	Dose (mg/m^2)	No. pts.	Previous therapy (%)	No. responses[a] CR	PR	Objective 95% CI response rate
5 day q 2–4 wk.	60	59	58	9	19	0.47 (0.34–0.60)
q.i.d. × 3 q 2–4 wk.	125–140	13	0	0	7	0.54 (0.25–0.81)
Weekly	200–300	36	68	1	7	0.22 (0.10–0.39)

[a]CR, complete response; PR, partial response.
From Ref. 11.

circumstances, study of more than one schedule in the clinic may be quite reasonable. If clinical antitumor activity then appears to be equal, the better schedule is the one that is better tolerated or more convenient.

DETERMINING THE LEVEL OF DRUG ACTIVITY OF INTEREST

The level of activity that a new drug must show to be of interest depends on the effectiveness of drugs already available for the particular disease in question. A new drug that causes a CR + PR rate in acute lymphocytic leukemia of 20% would have a low priority for first-line therapy, since many drugs with 40% complete response rates already are known. For the more resistant epithelial tumors of the adult, however, most investigators consider a response rate of 20% to be an appropriate cutoff, since agents with reproducible 20% response rates are in rather short supply for many of these tumors. Most trials are aimed at assuring that drugs with this level of activity will not be discarded. Toxicity also determines what level of activity is of interest. A relatively toxic drug such as cisplatin would be of less interest if it were not so active.

There are two obvious possible types of error that may occur in such studies (see Appendix 1). The first type is a false-positive result (type I or alpha error). This occurs when the results of the initial trial are more favorable than will be substantiated by further trials (12). Such errors are serious, since they may result in exposure of large numbers of patients to relatively ineffective treatment, as well as in costly and futile Phase III studies.

An even more serious error, however, is a false-negative evaluation in which an active agent may be missed (type II or beta error). The usual reason for this type of error is the inclusion of patients whose debilitated condition or heavy extent of prior therapy make them unlikely to respond. The only way to guard against this is to pay attention to the important prognostic factors for response when designing the trial and then to treat enough patients on the initial study, since one's confidence in an observed response rate is higher, the larger the sample size.

DETERMINING ACTIVITY OF DRUGS

Once the level of activity that is of interest has been decided on, one should design a trial that exposes the fewest possible patients to inactive therapy. The trial design should provide for stopping as soon as the data have shown that the response rate will not be higher than the response rate of interest. The method of Gehan and Schneiderman (13) for this calculation is described in Appendix 2. For a regimen that is actually 20% effective, there is a > 95% chance that one or more successes would be obtained in 14 consecutive cases. Thus, the initial cohort should be this size, if 20% is the level of interest.

In general, two trials with no responses in 14–20 patients with the same tumor type and no or minimal prior treatment should be adequate to decide that a new agent is inactive (2). If responses are seen after accrual of the initial cohort, more patients can be added until it is known with some predetermined precision (e.g., ± 20%) what the actual response rate is to that drug. In Appendix 3 a method is described for determining the standard error and confidence intervals for any particular response rate. These are also available in published tables (14). If a response occurs in the first 15 patients, the usual practice is to treat a second cohort of 20–25 patients. With 2 or fewer responses in 35 patients there is less than a 5% chance that the true response rate is 20% or greater.

It is most important to stop a trial early if a drug is found to be inactive. It may also be appropriate to stop a trial early if a drug is found to be extremely active, so that it can be moved quickly into definitive studies of efficacy. If one can define a level of activity at which further testing of the drug should definitely proceed, as well as a level at which the drug will be discarded as of no interest, then one can perform a Phase II trial using the multiple testing design described by Fleming (15) and presented in Appendix 4.

Large Phase II studies to define levels of activity very precisely are generally not indicated. Too much time spent studying a drug in this setting may delay its controlled evaluation in Phase III. In practice, however, a few more patients than are needed for evaluation may be entered in each cohort since < 100% of patients on a Phase II trial are likely to be evaluable for response.

RELIABILITY OF PHASE II TRIALS

The range of activity of a single agent in different trials in a single tumor type can be enormous; for 5-fluorouracil therapy of large bowel cancer, response rates range from 8 to 85% (16) (Table 5.2).

In addition to differences in dose and schedule of administration, there are other sources of variability in comparing responses from one study to another. These include (17):

1. Patient eligibility. The extent of disease, performance status, and amount of prior therapy should be similar if trials are to be compared.

TABLE 5.2. *Reported results of 5-fluorouracil therapy of large bowel cancer*

Trial	Patients treated	Objective response rate (%)
A	13	85
B	19	63
C	47	55
D	17	47
E	13	46
F	12	42
G	37	41
H	22	36
I	37	35
J	12	33
K	150	31
L	48	27
M	271	21
N	30	20
O	80	19
P	141	17
Q	358	17
R	87	12
S	22	9
T	11	9
U	12	8

From Ref. 16.

2. Response criteria. These should be carefully defined and the same from one study to the next.
3. Interobserver variability in response assessment.
4. Dosage modification and protocol compliance. Some investigators are more aggressive than others as to when drug should be given.
5. Reporting procedures. How are decisions made, for example, as to whether to exclude a particular patient from analysis?
6. Sample size. The confidence intervals for a particular response rate is extremely broad with small sample sizes.

RANDOMIZED PHASE II TRIALS

Interpretation of the uncontrolled Phase II trial is based on the assumption that measurable disease rarely, if ever, regresses spontaneously. This is a perfectly acceptable study design for showing that a drug has activity. The several sources of variability in results of Phase II trials have been discussed above. Randomized Phase II trials might be expected to reduce some of this variability and individual investigator bias. The major advantage to this design is that patients are centrally registered before treatment starts, and therapy for any individual patient is picked at random. In a centrally registered randomized study, therefore, differences obtained for the two agents will more likely represent real differences in toxicity or antitumor effects rather than differences in patient selection, response evaluation, or other factors noted above, since these factors will be handled in similar fashion for both arms of the study. The purpose of randomized Phase II designs is not a formal, rigorous comparison of two or more treatment arms, but rather a reduction in certain sources of variability that afflict Phase II trials.

Randomized Phase II Trials With Standard Control Arms

One type of Phase II design involves randomization between an investigational agent and an active standard treatment (17). The purpose of randomization here is not to determine whether the new agent is better or worse than the active control, but rather to help interpret the results with the investigational agent. If the new agent has an observed response of 25%, then the drug would probably be identified as having antitumor activity regardless of the magnitude of the response rate to the control treatment. However, if the new agent has a low observed response rate (e.g., < 10%), then one's conclusion about activity would depend on the response rate to the active control. If the control response rate is sufficiently large and if the sample size is adequate, then we would conclude that the new agent is inactive for this type of tumor. However, if the control rate was also unusually low we might conclude that patient selection for the trial had been unsatisfactory. Thus, a standard treatment can be a partial control for a false-negative result. For many resistant tumors, however, a better approach might be to limit entry to patients without prior treatment, since for such tumor types identification of a suitable active control may be difficult.

Randomized Phase II Trials Without Standard Control Arms

The second type of randomized design has two or more treatment arms, each of which involves an experimental agent. One could compare several schedules of a single agent or compare two or more experimental agents to one another. Such trials could be useful in developing priorities for future comparative Phase III studies. It should be emphasized that these comparative Phase II trials do not permit formal comparisons, but the results can be used in developing plans for introducing the investigational agents with the most promising Phase II results into front-line combinations. The potential utility of comparative Phase II trials is most obvious in cases involving analogs, different schedules of the same agent, different formulations of the same drug, or different agonists and antagonists of a physiologic substance.

If one wishes to develop precise comparative data about analogs, as is necessary if an analog appears to be much less toxic than the parent compound already in use, then one should probably begin the efficacy investigation of the new material with large-scale Phase III trials employing early stopping rules to handle the contingency that an analog could be totally ineffective.

One purpose of a randomized Phase II trial, then, is to rank the agents tested in order of importance for their further study. The direct method of statistical ranking and selection theory may be useful for this purpose (17). With the statistical selection theory criterion, one always selects for further study the treatment with the greatest response rate (or best value of the other primary endpoint used, e.g., lowest incidence of toxicity) regardless how small or nonsignificant its advantage over the other treatments seems to be. Conventional statistical designs used in clinical research require much larger numbers of patients, because they select a treatment as superior only when the data are incompatible with the hypothesis that the treatments are equivalent. Selection theory designs always select one treatment as superior, even if it may actually be equivalent to one or more of the others. The number of patients on each arm and the difference observed allow estimation of the probability that a real difference in fact exists. The concepts of significance level and power do not have direct applicability in selection theory.

CROSSOVER DESIGN FOR PHASE II STUDIES

In general, a crossover design for Phase II studies is less useful than a direct evaluation of a new agent, primarily because the effect of prior therapy in each arm is different and difficult to evaluate. If one does a crossover study with the first group of patients receiving drug A and then drug B and the second group of patients receiving drug B and then drug A, the patients who are treated with the drug on the crossover arm have received more prior therapy than those who entered on the trial per primum, and the analysis of response is complicated. It might conceivably be necessary to accumulate enough patients to look at response rates to A alone versus A after B, etc. In addition, if one gives both agents to all patients it is difficult to assess the contribution of either drug to survival.

Crossover trials may be acceptable in situations where the use of one treatment might affect the response to another so that it is important to look at the sequential effectiveness of the agents. In a recently reported breast cancer study (18), 5/15 patients who failed to respond to or progressed on tamoxifen had subsequent response to oophorectomy, while 2/18 patients who had relapsed or failed to respond after oophorectomy had partial responses after tamoxifen. Again, this Phase II design could assist in the ranking of agents during therapy. If sufficient patients were accrued to the trial one could see whether responses to A still occurred after failure on B and vice versa, before either treatment became too firmly established as the current standard and always had to represent first therapy. Crossover design may also be preferable to a strict sequential design in a situation where very few patients are available, such as in pediatric tumors.

SURVIVAL AS AN ENDPOINT IN PHASE II STUDIES

In the final analysis, a response is only meaningful to the patient if tumor shrinkage results in increased survival or improved quality of life. Because an untreated control group is generally not available, one cannot properly evaluate whether the new agent influences survival and this remains a question that is best addressed in Phase III studies. For diseases such as prostate cancer, where measurable disease is uncommon, a survival endpoint may even be the most effective way of evaluating antitumor activity (4).

Comparing survival in subsets of patients selected after the trial has been completed is not an adequate way of evaluating a new drug. Comparison of survival of responders to survival of nonresponders is not a valid way of demonstrating that treatment has had an impact on survival (19,20). Such comparisons are biased by the fact that responders must live long enough for a response to be documented. Also, responders may have more favorable prognostic factors than nonresponders, leading to a difference in survival regardless of treatment. It is even formally possible that treatment may shorten the survival of nonresponders rather than lengthening that of the responders. Figure 5.1 (19) shows an example in which non-small cell lung cancer responders survived longer than nonresponders, but the composite survival of the entire group is no different from an untreated historical control.

For similar reasons, comparison of response rate or survival in patients who were retrospectively categorized as having received full dose therapy versus those who received less than full dose, does not represent an indication of "dose response" in investigation of a new agent. Cortes et al. (21), in reporting the decreased rate of recurrence of osteosarcoma after an uncontrolled trial of postoperative adjuvant doxorubicin, note that patients who had no deviation from prescribed surgical or chemotherapeutic regimen had a lower incidence of recurrence than those who had

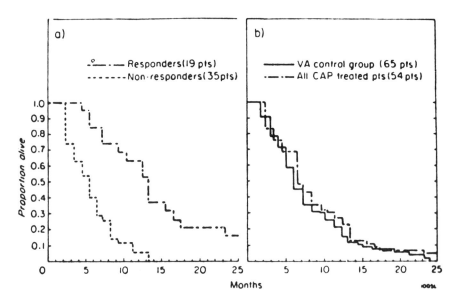

FIG. 5.1. Comparison of responders with nonresponders: A retrospective subset analysis which may produce misleading results. (From Ref.19.)

such deviations. They also note that deviations were less likely in patients with tibial and fibular lesions than in patients with femoral primaries, who are known to have a worse prognosis. They postulate that perhaps the patients with the more distal lesions were treated more vigorously ''because their doctors believed they had a better chance for cure.'' One has to ask why a certain subset of patients received and/or could tolerate the full dose. Were they better off to begin with? Were their physicians more philosophically committed to new drug studies and therefore less likely to become discouraged by some minor toxicity such as nausea? The question of whether high-dose therapy is more effective than low dose is a comparative one and must be asked prospectively in a Phase III setting.

PHASE II STUDIES IN CHILDREN

Most pediatric tumors are more responsive than adult tumors to available cytotoxic agents. This means that most of them have medically meaningful standard therapy, which must be given before a new agent is tried. For certain highly responsive tumors such as acute lymphatic leukemia, therapy given even after first relapse may be curative in about 15% of the patients, depending on whether the relapse occurred on or off therapy or in marrow or extramedullary sites (22). For many other tumors, standard therapy given after relapse may cause responses and prolong survival even if it does not cure. Nevertheless, it is important that Phase II studies be performed appropriately early in these patients, as soon as potentially curative therapy has been exhausted. In certain tumors such as disseminated neuroblastoma where initial response rate is high but cure is rare, a Phase II study may be justified as a front-line treatment. In patients where potentially curative therapy exists, a Phase II trial should be the second or third therapy tried, and probably no more than two Phase II agents should be studied in any single patient.

CONCLUSIONS

The purpose of a Phase II trial is to determine activity in a particular tumor type and obtain some estimate of how this new agent ranks relative to other agents available for treatment of this tumor. These trials should be conducted in such a fashion that for any individual patient the probability of benefit from the new agent will be maximized and that of toxicity minimized. This means that patients who have had multiple attempts at prior therapy and have a poor performance status should not be entered on such trials.

APPENDIX 1

Type I and Type II Error and Power

Type I error (alpha error) occurs when the null hypothesis has been rejected when it is in fact true (false positive). This occurs when the results of the initial trial are more favorable than will be substantiated by further trials. In clinical science today, alpha is usually set at 0.05, meaning that there will be a 5% chance that the positive result observed will be a "false positive" or random event. This is called *the significance level*.

Type II error (beta error) occurs when the null hypothesis is accepted when it is in fact false (false negative).

The power of a test is 1 − beta; that is, the probability of making the correct decision and concluding that new treatment is better than standard when it is actually better. Since the likelihood of a false-negative error goes down with increasing patient numbers, it is obvious that the power, its reciprocal, will go up under the same circumstances.

The null hypothesis will vary with the nature of the trial. For a Phase II trial the null hypothesis could be, "The response rate of drug A in tumor B is not higher than 20%." For a Phase III trial the null hypothesis could be, "Treatment A does not cause more than a 20% increase in the remission rate when compared with Treatment B." The degree of activity, or difference in activity, which one seeks to establish is selected for reasons which are discussed in the text.

The choice of error rates may also vary. In Phase II trials it is customary to set the probability of a false-negative conclusion at beta = 0.01 or 0.05, since if an effective drug is found to be negative in a Phase II trial, it is unlikely that the drug will be retested at a later date and an effective drug will have been missed. In Phase III trials, it is normally the Type I error, alpha, or the probability of a false-positive error which is preset to some specified low level, usually 0.05 or less. The choice of whether alpha or beta is to be fixed should depend on the type of study and type of treatments to be compared and should be reconsidered for each new trial.

It bears emphasizing that the decision to accept a level of 0.05 for alpha or beta is an arbitrary one, selected by the investigator. The decision as to what level of alpha and/or beta to accept is a factor in determining the number of patients required for a trial. The greater the error one is willing to accept, the smaller number of patients one will require (23).

APPENDIX 2

Patient Number Required for Phase II Trial
As Described by Gehan and Schneiderman (13)

In testing a new drug one hopes that it will be active; unfortunately, this is often not the case. Gehan and Schneiderman (13) describe the number of patients that must be entered sequentially on a trial without a response to tell when a trial can be stopped with a 90 or 95% assurance (power) that the response rate will not be higher than the predetermined level of interest.

Sample size (N) of a preliminary trial (Phase IIA) required to rule out given levels of therapeutic effectiveness and Type II error

Permissible Type II error (beta)	Level of therapeutic effectiveness (%)									
	5	10	15	20	25	30	35	40	45	50
5%	59	29	19	14	11	9	7	6	6	5
10%	45	22	15	11	9	7	6	5	4	4

When a regimen of 20% effectiveness or more is of interest and a beta error of 5% acceptable, then a trial with a minimum of 14 patients should be undertaken. For a regimen 20% effective or more, there is more than a 95% chance that one or more successes would be obtained in 14 consecutive cases. If you are interested in higher levels of effectiveness or if you are willing to tolerate higher levels of beta error, fewer patients could be placed on trial. If you wish to detect a drug with a 30% level of activity, and are not interested if the activity is lower, then only 9 patients need to be entered on trial. If no response is seen, the drug will not be studied further.

As noted in the text, the activity level of interest is arbitrarily selected prior to trial. For many relatively unresponsive solid tumors, a 20% level of activity is selected as the minimum level of interest.

APPENDIX 3

Standard Error and Confidence Intervals of a Response Rate

If one wishes to know the true response rate or proportion responding, p, then one starts with an estimate $\hat{p}$ which is the observed response rate in one's own study. This equals the number of patients responding divided by the number evaluable for response, N. It is assumed that the observed response rates will be normally distributed around the true response rate.

The precision of this estimate is measured by its standard error (SE). The 95% confidence interval (CI) is $p \pm 2$ SE.

The SE can be calculated by the formula:

$$SE_p = \sqrt{\frac{p \times 1 - p}{N}}.$$

Since N is the number of patients, it is obvious that the SE for any observed response rate is smaller, the larger the number of patients who have been studied. For example, if one has seen 4 responses in 8 patients then p is $4/8 = 0.5$ and $1-p = 1-0.5 = 0.5$.

$$SE_p = \sqrt{\frac{0.5 \times 0.5}{8}} \text{ or } \frac{0.5}{2.83} = 0.17.$$

The 95% CI for your response rate or $p \pm 2$ SE $= 0.5 \pm 0.34 = 0.16$–0.84. If, on the other hand, you have observed 8 responses in 16 patients, then your p is still 0.5, but

$$SE_p = \sqrt{\frac{0.5 \times 0.5}{16}} = \frac{0.5}{4} = 0.125,$$

and the 95% confidence limits are 0.5 ± 0.25 or 0.25–0.75. Thus, in the first instance one is not quite sure that the true response rate to the drug is more than 20%, but in the second instance, with a larger patient population, one feels more confident.

For a given sample size, as the level of response observed gets closer to 50%, the SE increases, and it is maximal at 50% response rate. Thus, any calculation to determine number of patients needed to detect a particular response rate will arrive at an adequate (albeit perhaps excessive) number if a response rate of 50% is anticipated before making calculations.

APPENDIX 4

Determination of Minimal and Maximal Numbers Needed in a Phase II Study as Determined by Fleming (15)

If one were testing a new drug which would be considered definitely promising if the response rate (p_A) were 30%, and not of much interest if the response rate (p_o) were less than 10%, then on the second line of the Table below, we can see that one could treat an original cohort of 15 patients. If no responses were seen, the trial would be terminated because there would be less than a 6% probability that the eventual activity would be 30%. If 5 responses were seen, the trial would also be terminated since the drug would have better than 10% activity with 99% confidence. If 1–4 responses were seen, the trial would be continued with the entry of another cohort of 10 patients. If, in the second analysis of all 25 patients, 3 or fewer responses were seen, the trial would be terminated because the likelihood of a 30% response would be minimal. If 6 or more were seen, the trial would also be terminated because the likelihood of a response that was more than 10% would be high. If 4 or 5 responses were seen, another cohort of 10 patients would be treated. If 6 or fewer total responses were seen, the drug would be rejected; if 7 or more were seen, further investigation would be pursued. This design has 0.94 probability of rejecting a drug with 10% true response rate and 0.93 probability of accepting a drug with 30% true response rate.

N	n_1	n_2	n_3	a_1	a_2	a_3	r_1	r_2	r_3	alpha	power
					$p_o = 0.05$ vs. $p_A = 0.20$						
40	20	20		0	4		4	5		0.052	0.922
					$p_o = 0.10$ vs. $p_A = 0.30$						
35	15	10	10	0	3	6	5	6	7	0.063	0.929
					$p_o = 0.20$ vs. $p_A = 0.40$						
45	15	15	15	1	7	13	8	11	14	0.057	0.907
					$p_o = 0.30$ vs. $p_A = 0.50$						
45	15	15	15	3	11	19	11	15	20	0.033	0.802

N = total number studied.
n_1, n_2, n_3, the size of the first, second, and third cohort.
a_1, a_2, a_3, the response at which the null hypothesis is accepted.
r_1, r_2, r_3, the point at which the null hypothesis is rejected.
p_o, response rate below which one is not interested in the drug.
p_A, response rate above which one is definitely interested in the drug.

REFERENCES

1. Estey, E., Hoth, D., Simon, R., et al. (1986): Therapeutic response in phase I trials of antineoplastic agents. *Cancer Treat. Rep.*, 70:1105–1115.
2. Wittes, R. E., Marsoni, S., Simon, R., and Leyland-Jones, B. (1985): The phase II trial. *Cancer Treat. Rep.*, 69:1235–1239.
3. Eisenberger, M. A., Simon, R., O'Dwyer, P. J., et al. (1985): A re-evaluation of nonhormonal cytotoxic chemotherapy in the treatment of prostatic carcinoma. *J. Clin. Oncol.*, 3:827–841.
4. Antman, K., Pomfret, E., Karp, G., et al. (1984): Phase II trial of etoposide in previously treated small cell carcinoma of the lung. *Cancer Treat. Rep.*, 68:1413–1414.
5. Eagan, R. T., Carr, D. T., Frytak, S., et al. (1976): VP 16-213 versus polychemotherapy in patients with advanced small cell lung cancer. *Cancer Treat. Rep.*, 60:949–951.
6. Wells, R. J., Feusner, J., Devney, R., et al. (1985): Sequential high dose cytosine arabinoside asparaginase treatment in advanced childhood leukemia. *J. Clin. Oncol.*, 3:998–1004.
7. Gasparini, M., Roesse, J., van Oosterom, A., et al. (1985): Phase II study of cisplatin in advanced osteogenic sarcoma. *Cancer Treat. Rep.*, 69:211–213.
8. Ling, V., Kartner, N., Sudo, T., et al. (1983): Multidrug resistance phenotype in Chinese hamster ovary cells. *Cancer Treat. Rep.*, 67:869–874.
9. Cooper, M. R., Pajak, T. F., Gottlieb, A. J., et al. (1984): The effect of prior radiation therapy and age on the frequency and duration of complete remission among various four drug treatments for advanced Hodgkin's disease. *J. Clin. Oncol.*, 2:248–255.
10. Goodell, B., Leventhal, B., and Henderson, E. (1971): Cytosine arabinoside in acute granulocytic leukemia. *Clin. Pharmacol, Ther.*, 12:599–606.
11. Radice, P. A., Bunn, P. A., Jr., and Ihde, D. C. (1979): Therapeutic trials with VP 16-213 and VM 26: Active agents in small cell lung cancer, non Hodgkin's lymphomas and other malignancies. *Cancer Treat. Rep.*, 63:1231–1239.
12. Simon, R. (1982): Design and conduct of a clinical trial. In: *Principles and Practice of Oncology*, edited by V. T. DeVita, Jr., S. Hellman, and S. A. Rosenberg, pp. 198–225, 1st ed. Lippincott, Philadelphia.
13. Gehan, E. A., and Schneiderman, M. A. (1982): Experimental design of clinical trials. In: *Cancer Medicine*, edited by J. F. Holland and E. Frei III, pp. 531–553, 2nd ed. Lea and Febiger, Philadelphia.
14. Scientific Tables. In: *Documenta Geigy*, edited by K. Diem, pp. 85*ff.*, 6th ed. Geigy Chemical Corporation, Ardsley, New York.
15. Fleming, T. R. (1982): One sample multiple testing procedure for phase II clinical trials. *Biometrics*, 38:143–151.
16. Moertel, C. G., and Thynne, G. S. (1982): Large bowel. In: *Cancer Medicine*, edited by J. F. Holland and E. Frei III, pp. 1830–1859, 2nd ed. Lea and Febiger, Philadelphia.
17. Simon, R., Wittes, R. E., and Ellenberg, S. S. (1985): Randomized phase II clinical trials. *Cancer Treat. Rep.*, 69:1375–1381.
18. Ingle, J. N., Krook. J. E., Green, S. J., et al. (1986): Randomized trial of bilateral oophorectomy vs. tamoxifen in premenopausal women with breast cancer. *J. Clin. Oncol.*, 4:178–183.
19. Tannock, I., and Murphy, L., (1983): Reflections on medical oncology: An appeal for better clinical trials and improved reporting of their results. *J. Clin. Oncol.*, 1:66–70.
20. Weiss, G. B., Bunce, H., and Hokanson, J. A. (1983): Comparing survival of responders and non-responders after treatment: A potential source of confusion in interpreting cancer clinical trials. *Controlled Clin. Trials*, 4:43–52.
21. Cortes, E. P., Holland, J. F., and Glidewell, O. (1981): Osteogenic sarcoma studies by the Cancer and Leukemia Group B. *Natl. Cancer Inst. Monogr.*, 56:207–209.
22. Rivera, G. K., Buchanan, G., Boyett, J. M., et al. (1986): Intensive retreatment for childhood acute lymphoblastic leukemia in first bone marrow relapse: A Pediatric Oncology Group Study. *N. Engl. J. Med.*, 315:273–278.
23. Sylvester, R. (1984): Planning cancer clinical trials. In: *Cancer Clinical Trials: Methods and Practice*, edited by M. E. Buyse, M. J. Staquet, and R. J. Sylvester, pp. 47–63. Oxford Unversity Press, Oxford.

CHAPTER 6

Design of Phase III Studies

Once Phase II studies have established that a new agent has activity in a particular disease, the next logical step is to determine whether the agent contributes significantly to the treatment of the disease. In other words, does the new agent, either alone or in combination, result in improved therapy for the patient? "Improved" can be defined in terms of endpoints relating to efficacy, toxicity, cost, convenience, quality of life, or any other factor that is relevant and quantifiable. No matter how it is formulated, such a question is explicitly a comparative one, since the judgment of whether therapy is "improved" or not is always with reference to some other treatment or to the untreated course of the disease. The question we are interested in is not merely whether one treatment is better than another, but how much better. The trials should yield reliable quantitative estimates of differences between treatments with respect to the endpoints of interest.

In the context of new drug evaluation, we call comparative clinical trials Phase III studies; this terminology emphasizes the orderly character of drug development. We have discussed in Chapter 5 the concept of randomized Phase II trials, which may be used to rank new therapies in their order of priority for further study. As we shall discuss below, the concept of the comparative clinical trial is a very general one, and the research questions that can be addressed by this methodology are certainly not limited to drugs. Comparative trials, by their nature, usually require a significant commitment of resources, and should only be mounted to address major therapeutic issues.

In this chapter we shall discuss the concerns that arise during the design of comparative trials. The next chapter deals with methods for analysis of these trials. A fully informative analysis is impossible without an adequate trial design, and a biostatistician is an essential collaborator throughout all stages of comparative trials from early planning through execution, analysis, and reporting.

RESEARCH QUESTIONS THAT CAN BE ADDRESSED
BY COMPARATIVE CLINICAL TRIALS

The major purpose of a comparative clinical trial is the detection and quantitation of clinically significant differences between treatments. The new therapy to be tested should be thought to differ in some significant way from the control or standard treatment, such that a clinically significant difference might result. This simple statement conceals some complex issues. What does "clinically significant" mean? With about 100,000 new cases of Stage II breast cancer in the U.S., U.K., and Western Europe per year, an absolute increase of only 8% in 5-year survival rates would benefit 8,000 women per year, a very considerable number. Thus, detection of small or modest differences in outcome might be defended as medically worthwhile, particularly for common diseases, since the impact on the public health may be substantial. On the other hand, one's enthusiasm for widespread application of a new treatment obviously depends on more than differences in a single endpoint. A nontoxic and inexpensive new therapy that results in an 8% increase in 5-year survival rates will be greeted very differently from one that exacts a high toxic or financial cost for the same outcome difference.

Relatively modest differences may be important for an additional reason that relates to the way in which treatment advances in oncology have cumulated. The history of advances in the treatment of Hodgkin's disease or acute lymphoblastic leukemia, for example, shows that major progress and the evolution of curative treatment strategies has resulted from the combination of individual stepwise improvements of modest magnitude. Unless a treatment advance is properly defined as such, however, it will be a very uncertain building block for further therapy development.

As implied previously, comparative clinical trials have also had a very important role in oncology outside the area of drug development. Before 1970, radical mastectomy was the standard surgical management for patients with breast cancer. As evidence mounted that breast cancer was often disseminated early in its course, the necessity for such extensive local surgery was increasingly questioned. From 1971 to 1974, physicians in the U.S. and Canada entered 1765 patients into a collaborative study under the aegis of the National Surgical Adjuvant Breast Project (NSABP). Women clinically free of axillary node involvement were randomized to either radical mastectomy, total mastectomy followed by radiation, or total mastectomy alone. The rate of treatment failure, both local and distant, was the same in all three groups at 5 years. These findings have helped define the appropriate surgical management of this disease and set the stage for further study of even more limited surgery in these patients (1).

Randomized clinical trials of new therapies may be structured in several ways, depending on the nature of the question one wishes to ask. The most common designs are illustrated below, where X indicates the new treatment under study; A, the standard treatment for the disease; and B, C, etc., other agents or modalities that have been used in treatment.

1. *A vs. No treatment:* It may be important to establish whether a therapy that has become standard for reasons other than scientific ones, does, in fact, have any effect on the natural history of the disease. This would be necessary if the new therapies one wished to test were not compatible in their toxicities with the older "standard," or if the survival with standard therapy was poor. The Brain Tumor

Study Group (2), in a comparative clinical trial that examined whether the therapy considered standard for the day was indeed effective, compared postoperative radio-therapy to no postoperative treatment in patients with Stage IV glioma. In the final analysis, there was a small but significant improvement in survival with radiotherapy when compared with surgery alone. Since radiotherapy is effective, it can serve as a meaningful baseline for all future studies of chemotherapy or chemotherapy + radiation (Fig. 6.1).

2. *A vs. X:* When pilot studies suggest that a new treatment may offer advantages over the current standard, the two treatments may be compared directly.

3. *A vs. AX (or AB vs. ABX, etc.):* Can a new treatment add significantly to standard therapy, which might be another drug, drug combination, or modality? An example of such a study might be the trial of surgery alone versus surgery plus 12 cycles of cyclophosphamide, methotrexate, and 5-fluorouracil in patients with node-positive breast cancer (3).

4. *A vs. AX vs. X:* This three-armed study would be the definitive way of combining the two questions asked above. Sometimes, however, investigators may not have enough confidence in the new therapy to give it alone in this fashion, and a three-armed study requires more patients per arm than a two-armed study. In the initial study of postoperative chemotherapy for Wilms' tumor, actinomycin alone was compared with vincristine alone and with the combination of the two drugs. The two-drug combination was so superior to either drug alone that it became the standard therapy (4). These data are shown in Fig. 6.2.

5. *ABC vs. AXC:* This design tests the substitution of X for B, which is suggested naturally when X is a chemical analog of B. One might, compare doxorubicin with another anthracycline in the combination therapy of breast cancer and be able to assess simultaneously the efficacy and toxicity of the analog and the parent com-pound in that situation. Trials of this design may be very difficult to interpret if the individual contribution of B to ABC has not been previously characterized. If

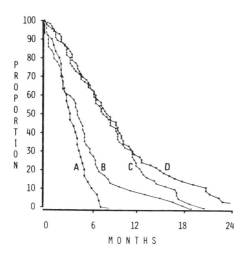

FIG. 6.1. Survival curves of brain tumor patients randomized to receive best conventional care only (*A*), BCNU (*B*), radiotherapy (*C*), and BCNU + radiotherapy (*D*). This study demonstrates that standard therapy (radiation) offered benefit over best conventional care alone (2).

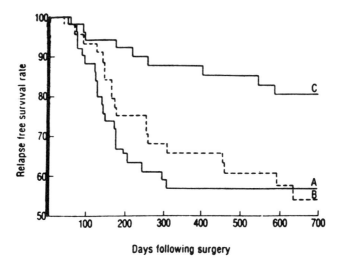

FIG. 6.2. Patients with Wilms' tumor were randomized to receive actinomycin (A), vincristine (B), actinomycin + vincristine (C). The combination is significantly superior to either drug alone (4).

it should turn out that AXC is equal in efficacy to ABC but less toxic, the reason could be either that X is equal in effectiveness to B and less toxic, or that both X and B are irrelevant to the efficacy of their respective combinations.

6. AB_{local} vs. A: This design might be particularly appropriate if one were assessing the contribution of radiation to chemotherapy. One could ask whether radiation therapy to bulky disease in patients with Hodgkin's disease added anything to local and/or systemic disease control if given along with chemotherapy. In assessing these trials it is important to assess sites of relapse to see whether local control was, in fact, achieved.

7. ABC vs. abc, etc.: This design describes comparisons of dosing or scheduling of particular agents. Pinkel et al. (5) compared full-dose or half-dose maintenance in acute lymphoblastic leukemia and found that the latter group had a significantly shorter remission duration (Fig. 6.3).

8. ABC vs. DEF: In this situation two combinations, both of which have been shown to have some activity in the disease are compared with one another to see which is better therapy. This is a relatively frequent design when a cooperative group has two successful pilot studies developed at individual institutions and they wish to know which one should be adopted as a baseline for future investigations. In the 1970s, the Children's Cancer Study Group (6) randomized 234 eligible patients to receive a 4-drug regimen (COMP) or a 10-drug combination (LSA_2-L_2). Patients were stratified by primary site of involvement, degree of spread, and histology. When all groups were considered together there was no difference in failure-free survival between the two regimens. However, analysis of subsets defined before the start of the trial showed that the 10-drug program was more effective

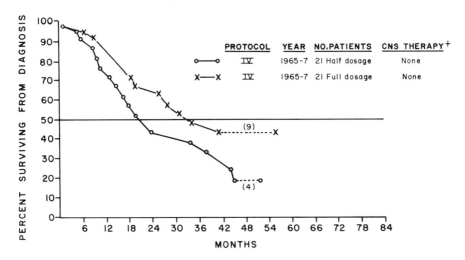

FIG. 6.3. Therapy of childhood lymphocytic leukemia. Full-dose maintenance therapy is more effective than half-dosage in a prospective randomized trial in acute lymphatic leukemia. (Redrawn from Ref. 5.)

than the 4-drug regimen in patients with disseminated lymphoblastic disease, whereas the 4-drug program was more effective in those with nonlymphoblastic disease. This type of trial design yields empirical information that can be very useful in patient management. It does not, however, help elucidate the factors contributing to the success of the individual regimens.

9. *ABC vs. AB:* The aim here is usually to see whether the deletion of one component of a combination results in an increase in therapeutic index by decreasing toxicity without decreasing therapeutic effect. In looking historically at the survival of patients with Wilms' tumor one could see that with surgery alone a certain proportion of patients survived. With the addition of radiotherapy, survival improved to 40–50%. When chemotherapy was added the survival improved to ≥ 80% (7). These successive treatment additions were applied in the order of their discovery rather than from considerations involving their relative merit. In 1969, the first National Wilms' Tumor Study (NWTS 1) was initiated to determine whether radiotherapy was still necessary for Group I patients who received chemotherapy. The 2-year disease-free survival in this group was already high (about 90%), and the idea of giving less therapy to these patients and possibly jeopardizing their survival was a clear risk. This risk was felt to be offset by the fact that radiotherapy to growing structures in very young children often results in severe musculoskeletal deformity. The initial report of this study (4) demonstrated that patients under the age of 2 did just as well in terms of relapse-free and overall survival when treated with actinomycin alone as when treated with actinomycin + radiation.

These designs may be used for various purposes. Each of them is suitable for demonstrating superiority in outcome of test over control treatment. Some of them (particularly No. 5) are often employed with the idea of demonstrating therapeutic equivalence between test and control. Under some circumstances the finding of equivalence may be clinically important, particularly if toxicity is simultaneously decreased. Such "equivalence" trials may also have commercial motivation since a pharmaceutical company must demonstrate the safety and effectiveness of a new agent in order to secure approval from the Food and Drug Administration to market a drug. One way of doing this is to show equivalence to known effective treatment. From a medical and scientific perspective, however, therapeutic superiority is always more important than equivalence. In addition, studies designed to demonstrate equivalence generally have very large sample size requirements.

As we shall explain in detail later, randomized clinical trials that attempt to define modest differences between treatments must necessarily be quite large. Differences in survival rates of < 10%, for example, are very difficult to detect in a single study, although they may be the most realistic differences to expect in many Phase III trials. As noted before, if the tumor is common, such as breast, lung, or colon cancer, detecting this sort of difference may be medically worthwhile. In such a setting, therefore, it seems important to design some major trials that have 90% power for detecting differences in survival rates on the order of 10–15%.

Comparative studies do not always have to include large numbers of patients in order to make an important contribution, as exemplified by a recent multiinstitutional trial in osteosarcoma (8). Prior to the 1970s, historical control data showed that about 20% of patients with localized disease would remain disease free at 2 years after amputation alone. Then a series of uncontrolled studies showed that disease-free survival improved to 40–80% with single drugs or drug combinations; during the same time period at the Mayo Clinic, however, the 2-year disease-free survival after surgery alone had risen to 40%. At this point many in the oncology community were unclear as to the benefit (or lack thereof) of postoperative adjuvant chemotherapy in osteosarcoma (9). In 1982, a randomized study of no postsurgical treatment versus high-dose multidrug chemotherapy in the postoperative period was begun. Because of the intense controversy surrounding the management of osteosarcoma, randomization proved to be very difficult; fewer than one-third of the eligible patients in this trial accepted randomization. After only 18 patients had been randomized in each arm, the trial was stopped because of the dramatic difference in relapse rate between the two arms. At the time of reporting there were 6/18 relapses on chemotherapy and 15/18 on observation (8) (Fig. 6.4). Thus, a randomized trial with 36 patients had helped settle a question whose answer remained controversial after several hundred patients had been treated in uncontrolled trials.

SELECTING PATIENTS FOR STUDY

The patients that should be studied have to be selected on the basis of the question you are asking. We have emphasized that patients on Phase I and II studies should

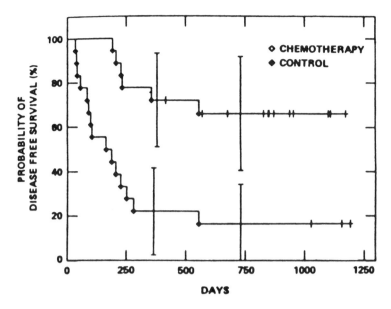

FIG. 6.4. Adjuvant chemotherapy in osteosarcoma (9). Life-table analysis of relapse-free survival after surgery in patients accepting randomization. Eighteen patients were assigned to adjuvant chemotherapy and 18 to observation alone. The difference in relapse-free survival was significant (< 0.001). Bars denote 95% confidence intervals at 1 and 2 years.

have the minimum amount of prior therapy consistent with ethical medical practice, and for Phase II studies patients must have measurable disease. In a Phase III trial, the critical point in design is that each arm of the study must be composed of comparable groups of patients. Measurable disease is not necessarily a requirement for patient entry, unless a comparison of response rates is a major goal of the trial. A postsurgical adjuvant chemotherapy trial would specifically include patients who have no measurable disease at the time they are placed on study, and this is perfectly appropriate as long as the proper endpoint (e.g., survival or disease-free survival) is selected. In the same way, patients may have received prior therapy as long as the amounts given to each group are comparable. A chemotherapy trial in a highly responsive tumor such as Hodgkin's disease might include both untreated patients and previously treated ones as long as the groups are stratified for these variables.

GENERALIZABILITY OF THE DATA

The results of clinical trials are most useful when their results can be generalized with reasonable confidence to the disease population at large. To know how generalizable results are likely to be, one must know how representative the patients studied are of all patients with the disease. One important indication of this is a numerical measure of how highly selected they are, i.e., how many of the patients seen with that diagnosis during the study period were entered in the trial? In addition, it is important to know how representative the study group is in terms of patient characteristics. Patients who are referred to a cancer center for a clinical trial may be healthier or sicker than patients with the same diagnosis in community hospitals, depending on local patterns of practice and referral. Some physicians may refer their sickest patients because they are so difficult to care for; others may refer patients who are in good general condition to give them every opportunity to receive experimental therapy. Even patients that are already being treated at a cancer center may not be considered for entry on a trial because of conscious or unconscious investigator bias. If an investigator has some reason for believing that a patient may do better with standard therapy, he may not enter that patient on the trial and "run the risk" of the patient's receiving experimental therapy. On the other hand, if the investigator considers the experimental treatment particularly promising, he may enter patients who are not really well enough to participate.

Gehan and Schneiderman have advocated maintaining a log book during the study period of all patients who have a confirmed diagnosis of the disease. The investigators should record data on the characteristics that possibly influence prognosis, such as age and stage of disease. If a patient is not entered into the study, the reason should be given. Even though many patients may not enter the study, a detailed log book permits the investigator to make statements about the characteristics of the population of patients with a confirmed diagnosis and the proportion of this population that has been selected for study. These data may be helpful in several ways. They may identify investigator bias. If many patients who appear otherwise eligible are not being entered on study, then one has to question the investigators' commitment to the question being posed or to the new treatment being explored. If only a small fraction of patients with the disease in question are in fact eligible for the protocol, then the selection criteria may have to be altered.

Finally, later analysis of this type of data can allow one to consider whether those patients who have agreed to enter a clinical trial have a different prognosis or different clinical characteristics than those who were excluded from the trial. Antman et al. (11) report that of 90 patients with sarcoma who were eligible for a randomized trial of adjuvant doxorubicin versus observation, 48 (53%) were not entered (24 by physician's choice and 24 by patient refusal). The disease-free survival of nonrandomized patients was inferior to that of randomized patients ($p = 0.15$). Some patients who were not randomized were treated with doxorubicin and others were not. Patients at high risk as defined by previously known prognostic factors appeared to avoid both randomization and adjuvant doxorubicin in this trial, resulting in a particularly inferior disease-free survival for the nonrandomized, untreated control group. This meant that no difference was observed between treatment groups in the randomized study ($p = 0.81$), while a trend toward an advantage for the doxorubicin arm was observed in the nonrandomized group ($p = 0.12$). If the patients in a clinical trial are not representative of the entire patient population because of patient or physician selection biases, the generalizability of the results to the entire patient population may be compromised.

APPROPRIATE CONTROLS

The word "control" describes the basis against which a treatment is to be evaluated. In a comparative trial we want to estimate quantitatively the degree of difference between test and control therapies. The most widely accepted method of planning a controlled study at the present time is concurrent randomization to the new treatment and some other treatment or no treatment.

There are two major advantages to randomization. First, patient allocation to treatment groups is unbiased; this guarantees the validity of the statistical tests of significance that are used to compare the treatments. A "significant" experiment is one in which more favorable outcomes occur in some treatment group (or groups) than would be expected by random assignment of patients to equally effective treatments. The process of randomization generates the significance test, and this process is independent of prognostic factors known or unknown (12). Second, randomization tends to balance treatment groups in covariates (prognostic factors) whether or not these variables are known.

The literature of the 1970s contains a great deal of discussion as to whether "historical" controls or controls from the literature are adequate (13–15). Proponents of retrospective studies using historical controls have asserted that such studies proceed more quickly and new knowledge is gained faster because all patients are assigned to a single treatment (10). They agree that to do this there should be a known, relatively constant response to the standard treatment and a detailed knowledge of the important prognostic factors in the disease so that appropriate matching can occur (15).

The use of historical controls is appealing in two particular circumstances. The first involves a new therapy that appears vastly more effective than any competing treatment; under these circumstances very large differences in outcome, so large as to be unprecedented, might well be convincingly attributed to the new treatment. The second circumstance involves a disease with a highly uniform and predictable natural history, stable over time; this might be a setting in which an increase in the cure rate with a new treatment might be reliably assessed even in the absence of randomized controls. Unfortunately, however, neither of these circumstances is often realized in practice. Treatment differences in oncology are most often moderate or small. The diseases are almost always variable in behavior, and the "natural" history or survival time from diagnosis can be affected as much by changes in diagnostic or staging techniques, referral patterns, and supportive care as by the specific treatment for the malignancy. Historical controls alone, therefore, have a very limited place in the rigorous evaluation of new treatments.

Pocock (16) has proposed that one may increase the power of a study by combining historical and randomized control groups, if the historical control group has been diagnosed, treated, and evaluated in an identical fashion to the proposed randomized control group and if the important patient characteristics and the majority of the treating physicians are the same. In addition, the two groups must be treated close in time to one another and there must be no other indications leading one to expect differing results between the randomized and historical controls. More rapid accrual on the new study might lead one to suspect more enthusiastic participation of investigators than in the previous study, so that the process of patient selection may have been different.

Clearly, "literature" controls would generally not meet these conditions. Pocock points out that with the increasing acceptance of randomized trials for the evaluation of new treatments, the occurrence of such acceptable historical data is also increasing. In his view, an example of such acceptable data might be sequential trials of different agents in the treatment of the same tumor by the same cooperative group. If the first trial consists of A vs. B, and A is better, then for the next trial (A vs. C), one might consider pooling data on both the historical and the concurrent arms given treatment A. However, even such closely matched controls are not without problems. Pocock himself (17) analyzed 19 instances under circumstances approaching those where a collaborative group carried one treatment over for two successive studies. For 4 of the 19 pairs of trials the differences in outcome between the first and second trial of the same treatment were statistically significant ($p < 0.02$). Farewell and D'Angio (18) elaborate on this point in an analysis of data from the first and second Wilms' tumor studies. In Study 1, regimen C (actinomycin + vincristine) was superior to either drug alone and gave a 2-year disease-free survival of 81%. Regimen C was therefore selected as the standard arm for Study 2, where two-drug therapy (C) was compared with three-drug therapy, regimen D (actinomycin, vincristine, and doxorubicin). However, in Study 2, regimen C gave a 2-year disease-free survival of only 70%. If they use only the historical controls who received regimen C in Study 1, then regimen D is not better than regimen C; however, if the concurrently randomized controls in Study 2 are used for comparison, then regimen D is significantly better than regimen C. An analysis of known prognostic factors revealed no obvious difference between historical and concurrent control groups. The investigators concluded that the use of historical controls is not reliable, even for a series of treatment studies in a particular disease. In the setting where the "best" treatment group in the most recent study becomes the control group for the following study, one may be particularly prone to have overestimated the efficacy of the "best" treatment. In a subsequent study, therefore, the results using historical controls and those using concurrent randomized controls could be different.

The Veterans Administration Cooperative Urological Research Group performed a large randomized clinical trial of 2313 patients with prostate cancer over a period of 7 years (12). A major aspect of the study was to compare survival in placebo-treated and estrogen-treated patients. For patients admitted in the last 2.5 years of the trial, no significant difference in the probability of death due to cancer was detected between patients treated with estrogen and those given the placebo. However, placebo-treated patients admitted in the first 2.5 years of the study had significantly shorter survival than the estrogen-treated patients admitted in the last 2.5 years ($p < 0.01$). Over the course of this study there had been no formal changes in admission criteria or the endpoint of interest (survival). If these placebo-treated patients from the earlier part of the study had been the only source of comparison (i.e., regarded as recent historical controls), an incorrect inference would have been drawn that estrogen treatment was superior to placebo. Close review of the data showed that patients admitted in the early part of the study were older and had less favorable performance status on admission. Adjustment for these two variables removed the apparent difference in survival. Thus, the difference was due not to treatment but to the noncomparability of the patients receiving the two treatments. Fortunately, in this instance data were available on variables that could explain the spurious difference in outcome. In another situation this might not have been the case.

Using a control group chosen by any method other than randomization requires the assumption either that the control and treatment groups are identical in all important variables except the treatment under study or that one can correct for all relevant differences. In the latter case one must assume that all factors affecting prognosis are known, and this is unlikely for any disease. When the value of a new therapy needs to be established, or the relative merits of existing therapies are in dispute, then a randomized clinical trial should be performed.

PERFORMING RANDOMIZATION

There are a number of ways of assigning patients to different treatment arms that do not represent randomization. Assignment by birthdate or hospital number, for example, may seem to be unbiased, but one can easily imagine otherwise. If the two arms contained mild and intensive therapy, respectively, and if the investigator knew in advance which arm the patient would receive, bias might well enter into his decision. He might have no qualms about entering very sick patients with even hospital numbers knowing they would get the less-intensive therapy, while those with odd numbers would be entered only if he considered them well enough to tolerate high doses of drug. This would result in a systematic imbalance of the two patient groups in performance status, which is such a powerful prognostic factor that the two groups would probably not be comparable. The likelihood of inducing such imbalance with prior knowledge of therapy is one reason why randomization is preferred. For the same reason, the process of randomization should not be performed by the physicians treating the patients. This should be done in a central office with the treatment lists prepared and the treatment assigned by someone other than investigator in the study, whether the trial involves one institution or many. A method for setting up a simple randomization scheme and a stratified scheme is described in Appendix 1.

Generally, randomization should take place as close as possible to the start of the treatment that is actually under investigation (19). If one is comparing two different maintenance regimens after a standard induction, randomization should take place once remission has been achieved. If one is comparing 10 weeks of therapy with 6 months of identical therapy, then randomization is probably best done at 10 weeks, which is the point at which the treatments diverge. This approach serves to reduce systematic biases in the treatment administered before the divergence of therapy in the two arms. It also reduces the impact of disqualifications of patients in early stages of the treatment.

It is often advisable, however, to have the patient agree to participate in the study and be registered at the beginning of all treatment with a consent to randomization at a later point. In an ongoing Pediatric Oncology Group study, patients with Hodgkin's disease receive four courses of chemotherapy and then, if complete response is achieved, they are randomized either to receive two more courses of chemotherapy or to receive radiotherapy. The patients consent to the study and are registered before the initial chemotherapy begins, but randomization does not take place until the response to chemotherapy becomes known. Registration of the patient at the beginning of the study allows one to collect the initial treatment data in a standard fashion. Late randomization once the response status of the patients is known avoids having too many nonresponders preassigned to one experimental treatment with an eventual imbalance in numbers and difficulty in analysis. Late randomization, however, does sometimes increase the anxiety of the patient and the investigator, both of whom want to know what the eventual treatment will be so that they can make plans for factors such as time lost from work, school, etc. This is so particularly if there is a significant difference in the nature and or schedule of the randomized treatments.

UNBALANCED RANDOMIZATION

Some biostatisticians advocate unequal allocation of patients to treatment arms within a trial. This is done when a great deal is known about one of the treatment arms and when, for comparison with other data, one wishes to maximize the number of patients receiving the new treatment. The chance of obtaining a statistically significant difference between the two treatments is not reduced much, as long as the chosen ratio is less extreme than 70:30 (20).

DESIGNS INVOLVING COMMON CONTROLS

In randomized multiinstitutional studies it is sometimes difficult to obtain agreement among all participants concerning the treatments to be used. A compromise design permits some institutions to select between doing a randomized study of treatments A and C and others to select doing a randomized study of treatments B and C. These two studies are conducted simultaneously, but at different institutions. This compromise is inferior to a simple randomization among the three treatments at all institutions. Schoenfeld and Gelber (21) have shown that unless one can assume that there are no differences among institutions in response to treatment, this design is very inefficient; with three treatments (one being the common control), this design requires twice as many patients as a straightforward three-way randomized design. Makuch and Simon (22) have pointed out that similar results for the common control treatment between the sets of institutions selecting the two options does not ensure that the other two treatments can be validly compared. Systematic differences among the institutions may still render the common control undesirable. For example, if the common control arm (treatment C) is a relatively less-aggressive therapy, the physicians at one institution might believe in more aggressive therapy and administer high doses of treatment A, while those at another institution might give only modest doses of treatment B. In the final analysis, both institutions would show the same result with treatment C, but the result of A might not be compared properly with B.

PROGNOSTIC FACTORS AND STRATIFICATION

The effect of various prognostic factors on response and survival cannot be overemphasized. For many kinds of cancer, the variability in prognosis among patients is greater than the size of treatment differences usually seen. Consequently, failure to understand and adequately account for patient heterogeneity easily leads to unreliable claims and inefficient trials (23). When there are known major prognostic factors for patients in a randomized study, the major prognostic strata should be randomized separately to assure equal distribution of these factors.

It is sometimes appropriate to stratify on the basis of tumor-specific factors such as estrogen receptors or histological classification. Alternatively, it may turn out that patient-related factors such as weight loss or performance status have a greater bearing on response, and sometimes are the most relevant bases for stratification. Simon (23) reviewed a series of clinical trials at seven tumor sites, all in patients with disseminated disease. He summarized the response as a function of initial ambulatory status. If the patients were initially ambulatory, 241/575 (0.42) responded. If they were initially nonambulatory, only 57/300 (0.19) responded.

The two most commonly used measures of functional performance, or performance status, in oncology are the Karnofsky scale (24) and the Eastern Cooperative Oncology Group [ECOG (Zubrod)] scale (25), which are scored as shown in Tables 6.1 and 6.2, respectively. Performance status is often a strong predictor of survival. Both scales described above seem to be reasonable measures of physical function and often highly correlated with patient outcome in clinical trials. Aisner and Hansen (26) have shown that performance status, extent of disease, and weight loss are the most important prognostic variables predicting survival in patients with inoperable lung cancer and that an imbalance in these by patient group could seriously affect the outcome of a study. When all factors were favorable, median survival was 72 weeks, if they were unfavorable, 6 weeks (Fig. 6.5). In this analysis, performance status emerged as a prognostic factor independent of disease status, and other studies have shown this as well. For many current trials, therefore, performance status is now used to stratify patients for trial entry and usually some minimal baseline level (e.g., 70) set below which patients are not entered on trial.

TABLE 6.1. *Karnofsky scale for assessment of performance*

Condition	Performance status
A. Able to carry on normal activity and work. No special care needed.	100—Normal. No complaints. No evidence of disease. 90—Able to carry on normal activity. Minor evidence of disease. 80—Normal activity with effort. Some signs of disease.
B. Unable to work. Able to live at home and care for most personal needs. Varying degree of assistance needed.	70—Cares for self. Unable to carry on normal activity or do active work. 60—Requires occasional assistance but is able to care for most of his needs. 50—Requires considerable assistance and frequent medical care.
C. Unable to care for self. Requires equivalent of institutional or hospital care.	40—Disabled. Requires special care and assistance. 30—Severely disabled. Hospitalization required though death not imminent. 20—Hospitalization necessary. Very sick. Active support necessary. 10—Moribund. Fatal processes progressing rapidly. 0—Dead.

From Ref. 24.

TABLE 6.2. *ECOG (Zubrod) performance scale*

Performance status	Definitions
0	Asymptomatic
1	Symptomatic, fully ambulatory
2	Symptomatic, in bed < 50% of the day
3	Symptomatic, in bed > 50% of the day, but not bedridden
4	Bedridden

From Ref. 25.

Site of metastasis may also be important, in addition to disease extent. Patients with malignant melanoma and multiple metastases had inferior survival to those with single metastases; in addition, those with a single skin or lymph node metastasis survived significantly longer than those with a single visceral lesion ($p < 0.001$) (27).

Prior therapy should also be considered as a stratifying variable. The generally negative effect of prior therapy on response has already been discussed. In some situations, however, previously treated patients may be more likely to respond. If a study in Hodgkin's disease were to compare MOPP and ABVD, and both pre-

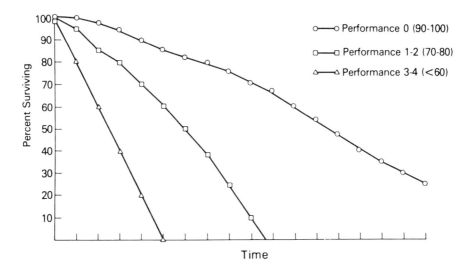

FIG. 6.5. Hypothetical survival curve modeled after data from the V.A. Lung Cancer study group. This graph illustrates the effect of performance status on survival time in unresectable patients with non-small cell lung cancer. (Reprinted from Ref. 26.)

viously untreated patients and radiotherapy failures were eligible, then entry to the two treatment arms should be stratified for prior radiotherapy, since it has been demonstrated that patients relapsing after a response to radiotherapy have a higher complete response rate to subsequent chemotherapy than those who are previously untreated (28).

Factors that are of clinical interest but have an unknown effect on response or outcome should not be used as a basis for stratification. If a factor is shown by retrospective analysis to be extremely important in prognosis, then it can be considered as a variable for stratification in future trials (19). Also, one should only stratify by factors that are reliably reported at the time of randomization. For instance, tumor pathology as defined by a reference panel may be an unsuitable variable if one has to wait several weeks for a centralized diagnostic review.

The greatest advantage of stratified over nonstratified randomization is that it safeguards against sizeable imbalances in major patient factors between the study arms. Specific strategies for stratification should result in approximately equal numbers of patients on each treatment arm within each stratum (see Appendix 1). If the treatment assignment and randomization is being done at a central office, then adjustments can be made serially for imbalances that might occur during the randomization procedure. Simon (29) has reviewed various stratification methods available and Zelen (30) has described a method particularly suitable for multiinstitutional trials.

The larger the sample size of a trial, the less important is stratification, since the chances of imbalance are progressively reduced. Even in the largest of trials, if interim analyses are required one should contemplate stratification. In any multiinstitutional trial, it is advisable to stratify or otherwise balance for institution since there may be subtle differences in the way patients are managed in each institution despite the adoption of a common protocol.

One should avoid stratifying for too many factors. In the first place, patient assignment becomes increasingly complex under these circumstances. Pocock and Simon (31) have shown that balance actually deteriorates if stratification is excessive. If there is extensive stratification, numerous strata will contain very few patients, and thus balance with regard to the most important factor or factors may be seriously impaired by the inclusion of factors of secondary importance. In practice, it is seldom advisable to stratify on more than three or four variables, even when more variables of prognostic value are known. A summary prognostic index based on several prognostic variables can be used as a single stratifying variable that will tend to achieve balance among the separate variables on which it is based (32).

DETERMINING ENDPOINTS

In designing a trial, we must decide what effect(s) we wish to assess. It is clear that various endpoints may be appropriate for comparisons of treatments under different circumstances. Tumor shrinkage, i.e., the percentage of patients who achieve complete or partial response, has certain advantages as an endpoint. It is a direct, semiquantitative expression of the antitumor effect of the experimental treatment and it is often rapidly observable. Since complete response is a prerequisite for long survival under many circumstances, this parameter may be a reasonable surrogate for survival. The use of response does, however, present certain difficulties. In Chapter 2 we discussed some of the problems in actually measuring tumor shrinkage accurately. Just as importantly, tumor shrinkage by itself is not a measure of direct therapeutic benefit to the patient, in the way that survival extension, relief of symptoms, or improved quality of life are. Thus, the recording of the relative percentage of patients responding to a particular regimen is often only one of the goals of a Phase III study.

In responding patients or in those rendered disease free by another modality prior to study entry, the disease-free interval (or disease-free survival) is sometimes a useful endpoint. The advantages of disease-free survival are (a) it provides a faster answer than overall survival, and (b) it is a reflection of the primary therapy of interest and not of any subsequent salvage maneuvers. Also, since living without evidence of cancer seems inherently more appealing than living with it, treatments that increase disease-free survival may have a positive impact on quality of life even if they do not increase survival itself very much. This is only true, of course, if the therapy is not so toxic that it overrides the effect of being disease free.

Whether disease-free survival is, in fact, a reliable surrogate for survival is a more complicated issue. First, if the increase in disease-free survival is small, the impact on survival may be negligible. Second, therapy used after relapse may have a substantial effect on survival. For example, adjuvant chemotherapy for Stage II testicular cancer produces a clear-cut improvement in disease-free survival compared with no adjuvant therapy. The effect on survival, however, is not significant, because patients who receive no adjuvant therapy and then relapse can be treated effectively at the time of relapse with chemotherapy (33).

The ultimate endpoint of interest in many Phase III trials will be overall survival. The endpoint here is objective and unambiguous, although it may not be the most appropriate in certain situations. For example, in highly responsive tumors such as acute leukemia, the analysis of the contribution of the initial therapy to overall survival may be confounded by the effects of successful subsequent therapy which, even if not curative, may prolong survival by several years in many patients (34). Here the observation most relevant to assessment of the comparative efficacy of the test and control treatments might well be relative disease-free survival on the initial treatment regimen, since here the effect sought is the contribution to ultimate cure. Overall survival also can take a long time to measure, often requiring years of careful and costly follow-up. Since it is the last endpoint to accrue in a clinical trial, comparative response rates, durations of response, and some preliminary assessment of toxicities and quality of life may all be at hand before a full, mature survival analysis is possible.

The trial should be designed in such a way that disease-specific mortality can be distinguished from mortality from other causes, although both of these should be looked at in any patient group. In addition, one must plan the study so that if a significant fraction of patients do, in fact, achieve long-term survival, late toxicities can be appreciated (see Chapter 3).

This discussion of survival, then, leaves us with the question of what are "medically significant" survival differences between two treatments? The obvious answer, namely than *any* survival difference is medically significant, is probably not true; an extremely toxic, complex, and expensive adjuvant therapy that increased the 5-year survival rate of a certain patient group from 50 to 53% would probably not be regarded as a medical advance by most physicians (assuming, of course, that the adjuvant treatment had no other beneficial effects). On the other hand, if the treatment were in the form of an inexpensive and nontoxic oral preparation, one might make a strong case that an improvement of this magnitude had real significance, particularly if the disease in question were a common one.

The practical problem is that the demonstration of small differences requires very large trials (see Appendix 2). For almost all cancers the required numbers of patients are beyond the accrual potential of nearly all single centers. And once the targeted differences fall below about 10 percentage points, the sample size requirements begin to challenge the capabilities of even large multicenter cooperative groups. For these very practical reasons, many clinical trials have been too small to target with reasonable power differences that are modest but still medically significant. The limited accrual potential of most clinical trials organizations has forced the targeting of differences that are often unrealistically large, (i.e., unlikely to be achieved by the therapy as given). Under these circumstances, any differences lacking statistical significance that emerge from the trial may be erroneously interpreted as good evidence for lack of a treatment difference. Such trials should really be interpreted as inconclusive rather than negative, since they were too small to detect all but the largest differences in the first place.

SAMPLE SIZE

In a Phase III trial it is just as important to decide how many patients should be studied as it is to decide what kinds of patients should be studied. The number of patients that will be needed for each endpoint depends on the expected difference between the standard and the experimental arm. The difference to be detected in the course of a study does not represent the difference we hope exists; it represents the size of difference that the study will be able to detect (35). In addition, it is the mark of a good trial design that a null result, if it occurs, will be of interest and the study will have sufficient power to establish it convincingly.

Comparing Success Rates

One of the most common and simple outcome variables in a clinical trial is the "success rate." The relative "success rate" of two therapies could then be compared. This type of analysis can be applied to remission rate or the duration of survival or remission at a specified period of time, for example, the proportion of patients alive after 2 years. Once each subject has been classified as a "success" or a "failure," each observation is simply a binary variable which can be compared using a chi-square type of analysis. In planning a trial where this sort of endpoint will be used, one must decide on an acceptable alpha and beta error (see definition under Phase II) and then whether to use a one- or two-tailed test for analysis. A conservative approach is to use two-sided significance levels, since one is generally interested in the possibilities that treatment A may be either better or worse than treatment B. In addition, it is better in the original planning to expect to accrue more patients than are needed to answer a question than to discover after the study has closed that not enough patients have been accrued. It is also common to attempt to establish an alpha of 0.05 (0.05 level of significance) and a beta of 0.10 or 0.05 (90–95% power). Once the conditions of the experiment have been established, a realistic estimate should be obtained of the level of improvement to be expected in the experimental arm over the control arm. If the expected success rate on the control arm is a complete response rate of around 20%, and the success rate in the experimental arm, anticipated from the Phase II studies, is approximately 35%, then one can anticipate how many patients should be entered on the study so that a difference with these specifications will be detected (see Appendix 2).

In making these estimates one should remember that promisingly high response rates in small uncontrolled studies are often not confirmed by subsequent Phase III studies. Ellenberg and Eisenberger (36) found that the average response rate for experimental regimens in the uncontrolled studies of treatment for head and neck cancer was 45%, 16 points higher than the average response rate of 29% for the same regimens in a controlled setting.

Comparing Duration of Response or Survival

For studies with survival or disease-free survival as endpoint, unless the curves show a clear plateau, then planning the trial based on comparing the entire curves is a better approach. Tables exist (35,37) that indicate the number of patients needed in each arm of a trial for any anticipated multiple of the control median survival that will be seen in the experimental treatment group. The detection of a doubling in the median, for example, from 6 months to 12 months of disease-free survival in disseminated lung cancer with a power of 0.90 and an alpha of 0.05 (two-sided) would require 88 adverse events, i.e., relapse or death in the two groups. In disease where relapse is rapid, this sort of large multiple of the median is all that would be medically significant. As the ratio of median survival between experimental and control group goes down (e.g., to 1.5), the number of events that has to occur goes up (in this case to 256 between the two groups). A ratio of 1.5 might be a reasonable difference to look for in a disease such as breast cancer where the initial survival might be 3 years in the selected patient group, the increase would be to 4.5 years, and the number of patients available for entry on study substantial. It should be pointed out that for many tumors, in order for 256 events to occur, many more than 256 patients will have to be entered on trial. Further description of this type of analysis is given in Appendix 3.

Rubinstein et al. (38) provide a technique for estimating the required length of accrual in a two-armed randomized trial using survival as the endpoint, when the failure rate is assumed to be exponential, and failures continue to occur until eventually all patients have failed. Sposto and Sather (39) have proposed another formulation that allows projection of patient numbers needed in an experiment where the survival curve may reach a plateau and adverse events no longer occur. This sort of model may be more appropriate to tumors where a significant percentage of cures can be expected with treatment.

In any clinical trial involving follow-up, it is almost inevitable that some patients will be lost from the study before the final outcome is observed. In addition to taking all possible steps to minimize losses to follow-up or inevaluable patients, one can also increase the planned accrual by a number of patients equal to the anticipated number lost or inevaluable. The effect on the analysis of data is discussed in the next chapter.

SEQUENTIAL DESIGN

In sequential trials (10), patients are paired within prognostic categories and each member receives one of the two treatments by random allocation. The differences between the responses in each pair are analyzed as the trial proceeds; entry of patients continues until a decision can be made about which treatment is superior. The plans for designing such trials are described by Armitage (40). The sequential design almost always has a single endpoint for evaluation compared with the fixed sample size study, which can be adapted to the analysis of multiple endpoints. A sequential design may require fewer patients than a fixed sample size study. This design, however, is not appropriate for most applications in oncology, where the endpoints of interest can only be determined after a long follow-up period. Because the design and strategy for continuation is more complex in the sequential design, problems in nonadherence to protocol and withdrawal from study affect the sequential design more than a fixed sample size study.

FACTORIAL DESIGN

A factorial design attempts to answer questions about two or more interventions simultaneously (19). The first factor represents the first two alternative treatment interventions, such as limb amputation or conservative tumor resection. The second factor represents two other alternative interventions superimposed upon the first, such as adjuvant chemotherapy or no further treatment. In such a 2 × 2 design there are actually four treatment groups (amputation alone, resection alone, amputation + chemotherapy, resection + chemotherapy). Proponents of such designs (41), suggest that the effect of each treatment factor can be addressed using all of the patients and pooling with regard to the other factor (or with the influence of the other factor accounted for in the analysis, but not separate analysis for each level of the other factor).

The validity of such an analysis depends on the assumption that the two treatment variables are not interrelated in any way. In other words, if adjuvant chemotherapy is beneficial for amputees, then it is also beneficial for resected patients, and the difference in efficacy of the two surgical procedures is either concurrently positive, negative, or zero, both for patients receiving adjuvant chemotherapy and for those not receiving further treatment. If these assumptions are not satisfied then the study must be analyzed by the simultaneous comparison of all four treatment groups. One can easily imagine, in the example above, that if resection involved the insertion of an internal prosthesis, then this group of patients might have more postoperative complications that might require delays and reduction in doses of chemotherapy. Under these circumstances it would not be really valid to pool both chemotherapy groups of patients. The risk in planning such a study is that the projected number of required patients will be sufficient only for pooled two-group comparisons, yet the data may suggest that such an analysis is not adequate. Also, the number of patients required to determine whether such an interaction is present may be greater than the number required to perform two-group comparisons. Thus, the factorial design offers the possibility of increased efficiency, but with some risk of difficulty in interpretation.

CROSSOVER DESIGN

The usefulness of this approach, as discussed under phase II, for the evaluation of drugs in general is limited by the fact that the condition of the patient changes with time, and the effect of a treatment may be influenced by previous treatments or conditioned by previous responses. Use of the crossover design except in special circumstances is not recommended.

ASSURING ADEQUATE PATIENT ACCRUAL

Once the required number of patients is determined, the investigator must verify that there will be *enough* patients available to complete the trial. Probably the single most common cause of an uninterpretable result in a clinical trial is the accrual of too few patients to make a definitive statement. Freiman et al. (42) reviewed 71 "negative" trials and found that the majority of the trials reported had too few patients to detect risk reductions of 25 or even 50%; such studies are inconclusive, not negative, and represent a distressing waste of time, effort, and resources.

The lack of sufficient numbers of patients to carry out a study to completion may be due to either an overestimate of the expected difference between treatments, or to an overestimate in the expected patient accrual rate. One should ascertain in advance, as accurately as possible, the number of patients who will be available. This figure is often grossly overestimated, particularly in multicenter trials. The most useful statistic is usually the accrual rate for the same tumor on a previous trial, but even this may not predict, if, for some reason, the level of enthusiasm among investigators is much higher or much lower for the current trial than the previous one. Because not all patients will be evaluable for the endpoints of major interest, one should probably accrue a patient total which is 15–20% larger than the minimum necessary for analysis.

The rate of accrual is also important. When possible, the rate should be sufficient to complete entry by 2–3 years. After this period of time, interest in the protocol usually begins to wane and the entry rate may decrease. In addition, if the trial runs too long, other more promising therapies may appear and the original protocol may never be completed, even though the question it asked may be important to the overall strategy for cure in the particular disease. It is also possible that the answer to a question may no longer be relevant if a study goes too slowly. A protocol comparing 1000 cGy with 2000 cGy as treatment for Stage I Wilms' tumor would not provide an answer of much interest if in the interim no radiation at all had been shown to be the proper amount.

The lessons from our frequent experience with trials of inadequate power are plain. First of all, trials that can realistically expect to detect only modest differences in therapeutic outcome should not be mounted when the inadequacy of patient numbers makes an inconclusive result highly likely; to do so is a waste of time and resources. Second, investigators and sponsoring agencies must insure that trials target realistic differences in outcome and that the necessary accrual be achieved within a reasonable time frame.

APPENDIX 1

Balanced Randomization

To design a randomization plan for a study, select any table of two-digit random numbers. If you will randomize 100 or fewer patients in your study, then assign the numbers 00–49 to be treatment A and 50–99 to be treatment B. An example of a sequence of letters which might be derived is:

BBBBABAABBBBBABABBBABABABBAABA.

Your random treatments could be assigned to the group as a whole using this scheme, although with the small number here, you would end up with 19 patients on B and 11 on A.

If you wish to make this a stratified randomization, you decide how many factors will be used for stratification. Decide on some arbitrarily sized blocks of patients, at the end of which the groups will be matched. Let us say that two treatments are being compared, that patients will be matched in blocks of six and you expect 30 patients in each of four strata. Then you could take the above series of 30 letters to prepare your list for one stratum. Within each block of six, as soon as there were three of one letter, you would complete the block with the other letter. Thus, for this example, if "/" marks are inserted at the point at which the blocks have to be evened up to get three As and three Bs in each block of six, the pattern would look like this:

BBB / / /   BABAAB   BBB / / /   BABAB /   BBAB / /
BBBAAA   BABAAB   BBBAAA   BABABA   BBABAA

Within the blocks, the sequence of treatments are random, but after each block of 6 patients within the stratum, the treatment groups overall contain equal numbers of patients on each treatment. Different sized blocks of patients can be used. It is critically important that the actual randomization sequences be prepared and the randomization itself be administered centrally, by an individual who is not a participant in the trial.

APPENDIX 2

Comparing Success Rates

When the smaller response rate is thought to exceed 50% the table given here should be used with regard to comparing failure rates (100% minus the response rate) (19).

Number of patients required on each of two treatments to compare success rates

Smaller success rate	Larger minus smaller success rate				
	0.10	0.20	0.30	0.40	0.50
0.05	206	74	42	27	19
0.10	285	92	48	30	21
0.15	354	106	53	33	22
0.20	411	118	57	34	22
0.30	495	134	62	36	22
0.40	537	139	62	34	21
0.50	537	134	57	30	17

Alpha = 0.05, beta = 0.10, two-sided test.

As an example, if one knows in the control arm that there will be only 5% of patients with Stage IV glioma alive at 2 years after radiotherapy alone, then one could consider this the control success rate and estimate how many patients it would take to detect a desired level of improvement with a new experimental treatment. From the above table we see it would require, for example, 74 patients in each arm to detect an improvement from 5% to 25% survival at 2 years in patients with Stage IV gliomas.

If there are more than two groups in the study, and if one assumes that the success rate for the additional group(s) will fall somewhere between the extremes of the two groups already under discussion, then George (37) has developed factors for multiplying the numbers already given. The factor one uses to multiply the number of patients in each arm for a three-arm study is 1.20, four-arm 1.35, five-arm 1.47, and six-arm 1.57 (for an alpha = 0.05, beta = 0.10). Thus, each arm of the three-armed study will have to be larger than either arm of a two-armed study, and the total number of patients required to compare K groups simultaneously is always greater than K times the number of patients required in each group for a comparison of two groups. Thus, to detect an improvement in response from 10 to 50% with an alpha of 0.05 and beta of 0.10 in a two-armed study would require 27 patients in each group for a total of 54. If one introduces a third patient group (perhaps a second treatment if the first two groups were treatment A and no treatment), then the number of patients required in each group is 1.2 × 27 or 32, for a total of 96. This requirement for larger patient numbers should be weighed against the possibility of greater information at the time of final analysis from the comparisons between treatments.

APPENDIX 3

Comparing Survival Distributions

In general, for studies with survival or disease-free survival as endpoint, unless the curves show a clear plateau, then planning the trial based on comparing the entire curves is a better approach than comparing success rates. This would be natural, for example, in disease where survival is very short. In planning to use such an analysis it is important that the protocol define the time when the period begins as well as when it ends. Survival time can be measured from the date of randomization. Remission duration will have to be measured from the date remission was achieved. George (37) has also given tables showing the numbers of patients required on each treatment arm to compare survival distributions:

Number of deaths required on each of two treatment arms to compare survival distributions

	Ratio of medians: larger to smaller					
Ratio	1.2	1.5	1.8	2.0	3.0	4.0
N	633	129	62	45	18	12

Alpha = 0.05, beta = 0.10, two-tailed test.

Again, if there are more than two groups the number per arm will be increased. It is clear that it will take very large trials to detect differences with an increase much less than twice the control medium.

The above chart refers to deaths. Exactly the same kind of relationship holds between relapse and disease-free survival. If not all patients are followed until failure, more than 45 patients will be required on each arm in order that 45 events occur within a period that is resonable for analysis. Tests are usually made at various times during the study when many patients are still alive (or censored, in statistical terminology) and the effect of censoring on the power of tests must be clearly understood.

REFERENCES

1. Fisher, B., Montague, C., Redmond, C., et al. (1977): Comparison of radical mastectomy with alternative treatments for primary breast cancer. A first report of results from a randomized clinical trial. *Cancer*, 39:2827–2839.
2. Walker, M. D., Alexander, E., Jr., Hunt, W. E., et al. (1978): Evaluation of BCNU and/or radiotherapy in the treatment of anaplastic gliomas: A cooperative clinical trial. *J. Neurosurg.*, 49:333–343.
3. Veronesi, U., Zucali, R., and Luini, A. (1986): Local control and survival in early breast cancer: The Milan trial. *Int. J. Radiat. Oncol. Biol. Phys.*, 12:717–720.
4. D'Angio, G. J., Evans, A. E., Breslow, N., et al. (1976): The treatment of Wilms' tumor. Results of the National Wilms' Tumor Study. *Cancer*, 38:633–646.
5. Pinkel, D., Hernandez, K., Borella, L., et al. (1971): Drug dosage and remission duration in childhood lymphatic leukemia. *Cancer*, 27:247–256.
6. Anderson, J. R., Wilson, J. F., Jenkin, D. T., et al. (1983): Childhood non-Hodgkin's lymphoma: The results of a randomized therapeutic trial comparing a 4-drug regimen (COMP) with a 10-drug regimen (LSA$_2$-L$_2$). *N. Engl. J. Med.*, 308:559–565.
7. Belasco, J. B., Chatten, J., and D'Angio, G. F. (1984): Wilms' tumor. In: *Clinical Pediatric Oncology*, edited by W. W. Sutrow, D. J. Fernbach, and T. J. Vietti, pp. 588–621, 3rd ed. Mosby, St. Louis.
8. Link, M. P., Goorin, A. M., Miser, A. W., et al. (1986): The effect of adjuvant chemotherapy on relapse-free survival in patients with osteosarcoma of the extremity. *N. Engl. J. Med.*, 314:1600–1606.
9. Carter, S. K. (1984): Adjuvant chemotherapy in osteogenic sarcoma: The triumph that isn't? *J. Clin. Oncol.*, 2:147–148.
10. Gehan, E. A., and Schneiderman, M. A. (1982): Experimental design of clinical trials. In: *Cancer Medicine*, edited by J. F. Holland and E. Frei III, pp. 531–553, 2nd ed. Lea and Febiger, Philadelphia.
11. Antman, K., Amato, D., Wood, W., et al. (1985): Selection bias in clinical trials. *J. Clin. Oncol.*, 3:1142–1147.
12. Byar, D. P., Simon, R. M., Friedewald, W. T., et al. (1976): Randomized clinical trials: Perspectives on some recent ideas. *N. Engl. J. Med.*, 295:74–80.
13. Chalmers, T. C., Block, J. B., and Lee, S. (1972): Controlled studies in clinical cancer research. *N. Engl. J. Med.*, 287:75–78.
14. Ingelfinger, F. J. (1972): The randomized clinical trial. *N. Engl. J. Med.*, 287:100–101.
15. Gehan, E. A., and Freireich, E. J. (1974): Nonrandomized controls in cancer clinical trials. *N. Engl. J. Med.*, 290:198–203.
16. Pocock, S. J. (1976): The combination of randomized and historical controls in clinical trials. *J. Chronic Dis.*, 29:175–188.
17. Pocock, S. J. (1977): Randomized clinical trials (letter). *Br. Med. J.*, 1:1661.
18. Farewell, V. T., and D'Angio, G. J. (1981): A simulated study of historical controls using real data. *Biometrics*, 37:169–176.
19. Simon, R. M. (1982): Design and conduct of clinical trials. In: *Cancer: Principles and Practice of Oncology*, edited by V. T. DeVita, Jr., S. Hellman, and S. A. Rosenberg, pp. 198–225, 1st ed. Lippincott, Philadelphia.
20. Peto, R., Pike, M. C., Armitage, P., et al. (1976): Design and analysis of randomized clinical trials requiring prolonged observation of each patient. 1. Introduction and design. *Br. J. Cancer*, 34:585–612.
21. Schoenfeld, D. A., and Gelber, R. D. (1979): Designing and analyzing clinical trials which allow institutions to randomize patients to a subset of the treatments under study. *Biometrics*, 35:825–830.
22. Makuch, R., and Simon, R. (1978): Sample size requirements for evaluating a conservative therapy. *Cancer Treat. Rep.*, 62:1037–1040.
23. Simon, R. (1984): Importance of prognostic factors in cancer clinical trials. *Cancer Treat. Rep.*, 68:185–192.
24. Karnofsky, D. A., and Burchenal, J. H. (1949): The clinical evaluation of chemotherapeutic agents in cancer. In: *Evaluation of Chemotherapeutic Agents*, edited by C. M. Macleod, pp. 191–205. Columbia University Press, New York.

25. Zubrod, G. C., Schneiderman, M., Frei, E., III, et al. (1960): Appraisal of methods for the study of chemotherapy of cancer in man: Comparative therapeutic trial of nitrogen mustard and triethyl-enethiophosphoramide. *J. Chronic Dis.*, 11:7–33.
26. Aisner, J., and Hansen, H. H. (1981): Commentary: Current status of chemotherapy for non-small cell lung cancer. *Cancer Treat. Rep.*, 65:979–986.
27. Berdeaux, D. H., Moon, T. E., and Meyskens, F. L., Jr. (1985): Clinical–biological patterns of metastatic melanoma and their effect on treatment. *Cancer Treat. Rep.*, 69:397–401.
28. Cooper, M. R., Pajak, T. F., Gottlieb, A. J., et al. (1984): The effects of prior radiation therapy and age on the frequency and duration of complete remission among various four-drug treatments for advanced Hodgkin's disease. *J. Clin. Oncol.*, 2:748–755.
29. Simon, R. (1979): Restricted randomization designs in clinical trials. *Biometrics*, 35:503–512.
30. Zelen, M. (1974): The randomization and stratification of patients to clinical trials. *J. Chronic Dis.*, 27:365–375.
31. Pocock, S. J., and Simon, R. (1975): Sequential treatment assignment with balancing for prognostic factors in the controlled clinical trial. *Biometrics*, 31:103–115.
32. Byar, D. P. (1984): Identification of prognostic factors. In: *Cancer Clinical Trials: Methods and Practice*, edited by M. E. Buyse, M. J. Staquet, and R. H. Sylvester, pp. 423–443. Oxford University Press, Oxford.
33. Pizzocaro, G., Zanoni, F., Milani, A., et al. (1986): Orchiectomy alone in clinical Stage I non-seminomatous testis cancer. A critical appraisal. *J. Clin. Oncol.*, 4:35–40.
34. Leventhal, B. G., Levine, A. S., Graw, R. G., Jr., et al. (1975): Long term second remissions in acute lymphatic leukemia. *Cancer*, 35:1136–1140.
35. Simon, R. (1985): Size of Phase III cancer clinical trials. *Cancer Treat. Rep.*, 69:1087–1093.
36. Ellenberg, S. S., and Eisenberger, M. A. (1985): An efficient design for Phase III studies of combination chemotherapies. *Cancer Treat. Rep.*, 69:1147–1152.
37. George, S. L. (1984): The required size and length of a phase III clinical trial. In: *Cancer Clinical Trials: Methods and Practice*, edited by M. E. Buyse, M. J. Staquet, and R. J. Sylvester, pp. 287–310. Oxford University Press, Oxford.
38. Rubinstein, L. V., Gail, M. H., and Santner, T. J. (1981): Planning the duration of a comparative clinical trial with loss to follow up and a period of continued observation. *J. Chronic Dis.*, 34:469–479.
39. Sposto, R., and Sather, H. N. (1985): Determining the duration of comparative clinical trials while allowing for cure. *J. Chronic Dis.*, 38:683–690.
40. Armitage, P. (1975): *Sequential Medical Trials*. Charles C Thomas, Springfield, Illinois.
41. Pocock, S. J. (1979): Allocation of patients to treatment in clinical trials. *Biometrics*, 35:183–197.
42. Freiman, J. A., Chalmers, T. C., Smith, H., Jr., and Keubler, R. R. (1978): The importance of beta, the type II error and sample size in the design and interpretation of the randomized control trial: Survey of 71 "negative" trials. *N. Engl. J. Med.*, 299:690–694.

CHAPTER 7

Analysis of Comparative Trials

The previous chapters have addressed some of the conceptual and statistical problems in the design of comparative trials. This chapter will discuss the difficulties that occur once the trial is underway and after its completion. In considering the analysis of comparative trials we will discuss some of the theoretical and practical issues in analysis as well as some common difficulties in interpreting the analyses.

COMPARISON OF PROPORTIONS RESPONDING ON EACH ARM OF A STUDY

If the study has been designed so that each observation is a binary variable, i.e., the result for each patient can be expressed as the answer to a yes/no question, then a chi-square analysis of the data can be done. An example of such a question would be: Did the patient achieve remission with treatment A? The answer for each patient is either Yes or No and one ends up with a proportion of patients on treatment A who have achieved remission and can be considered "successes" with the remainder considered failures. One can then compare this with the proportion of patients who achieved remission with treatment B and see whether the proportion is different from that which would be predicted by chance if the two treatment arms were identical. A sample calculation of a chi-square analysis of proportions of successes in two treatment arms is given in Appendix 1. The significance of the result of a chi-square analysis can only be assessed if one knows the degrees of freedom, i.e., the number of independent variables entered into the calculation. This issue is discussed in Appendix 2.

One can also do a chi-square analysis to compare disease-free survival on different treatment arms at a specific point in time, for example, is the proportion of patients in remission on arm A higher than that in remission on arm B at 2 years? This might be a particularly useful comparison in a situation where, although the majority of patients had not benefited from the therapy, there was a small group of long-term survivors after treatment. Obvious weaknesses of this approach are (a) its sensitivity to the (arbitrary) choice of the time point; in fact there is a temptation to choose the time point for analysis as the point at which the data look the most different, which may require more complicated analytical techniques (1), and (b) its relative inefficiency since information from the entire curve is not being used.

104

CONSTRUCTION OF SURVIVAL CURVES

If one wishes to compare survival curves rather than just answer the Yes/No binary question, generally one would not want to wait until all the patients have died or relapsed. "Actuarial" (2) or a life-table estimates (3) of the data are commonly employed in this situation. To construct a life table each patient is considered as part of the proportion only for the period for which they have been followed. In other words, a person who has been followed and is still in remission at 6 months is considered in the proportion remaining in remission at 6 months, but is "censored" beyond that point; that is, he makes no contribution either to the numerator or the denominator when the fraction estimated still to be in remission at 9 months is calculated. The raw data for two groups of patients with the survival curve constructed from these data are shown in Fig. 7.1. The method for constructing these curves is shown in Appendix 3.

The projected survival curves constructed from these data have vertical "tick" marks at each point where a patient still survives. The median survival time, that is, the time when the proportion of patients surviving is 0.5, is not indicated exactly but is somewhere between 10 and 15 months for the Group A patients and is somewhere beyond 35 months for the Group B patients. This is longer than the median of 9.5 months for Group A and 19 months for Group B which would be arrived at by taking the midpoint of the actual numbers. This is because a number of the observations have been censored. Comparing medians can be a useful first look at whether one set of data is different from another, but one should remember to construct life tables from the data before performing this maneuver if there is a significant number of censored observations.

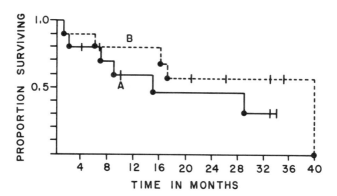

FIG. 7.1. Life-table curve for two theoretical groups of patients. The actuarial survival curve is constructed from the following data by the method described in Appendix 3. Survival data in months for two groups of patients:

Treatment A: 1, 2, 4+, 7, 9, 10+, 15, 29, 33+, 34+
Treatment B: 1, 6, 7+, 16, 17, 21+, 26+, 33+, 35+, 40

A plus sign indicates that the patient is still alive at the designated time of last follow-up.

The life-table estimates of the survival curve at the ends of successive intervals can be joined by straight lines to make the curve easier to look at, but it is not good practice to draw a smooth line through the steps of an actuarial curve. The steps conventionally are used to indicate that it is an actuarial (i.e., projected) curve rather than one based on data which is already complete (i.e., where all patients have either relapsed or died). Survival curves based on small numbers of patients can exhibit large drops as a result of single (or very few) events. This occurs simply because the curve is calculated on the basis of the proportion of patients surviving at a particular point in time. Note for example, how the curve for Group B falls precipitously to 0 when 1 patient relapses at 40 months, despite the fact that, up to that point, it looked as though there was a reasonable plateau with more than 50% of the patients in remission. This is because the 1 patient who relapsed represented 1/1 or 100% of those followed for this length of time on this treatment. The tails of survival curves plotted from actuarial analyses of small numbers of patients are often extremely unstable and should not be taken as an accurate indicator of how a large population on the same treatment would behave at similar points in time.

Many life tables are constructed with a tick mark indicating the time of follow-up of each censored patient. If a trial is so big that it would be impossible to show a distinct point for each patient, an alternative is to write at several different times along the foot of the life table the number of patients with trial times of at least those magnitudes (1). An example of such a large trial is shown in Fig. 7.2 (4).

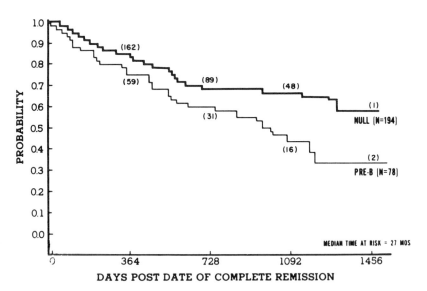

FIG. 7.2. Duration of continuous complete remission for patients with "null" and pre-B-cell acute lymphocytic leukemia ($p = 0.004$). The number of patients who remain at risk at various points in time are noted in parentheses (from ref. 4).

COMPARISON OF SURVIVAL CURVES

The Log Rank Test

The life table can provide a visual description of the survival data. Statisticians have devoted much attention to the problem of how to evaluate whether two survival curves differ significantly from each other. Unfortunately, no general techniques exist that are applicable to all kinds of curves. If, however, two curves exhibit risks of death whose logarithms are in a fixed ratio at all time points, it turns out that the log rank test is the optimal test of statistical significance for differences between the curves. This technique was first described by Mantel (5) in 1966 and depends on the following principle. Of the patients under observation on a particular day after randomization, if two-thirds are in treatment Group A and one-third in treatment Group B, then on average two-thirds of the deaths on that day would be expected in A patients and one-third in B patients. The number actually *observed* at each point (which is known) can then be compared with the number *expected* (which can be calculated). The number of events observed and those expected at each time interval are added together and the cumulative tools compared by the method shown in Appendix 4. A detailed discussion of the considerations that go into making these measurements is given by Peto et al. (1).

The log rank test is optimal under the assumption of proportional hazards. This means that the mortality rate per unit time (hazard rate) in one curve is a constant multiple of the other (constant difference on a log scale). To the extent that the curves to be tested do not exhibit proportional hazards, the log rank test will be less ideal, though it may still be useful. In some cases, however, if the curves depart sharply from proportional hazards behavior, use of the log rank test may be inappropriate. In Fig. 7.3 (6), for example, a complicated situation exists where one treatment is evidently to be preferred in the early posttreatment period, while another is superior later on. This result was obtained in the study of intensive chemoradiotherapy in gastric cancer, where therapy resulted in a significant number of early toxic deaths, but eventually a higher proportion of long-term survivors. In this situation it is unlikely that any single statistical analysis will be adequate, and analysis by multiple periods may have to be performed before the curves can be completely compared for their significance. Clearly, adequate survival analysis is a complex subject and should not be undertaken without the assistance of someone with technical statistical expertise.

Confidence Intervals

Another way of expressing the difference between groups of patients is with confidence intervals (7). Rather than dealing with the response rate observed in a single study, one can calculate an interval that has a specified probability of containing the true response rate, as discussed in Chapter 5. It is also possible for a

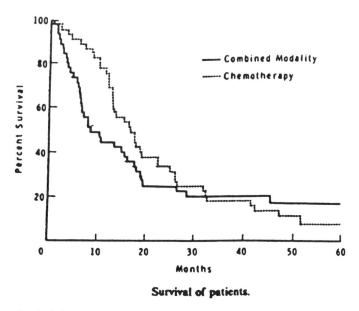

Survival of patients.

FIG. 7.3. Survival of two patient groups with gastric cancer. Therapy resulted in a significant number of early toxic deaths, but eventually a higher proportion of long-term survivors. The hazards are not proportional on these curves (from ref. 6).

comparative study to calculate an interval for the difference between response rates that will, with a high probability, contain the true difference between response rates (see Fig. 6.4). Such calculations may be particularly useful when lack of "statistical significance" is seen in small studies (7). Calculation of confidence intervals in this setting may give a supplemental feel as to whether an important difference might emerge if the trial were expanded or repeated.

SOURCES OF BIAS IN THE ANALYSIS OF SURVIVAL CURVE DATA

The calculation of the survival curve depends on (a) correct recording of time of entry to the study; (b) correct recording of time of loss to follow-up or death; and (c) the assumption that a patient's chance of being lost or withdrawn is unrelated to his risk of dying. The frequent failure to satisfy these three conditions may lead to serious bias in the survival curve and sometimes to bias in the comparisons of treatments (3).

For purposes of analysis, the time of entry onto the study may be the time of registration on study, if the endpoint is overall survival; or it may be the point of randomization, which, as we have discussed earlier, may have been delayed for some time after registration. It may also be the time of achieving remission if we are going to analyze disease-free survival. This situation could easily apply if one were analyzing a randomized maintenance therapy in a group of patients who all received identical induction. A common error in defining date of entry occurs when patients are subclassified after the original classification has occurred, and then the subgroup is compared with the patient group as a whole. For example, if the survival of patients with acute nonlymphocytic leukemia receiving bone marrow transplantation in complete remission were compared with those patients receiving conventional chemotherapy, one must realize that no patient who dies during the initial induction period is included in the bone marrow transplant group (since all patients had to be in complete remission to be transplanted), whereas all patients are included in the chemotherapy arm. Thus, the overall survival for the conventional chemotherapy group may appear less favorable, unless the study is structured and the data anaylzed in an unbiased fashion. In other words, the date of entry for this analysis must be a comparable time after remission has been achieved for both the chemotherapy and the transplant group.

Correct recording of time of the event to be analyzed, usually relapse or death, is also critical. Patients in each arm of treatment must be followed at comparable intervals and with comparable tests if these comparisons are to be valid. If you are comparing treatment to a no-treatment control and you see your treated patients monthly for therapy but the no-treatment control patients only every 3 months, you will, in general, detect relapses a few months earlier in the treated patients, and fewer of them will be lost to follow-up.

EXCLUSIONS, LOSSES, AND REMOVAL OF PATIENTS

Patients may be excluded from a trial because they do not meet the eligibility criteria. This may affect the generalizability of the resulting treatment comparison, but because the determination is made prior to randomization, it does not confound the final analysis. On the other hand, if a patient is not evaluable after randomization, the validity of the entire comparison is threatened. For any final report of a study, an analysis including all patients by the treatment to which they were randomized must be included. It may also be of interest to analyze outcome according to the treatment actually received, but the primary analysis is according to the assigned treatment, since that is the only way that comparability of the treatment groups is assured. Removals after randomization for any reason may bias the treatment comparison between the two randomized groups, because in many cases, the removals are not random.

A review of the articles published in *Cancer Treatment Reports* in 1984 disclosed that, in general, the inevaluability rate of the trial increases with increasing sample size. These data are shown in Table 7.1. The reasons given for inevaluability were:

Ineligible (31)
Early death (135)
Major protocol violation (31)
Patient refused therapy (13)
Evaluable for toxicity only (9)
Lost to follow-up (7)

TABLE 7.1. *Evaluability of patients in trials reported in* Cancer
Treatment Reports, *1984*

No. pts. in trial	< 20	21–40	> 40
No. trials	17	27	12
Total no. pts.	285	743	991
No. evaluable	281	642	817
% evaluable	0.99	0.86	0.82

Insufficient data (24)
Unknown (37)

Following is a discussion of how each of these reasons for inevaluability may result
in bias.

Exclusion Because of Ineligibility

Patients who are found retrospectively not to satisfy the eligibility criteria are
often removed from analysis (8). As an egregious example, suppose a patient with
bronchitis was mistakenly randomized on a lung cancer protocol. Should such a
patient be removed from analysis? Removing such a patient will not bias the
treatment comparison provided the detection of this eligibility violation was unrelated to treatment assignment. To avoid such an association, it is important to
use uniform standards on both treatment arms to review for such protocol violations.
In the example given, if the patient were assigned to a no-treatment arm and had
lived so long that the original diagnosis was questioned by the investigator and the
pathology was reviewed on only this patient, then this would not be reasonable.
The pathology on all patients should be reviewed to assure that other such patients
had not been included in the study.

Some badly flawed protocols declare patients ineligible on the basis of events
following randomization. For example, suppose resected lung cancer patients are
randomized to adjuvant chemotherapy or no further treatment (control) with the
stipulation that chemotherapy begin within 30 days following surgery. A proper
analysis of this trial should compare the outcome of the control group with that of
all the patients assigned to chemotherapy whether or not they were able to begin
chemotherapy within the designated period. Otherwise, if patients beginning chemotherapy after 30 days are considered ineligible for analysis, the comparison may
be severely biased, since all the patients receiving no further therapy would then
be compared only with those chemotherapy patients who were well enough to receive
chemotherapy within 30 days after surgery.

Exclusion for Death or Toxicity

Early death of more than an occasional patient on study generally means that the
investigators are entering patients who were too sick initially or who had too low

a performance status. The damaging effect of this practice on the conduct of the study has been discussed in Chapter 6. In a multiinstitutional trial this may reflect differences in institutional policy and may indicate more widespread differences in treatment philosophy. For example, physicians who consider intensive experimental therapy appropriate only for very ill patients might be hesitant to give the therapy at all, with consequent delay of potentially successful therapy and a disproportionate number of early deaths on one experimental arm.

If the principal endpoint of interest is survival rather than response or response duration, then patients who are evaluable for toxicity but not for response should not be excluded from the analysis of survival. The biases that are introduced by this kind of exclusion are obvious. If a randomized trial is comparing experimental therapy to no therapy, then patients dying from experimental therapy should be included in the survival analysis; they should *not* be considered "evaluable for toxicity only." The same applies if one is comparing treatments A and B. One can easily see that certain kinds of severe toxicities might well appear more frequently in one subset of patients on one of the therapies (e.g., elderly patients receiving anthracyclines). The exclusions of such early deaths from the survival analysis would clearly introduce unacceptable biases into the analysis.

Exclusion Because of Failure to Comply with Treatment Plan or Loss to Follow-up

Another common justification for removals is failure to comply with the intended treatment, as when physicians fail to give or patients refuse to take all or part of their chemotherapy following randomization. In essence, this represents a form of retrospective subset analysis. A most interesting description of the problems inherent in this type of analysis was published some years ago by the Coronary Drug Project Research Group (9). The Coronary Drug Project was carried out as a double-blind experiment to evaluate the efficacy and safety of several lipid-lowering drugs in the long-term treatment of coronary heart disease. The 5-year mortality in 1103 men treated with clofibrate was 20.0% as compared with 20.9% in the 2789 men given placebo ($p = 0.55$). Good adherers to clofibrate (patients who took 80% or more of the protocol prescription during the 5-year follow-up period) had a substantially lower 5-year mortality than did poor adherers to clofibrate (15.0% versus 24.6%; $p = 0.00011$). However, similar findings were noted in the placebo group, i.e., 15.1% mortality for good adherers and 28.3% for poor adherers ($p = 4.7 \times 10^{-16}$). Thus, survival appeared to be related somehow to patient behavior rather than to the agent administered. Further analysis of these data has not yet presented an obvious explanation for this observation in terms of previously known prognostic factors. These findings and various other analyses of mortality in the clofibrate and placebo groups of the project show the serious difficulty, if not impossibility, of evaluating treatment efficacy in subgroups determined by patient responses to the treatment protocol after randomization. It cannot be emphasized too strongly that randomization assures comparability of patient groups as a whole, not of subsets (10).

Losses to follow-up after randomization may also have a profound effect on the analysis because these losses may occur in a nonrandom fashion. Gail (8) has presented a summary of hypothetical survival data of adjuvant chemotherapy against placebo in which 20% of patients are lost to follow-up on each treatment. If 80 patients were entered on each arm and of those followed there are 35 deaths within the first year in the adjuvant chemotherapy group and 40 in the placebo group, one might presume a slight benefit for adjuvant therapy. In this particular example, when they retrieved the data on the "lost" patients they proposed that 15/20 patients lost to follow-up in the chemotherapy group had died, while only 10/20 lost to follow-up in the placebo group had died. Thus, the mortality in both groups was equivalent, but the patients lost from the chemotherapy group were sicker than those lost from the placebo group. This kind of differential loss to follow-up may introduce a bias. The fact that 80% of the patients were followed on both treatment groups does not guarantee that the two followed groups are comparable, even though the patients were initially randomized to insure comparability. These considerations emphasize the importance of trying to discover the fate of *every* patient prior to the final analysis of the data, even if they have moved to another area or transferred their care to another physician.

In essence, then, all patients should be available for analysis once they have been entered on trial and none should be declared "inevaluable." Certainly, an inevaluability rate of $> 10\%$ should raise serious questions about the conduct of the trial.

INTERIM ANALYSES

One might think it desirable for the investigator to be on top of the data at all times. Clearly, evolving data in a comparative trial must be monitored, if only because it would be unethical not to look for signs of undue risk to participating patients. In practice this means that it is necessary to generate the observed distributions of toxic effects, tumor shrinkage, disease progression times, and survival times on a regular basis, perhaps every 4–8 months depending on accrual, and to terminate an arm or even the entire study if there is good evidence of substantial damage to patients. However, there are both procedural and statistical problems with interim analyses for the endpoints of efficacy (11).

Procedural Problems

Most interim analyses are very superficial compared with the final report. There can be major problems with the analysis of both toxicity and response rate during the course of a study. Differential delays in the submission of data may lead to unbalanced reporting of toxicity. Investigators may be more likely to report deaths or severe toxicities on the experimental arm than on the standard treatment arm because they are more familiar with managing the complications of the standard therapy.

At the same time, appreciation of the true relative effect of the different treatments under consideration may be obscured by possible imbalances in the prognostic characteristics of the patients assigned to the different treatment groups. The likelihood of substantial imbalance will be minimized if balanced stratification for the most important prognostic factors has been included in the initial trial design, so that even if the groups are small, they are probably comparable. Analysis of treatment outcome in subsets of patients may not be possible at all in interim analyses, since presumably the trial has been designed to accrue in toto the minimum number of patients required for this analysis, but the balanced stratification will allow one to compare treatment groups overall.

Unanticipated biases in patient evaluation may occur after the study is underway. For example, in a randomized study of regional chemotherapy by implantable pump versus intravenous chemotherapy, surgeons might consider patients ineligible in whom they were unable to implant the pump for various physical reasons. Since the intravenous chemotherapy group includes all patients, including those who might have been declared ineligible by the surgeons, there are systematic biases introduced into the evaluation data for the two treatment groups that must be addressed before the treatment comparison can be properly interpreted. Obesity, for example, which might be a factor making it difficult to implant a pump has been shown to be an adverse prognostic factor for some types of chemotherapy (12).

Statistical Problems

False-positive Results

(a) Frequent repetition of a single test has a very high chance of generating a p value < 0.05 at some time during the trial even when there is no difference among the distributions being compared. The mathematical likelihood of this result can be calculated and is shown in Table 7.2 (13).

TABLE 7.2. *Overall probability (%) of achieving a result with a given nominal significance after L repeated tests when there is no difference in the effects of two treatments*

Nominal significance level (p)	No. repeated significance tests (L)								
	1	2	3	4	5	10	25	50	200
0.01	1	1.8	2.4	2.9	3.3	4.7	7.0	8.8	12.6
0.05	5	8.3	10.7	12.6	14.2	19.3	26.6	32.0	42.4
0.10	10	16.0	20.2	23.4	26.0	34.2	44.9	52.4	65.2

The first column of this table is merely a definition of the significance level. If you perform one analysis you have a 5% chance of coming up with a difference with $p = 0.05$ between two arms when none exists. However, as you can see, on a chance basis alone, if you do five analyses, your likelihood of getting $p < 0.05$ when no difference exists is 14%. Because this phenomenon has been known to clinical trials investigators for some time, considerable work has already been done to develop appropriate methods for interpreting a series of interim analyses (14,15). In a very general way, the assumption is that if one is looking for $p < 0.05$ in the final analysis, one would stop the trial after an interim analysis only if the difference between the two arms were significant at a p value higher than that, say $p < 0.01$, depending on the number of analyses planned.

It is important for the use of these procedures that the maximum number of tests of the data and the number of observations to be collected between successive tests be fixed in advance. One should not just examine the data in an impulsive or unplanned fashion. These procedures, however, do allow one to terminate a trial early when one treatment performs markedly better than the other.

(b) Testing for several different outcome variables (e.g., survival, tumor decrease, time to disease progression, incidence of special toxic effects, various quality of life measures) has a very high chance of generating at least one value that is less than 0.05 even when there are no real differences in the distribution of any of the variables among the treatment groups being compared. If 20 variables are examined, then it is quite likely that at least one factor would differ significantly between the two arms at the 0.05 level.

False-negative Results

To interpret negative results properly we must know (a) whether the most powerful statistical test for the problem has been used, and (b) whether covariate analyses (16) have been done to assess the association of treatment with the responses or survival variables after adjustment for the effects of other important variables that might not be evenly distributed among the treatment groups (12).

Dissemination of Interim Analyses

Many advocate that information on treatment efficacy should not be given out in routine general reports distributed to all study investigators until after patient accrual ends. Blinding the arms of the study for interim reports will not solve the problem since it will still be obvious whether the treatments are identical or whether one arm appears inferior. If one arm appears inferior, even if the investigators do not know which one it is, patient accrual may be affected because they may be afraid to take the chance that their patient might get the inferior arm. This may lead to failure to complete accrual to the study so that the final result may well be inconclusive. Multidisciplinary monitoring committees responsible for the ethical conduct of the trial may be constituted to perform these interim analyses, so that the individual investigators can be assured that their patients are not being placed at excessive risk of treatment failure or toxicity on any individual arm of a study. Within the cooperative cancer study groups in the United States such committees, where they exist, usually consist of the principal investigators and the statisticians. In groups where there are no such formal committees, the statistical office performs this function. Certain large trials in other subspecialties such as cardiology, routinely employ data monitoring committees composed of individuals not involved in the study design or conduct to keep an eye on the data. This may help to eliminate bias.

TREATMENT–COVARIATE INTERACTIONS

The aim in any clinical experiment is to determine whether the effect observed is in fact related to the treatment. We must, therefore, assure ourselves that there is not some other explanation. It is sometimes the case that treatments affect different kinds of patients differently. If we are comparing treatments A and B, it might happen that treatment A is much more effective than treatment B in males, but no difference is observed in females, or it may even be that treatment B is superior for females. In statistical language, such a situation is called an interaction between treatment and a covariate (in this example, gender) (17). We may have already known about the significance of gender when planning the trial and stratified the patient groups appropriately; however, when the data have been collected it is important to look at them retrospectively and see whether there are other possible subgroups of patients which should be considered independent of the group as a whole. Deciding how to do this properly is often a difficult problem in clinical trials. Indiscriminate examination of many different subsets for differential treatment effects is likely to produce spurious results simply by chance alone. In general, the important subsets should be decided on when the trial is still in its planning stages. Of special importance are the covariates that are known or suspected to be of significance or those that are bolstered by some reasonable hypothesis. If the sample size of the trial is too small for a powerful overall analysis of treatment effect, the analysis of treatment–covariate interactions is unlikely to be productive.

In order to decide whether a variable is correlated with prognosis one can construct actuarial survival curves for each category and compare them for statistical significance. An example of such a calculation demonstrates the prognostic importance of renal function at the time of randomization on the likelihood of achieving remission with two hypothetical treatments A and B (1). After having identified the possibly important individual prognostic factors from analysis of the data at hand and from the appropriate literature, the next step is to examine the effects of the variables when more than one is evaluated simultaneously. To do this one performs regression analyses.

Regression analysis is the study of the relationship of one variable Y to another variable X. Often, in clinical oncology the variable Y might be survival time or remission duration and the variable X might be some other measurable continuous function such as age at diagnosis. This type of analysis of two factors can be adapted to a linear regression model. If Y is a binary outcome, such as remission or no remission, then the logistic model of Cox (18) is often used. If the feature to be used as the Y variable is a time variable where some of the observations are censored, then the proportional hazards model of Cox (19) can be employed. Once individual variables have been identified that correlate with outcome, multivariate logistic methods can be used to identify the most important factors. For example, in acute leukemia, outcome might be correlated with white count elevation and liver and spleen size at the time of diagnosis if each were analyzed separately. However, if the data were already analyzed for the importance of white count, then the size of the liver and spleen might add nothing further to the correlation, since all three of these might be measures of tumor load with the white count being the most accurately measured.

Regression models are used for both inference and prediction (17). First one inspects the data to identify factors that appear to determine the response to therapy (inference). Once these factors have been identified, they may be incorporated into future studies for a variety of purposes: to identify poor risk subsets of patients on which to focus future studies, to determine stratification criteria for future trials, to improve the precision of treatment comparisons for randomized trials, to compare results from different institutions, or to select a nonrandomized control group.

When using statistics for any sort of analysis it is important to use common sense as well. One might wish to analyze the number of courses that have been given at full dose, or the number that have been reduced or omitted due to toxicity to see if this affected survival. If one takes the date of entry as the date of first treatment, then one might find that the patients who have had many dose reductions have lived longer than those who have not. The reason for this could be simply that the patient has to have lived quite a long time to be able to have a large number of dose reductions. On the other hand, if patients who had to have their doses reduced died earlier than those who received full dose, this might be because the patients whose doses were reduced were sicker at the beginning of the study. In this sense, dosage reduction served as a prognostic factor rather than a causal event for poor survival. This particular distinction is often extremely difficult to make.

Freireich (20) has adapted detailed multivariate logistic regression to identify those factors most important for predicting response to a given treatment. In an analysis of leukemia patients treated between 1973 and 1977, approximately 40 variables were selected that correlated with response to treatment with combination chemotherapy regimens including anthracyclines and cytarabine. A regression coefficient was calculated for the degree of association or the predictive value of each variable and expressed quantitatively by the log likelihood value. The variables were ordered by their degree of predictive power. For this particular analysis, the age of the patient at diagnosis ranked first. Degrees of interrelation between the variables were assessed by investigating those variables other than the highest ranking one (in this case age) that, if added to age, produced the best prediction of response. After this was done, all the variables other than age were ordered in terms of their contribution to age in making good predictions. In this fashion, a second variable was chosen (cytogenetic findings), and then the procedure was repeated to investigate which of the residual variables if added to the first two variables produces the greatest increase in predictive power. Having once generated such a table of data, it becomes possible to construct a regression equation that allows computation of the probability of response for each individual patient.

The difficulty with this sort of analysis for planning future studies is that the same factors may not apply even for the same disease with a different treatment (discussion published with Ref. 20). If one therapy were particularly intensive and elderly patients tolerated it poorly, then age might be more important as a prognostic factor for this treatment than for a less-intensive regimen. As treatment improves and higher percentages of patients respond to the therapy, then prognostic indicators become less important. At the extreme, for treatment that is uniformly curative, it does not matter what characteristics the patient had at the beginning of treatment.

One important use of covariate analysis is to help determine how much data need to be collected at the time a patient goes on study. If one is using 24 monoclonal antibodies to type leukemia cells and only 6 contribute prognostically important information by covariate analysis, one may be able to restrict the required tests performed on each patient.

POOLING DATA

Well-informed physicians usually draw conclusions about the value of a certain therapy by considering all the available evidence. In cases where treatment effects may be modest or small, the problem may be particularly vexing, since the available randomized clinical trials may individually not be large enough to detect small but still medically worthwhile differences with reasonable power.

To increase the reliability of inference under these circumstances, statisticians and physicians have developed methods for combining results from independent trials that are similarly designed and targeted to similar patient populations. The techniques used to do this are often referred to as "meta-analysis," "pooling," or "statistical overviews."

In recent years Peto and his colleagues at Oxford have been the most vocal proponents of statistical overviews. They have expressed the view that the most reliable and least biased answer is likely to emerge from an overview that includes *all* randomized trials, published and unpublished. For each separate trial one calculates O (number of observed events) and E (number of expected events) for treatment A, and O and E for treatment B. Finally, one adds all the O's for treatment A to get an overall O_A, and the E's for treatment A to get an overall E_A and does the same for B. Comparison of O_A with E_A and O_B with E_B in the usual way (see Appendix 5) will lead to a p value testing whether A and B are statistically significantly different from each other.

TABLE 7.3. *Pooled data from patients in 15 randomized trials*

Allocated therapy	Total	Deaths	% Deaths	
Control	7970	804	10.1	
Beta blocker	8378	670	8.0	$p < 0.0001$

From ref. 21.

In pooling results from several trials, it is important to be sure that the individual trials pooled have been truly randomized, that complete data are available from all of the trials, and that the treatment regimens to be pooled are reasonably comparable to one another. Yusuf et al. (21) have published an overview analysis of 15 randomized trials of beta blockade during and after myocardial infarction in which this technique was used. Only 3 of these trials had shown a significant difference between treated and control groups when analyzed separately, but when analyzed together they had a large combined total of patients as shown in Table 7.3.

This same group of investigators has studied several factors in the treatment of breast cancer with this method. In looking at the effect of radiation therapy after surgery, they found that for the first 10 years there was no obvious effect but that after 10 years, the radiotherapy group had a significantly worse survival than the surgery alone group (22).

The concept of statistical overviews is quite controversial at present. Many investigators are deeply disturbed by the notion that the pooling process makes no clear distinction between data of excellent quality and data from groups that do not pay meticulous attention to quality assurance procedures. Others are troubled by the medical meaning of results from overviews; it seems clear that the medical value of meta-analyses depends largely on the similarity of the treatments and the patient populations that are being combined. Fuller discussions of some of the problems in the interpretation of overviews are available elsewhere (23,24). Whatever the values and the problems inherent in analyses of this type, all agree that although a single trial may not replace a well-done review, by the same token a review, no matter how well done, cannot replace well-performed individual trials of adequate size (25). It seems likely, however, at least in carefully defined circumstances, that quantitative overviews can aid in the evaluation of therapy.

APPENDIX 1

Chi-square Test

The chi-square test is designed to compare the difference between the number of events observed (O) and the number of events expected (E) in each arm of a study on the basis of a null hypothesis that there is no difference between the arms, and that each arm will have the same proportion of responses as it does patients. The number of events observed is known. The number expected in arm A is the total number of events multiplied by the number of patients in arm A over the total number of patients. This difference ($O - E$) is then squared and divided by the expected number. The sum of all such terms, one for each category (26) is:

$$\chi^2 = \frac{(O - E)^2}{E} \, .$$

For a two-armed study

$$\chi^2 = \frac{(O_A - E_A)^2}{E_A} + \frac{(O_B - E_B)^2}{E_B}$$

The assessment of the proportion of successes and failures can be generalized to the following formula (27):

	Success	Failure	Total
Therapy A	S_A	F_A	N_A
Therapy B	S_B	F_B	N_B
Total	$S_A + S_B$	$F_A + F_B$	$N_A + N_B = N$

Then the general formula for the χ^2 statistic is:

$$\chi_1^2 = \frac{(S_A \cdot F_B - S_B \cdot F_A)^2 \cdot N}{(S_A + S_B) \cdot (F_A + F_B) \cdot N_A \cdot N_B}$$

The subscript on the χ^2 denotes 1 *df* (see below).

If we take a specific case in which with treatment A, 7 of 41 patients achieved a response and with treatment B, 14 of 39 achieved a response, then the analysis goes as follows.

	Success	Failure	Total
Therapy A	7	34	41
Therapy B	14	25	39
Total	21	59	80

By chance alone, if the treatments are equivalent, one would expect 41/80 or 51.2% of the responses to occur on therapy A and 39/80 or 48.8% of the responses to occur on therapy B since that is the proportion of the total patients assigned to each group. One can see that the proportion of responses on therapy B is higher than that, namely 14/21 or 66.6% of the responses; but in order to find out whether this difference is statistically significant we do the following χ^2 analysis and the formula appears:

$$\chi_1^2 = \frac{(7 \cdot 25 - 14 \cdot 34)^2 \cdot 80}{21 \cdot 59 \cdot 41 \cdot 39} = 3.07$$

With 1 df the values for χ^2 are:

p	Two-sided test
< 0.05	> 3.84
< 0.02	> 5.42
< 0.01	> 6.63
< 0.001	> 10.80

Thus, with a two-sided test in our example $p > 0.05$; that is, there is a greater than 5% chance that the difference between the observed responses and the expected responses on the two arms of treatment would have happened by chance alone. A one-sided test would have been less stringent, but even though we know the direction of the actual difference (in this case that A appeared better than B), it is still more appropriate that a two-sided test be used.

In this example the 4 cells, i.e., the intersections of rows and columns, contained 7, 34, 14, and 25 patients, respectively. The Fisher's exact test is appropriate when the numbers are too small for the χ^2, i.e., when any cell contains less than 5 observations (26).

APPENDIX 2

Degrees of Freedom

The degrees of freedom are the number of independent differences being considered in the course of the test. When two or more sample distributions are compared and the data are arranged in r rows and c columns, the $df = (r - 1) \times (c - 1)$. For the example given in Appendix 1, there is only 1 df: $(2 - 1) \times (2 - 1) = 1$. This reflects the practical observation that once we know the total of each row and each column, we need to know only a single number in one "cell" that is the intersection of a row and a column in order to fill in each of the other 3. If we were comparing 3 or more treatments the degree of freedom would increase. The larger the number of degrees of freedom, the larger must be χ^2 for a given level of significance. Tables are available in the Bahn textbook (26).

APPENDIX 3

Actuarial Survival Curves

The method of calculating the actuarial survival follows immediately from the observation that to survive a year, a patient must survive the first day and the second and the third and so on to the 365th day. The separate probabilities of surviving each day are calculated and multiplied together (1).

For day 100, patients who died before day 100, those lost to follow-up before day 100, and those who entered the study less than 100 days ago contribute no information on the probability of surviving from the 100th to the 101st day and $E_{(100)}$, the estimated probability of surviving the 100th day for patients who have already survived 99 days is:

$$E_{(100)} = \frac{\text{No. at risk on day 100} - \text{no. deaths on day 100}}{\text{No. patients at risk on day 100}}$$

In many studies patients are followed up periodically, and the exact day when a patient was lost to follow-up cannot be accurately determined. If patients are seen every 3 months, for example, several deaths and losses to follow-up may occur between successive follow-ups and the number "at risk" when a particular death occurred will not be known exactly. A reasonable approximation is to average the numbers; thus, the number "at risk" in an interval is taken to be the number at risk at the start of the interval minus half the number lost during the interval.

As an example we shall construct survival curves for two hypothetical treatment groups.

Survival in months of patients after treatment

Treatment A:	1, 2, 4+, 7, 9, 10+, 15, 29, 33+, 34+
Treatment B:	1, 6, 7+, 16, 17, 21+, 26+, 33+, 35+, 40

A plus sign denotes that the patient is still alive at the designated time of last follow-up. Patients who are alive will have their data considered for the period of time for which they have been on study, but they will be "censored" after that; that is, they will not contribute to the numerator or the denominator of the proportion surviving the next time period.

For these graphs:

p_X is the proportion of patients at risk who have survived the interval;
p_Y is the cumulative proportion of patients who survived the previous interval;
p_C is the cumulative proportion of patients surviving the current interval, i.e., the number which is placed on the graph for that interval.

Life-table analysis for patients in arm A

Time (mos.)	No. at risk	Deaths	Censored	Survive	$p_X \times p_Y = p_C$
Start	10	0	0	10/10	1.00 1.00
1	10	1	0	9/10	0.90 × 1.00 = 0.90
2	9	1	0	8/9	0.89 × 0.90 = 0.80
4	8	0	1	8/8	1.00 × 0.80 = 0.80
7	7	1	0	7/8	0.88 × 0.80 = 0.70
9	7	1	0	6/7	0.86 × 0.70 = 0.60
10	6	0	1	6/6	1.00 × 0.60 = 0.60
15	5	1	0	4/5	0.80 × 0.60 = 0.48
29	3	1	0	2/3	0.66 × 0.48 = 0.32
33	2	0	1	2/2	1.0 × 0.32 = 0.32
34	1	0	1	1/1	1.0 × 0.32 = 0.32

Life-table analysis for patients in arm B

Time (mos.)	No. at risk	Deaths	Censored	Survive	$p_X \times p_Y = p_C$
Start	10	0	0		1.00
1	10	1	0	9/10	0.90 × 1.00 = 0.90
6	9	1	0	8/9	0.90 × 0.90 = 0.80
7	8	0	1	8/8	1.00 × 0.80 = 0.80
16	7	1	0	6/7	0.86 × 0.80 = 0.68
17	6	1	0	5/6	0.83 × 0.68 = 0.57
21	5	0	1	5/5	1.00 × 0.57 = 0.57
26	4	0	1	4/4	1.00 × 0.57 = 0.57
33	3	0	1	3/3	1.00 × 0.57 = 0.57
35	2	0	1	2/2	1.00 × 0.57 = 0.57
40	1	1	0	0/1	0 × 0.57 = 0

These results are shown graphically in Fig. 7.1.

APPENDIX 4

Log Rank Test

Let us construct a log rank analysis for the two groups of patients for whom we already have the life-table analysis. As before, the survival data at the time of constructing the curve are as follows:

$$\text{Group A} \quad 1, 2, 4+, 7, 9, 10+, 15, 29, 33+, 34+$$
$$\text{Group B} \quad 1, 6, 7+, 16, 17, 21+, 26+, 33+, 35+, 40$$

By life-table analysis you remember that the median survival for Group A is somewhere between 10 and 15 months and for Group B is not reached until after 35 months with the cumulative proportion surviving at $35+$ months being 0.57. Of course this falls to 0 with our last relapse as we have seen, but one might expect a difference in the overall analysis of survival with this twofold difference in the medians.

To estimate the significance of the difference between the two groups where the event to be analyzed is death, we need to discover what the estimated risk of death is for either group at any time period, and then compare this with the observed number of deaths. In essence, the number of "events" in any time period is multiplied by the proportion of patients at risk in each group during each time period (1,5,28). This calculation is performed in the following manner:

Calculation of expected risk of death for arms A and B

Time	No. of events observed (O)	No. at risk Total (N_r)	A (N_A)	B (N_B)	No. of events expected $E_A = \dfrac{O \cdot N_A}{N_r}$	$E_B = \dfrac{O \cdot N_B}{N_r}$
1,1	2	20	10	10	1.00	1.00
2	1	18	9	9	0.50	0.50
4+	0	17	8	9	0	0
6	1	16	7	9	0.44	0.56
7,7+	1	15	7	8	0.46	0.54
9	1	13	6	7	0.46	0.54
10+	0	12	5	7	0	0
15	1	11	4	7	0.36	0.64
16	1	10	3	7	0.30	0.70
17	1	9	3	6	0.33	0.67
21+	0	8	3	5	0	
26+	0	7	3	4	0	
29	1	6	3	3	0.50	0.50
33+	0	5	2	3	0	
34+	0	3	1	2	0	
35+	0	2	0	2	0	
40	1	1	0	1	0	1.00
Total	11				4.35	6.65

We now know the total extent of exposure to the risk of death in each group and we can then complete our formula:

Definitions	Number
O_A = Observed number of deaths in Group A	6
E_A = Extent of exposure to risk of death in Group A	4.35
O_B = Observed number of deaths in Group B	5
E_B = Extent of exposure to risk of death in Group B	6.65

To check for arithmetical accuracy make sure that $O_A + O_B = E_A + E_B$. We see that in our example both these sums are 11.

Calculate:

$$\chi^2 = \frac{(O_A - E_A)^2}{E_A} + \frac{(O_B - E_B)^2}{E_B}$$

$$\chi^2 = \frac{(6 - 4.35)^2}{4.35} + \frac{(5 - 6.65)^2}{6.65} = 1.250$$

and the two results are not statistically significantly different from one another despite the rather marked difference in projected median values.

For significance levels for χ^2, see Appendix 1.

APPENDIX 5

Calculation of χ^2 from Pooled Data (1)

Data extracted from three trials cited in the paper by Yusuf et al. (21)

Trial	Death/no. randomized	
	A (Control)	B (Beta blocker)
P	3/39	3/38
Q	14/116	7/114
R	11/93	5/69

Trial	No. of events observed (O)	No. at risk			No. of events expected	
		Total (N_r)	A (N_A)	B (N_B)	$E_A = \dfrac{O \cdot N_A}{N_r}$	$E_B = \dfrac{O \cdot N_B}{N_r}$
P	6	77	39	38	3.04	2.96
Q	21	230	116	114	10.59	10.41
R	16	162	93	69	9.19	6.81

	O vs. E for pooled trials			
	A		B	
	O	E	O	E
P	3	3.04	3	2.96
Q	14	10.59	7	10.41
R	11	9.19	5	6.81
Total	28	22.82	15	20.18

$$\chi^2 = \frac{(28 - 22.82)^2}{22.82} + \frac{(15 - 20.18)^2}{20.18} = 2.48 = p > 0.05 \text{ with 1 } df$$

This is the first 3 of 15 trials in one example by Yusuf et al. to illustrate the method by which the data were pooled. Only 3 of the trials in themselves gave statistically significant results (none of which are cited above), but when all 15 were pooled the difference between beta blocker and no beta blocker in this situation was significant at a $p < 0.0001$.

REFERENCES

1. Peto, R., Pike, M. C., Armitage, P., et al. (1977): Design and analysis of randomized clinical trials requiring prolonged observation of each patient, II. Analysis and example. *Br. J. Cancer*, 35:1–39.
2. Kaplan, E. L., and Meier, P. (1958): Nonparametric estimation from incomplete observations. *J. Am. Statist. Assoc.*, 53:457–481.
3. Peto, J. (1984): The calculation and interpretation of survival curves. In: *Cancer Clinical Trials: Methods and Practice*, edited by M. E. Buyse, M. J. Staquet, and R. J. Sylvester, pp. 361–380. Oxford University Press, Oxford.
4. Crist, W., Boyett, J., Roper, M., et al. (1984): Pre-B cell leukemia responds poorly to treatment: A Pediatric Oncology Group study. *Blood*, 63:407–414.
5. Mantel, N. (1966): Evaluation of survival data and two new rank order statistics arising in its consideration. *Cancer Chemother. Rep.*, 50:163–170.
6. Schein, P. S., for the Gastrointestinal Tumor Study Group (1982): A comparison of combination chemotherapy and combined modality therapy for locally advanced gastric carcinoma. *Cancer*, 49:1771–1777.
7. Simon, R. (1986): Confidence intervals for reporting results of clinical trials. *Ann. Intern. Med.*, 105:429–435.
8. Gail, M. H. (1985): Eligibility exclusions, losses to follow-up, removal of randomized patients, and uncounted events in cancer clinical trials. *Cancer Treat. Rep.*, 69:1107–1113.
9. Canner, P. L., for The Coronary Drug Project Research Group (1980): Influence of adherence to treatment and response of cholesterol on mortality in the coronary drug project. *N. Engl. J. Med.*, 303:1038–1041.
10. Simon, R. (1982): Patient subsets and variation in therapeutic efficacy. *Br. J. Clin. Pharmacol.*, 14:473–482.
11. O'Fallon, J. R. (1985): Policies for interim analysis and interim reporting of results. *Cancer Treat. Rep.*, 69:1101–1104.
12. Wiernik, P. H., and Serpick, A. A. (1970): Factors affecting remission and survival in adult acute nonlymphocytic leukemia (ANLL). *Medicine*, 49:505–513.
13. Summarized in McPherson, K. (1984): Interim analysis and stopping rules. In: *Cancer Clinical Trials: Methods and Practice*, edited by M. E. Buyse, M. J. Staquet, and R. J. Sylvester, pp. 407–422. Oxford University Press, Oxford.
14. O'Brien, P. C., and Fleming, T. R. (1979): A multiple testing procedure for clinical trials. *Biometrics*, 35:549–556.
15. Pocock, S. J. (1982): Interim analyses for randomized clinical trials: The group sequential approach. *Biometrics*, 38:135–162.
16. Byar, D. P. (1984): Identification of prognostic factors. In: *Cancer Clinical Trials: Methods and Practice*, edited by M. E. Buyse, M. J. Staquet, and R. J. Sylvester, pp. 423–443. Oxford University Press, Oxford.
17. Simon, R. (1984): Use of regression models: Statistical aspects. In: *Cancer Clinical Trials: Methods and Practice*, edited by M. E. Buyse, M. J. Staquet, and R. J. Sylvester, pp. 444–466. Oxford University Press, Oxford.
18. Cox, D. R. (1970): *The Analysis of Binary Data*. Methuen, London.
19. Cox, D. R. (1972): Regression models in life-tables (with discussion). *J. R. Statist. Soc. (b)*, 34:187–220.
20. Freireich, E. J. (1983): Methods for evaluating response to treatment in adult acute leukemia. *Blood Cells*, 9:5–20.
21. Yusuf, S., Peto, R., Lewis, J., et al. (1985): Beta blockade during and after myocardial infarction: An overview of the randomized trials. *Progr. Cardiovasc. Dis.*, 27:335–371.
22. Cuzick, J., Stewart, H., Peto, R., et al. (1987): Overview of randomized trials of postoperative adjuvant radiotherapy in breast cancer. *Cancer Treat. Rep.*, 71:15–25.
23. Simon, R. (1987): Overviews of randomized clinical trials. *Cancer Treat. Rep.*, 71:3–5.
24. Wittes, R. (1987): Problems in the medical interpretation of overviews. *Statist. Med.*, 6:269–280.
25. Yusuf, S., Collins, R., and Peto, R. (1984): Why do we need some large, simple randomized trials? *Statist. Med.*, 3:409–420.

26. Bahn, A. K. (1972): *Basic Medical Statistics*, Grune and Stratton, New York.
27. Bartolucci, A. A. (1984): Estimation and comparison of proportions. In: *Cancer Clinical Trials: Methods and Practice*, edited by M. E. Buyse, M. J. Staquet, and R. J. Sylvester, pp. 337–360. Oxford University Press, Oxford.
28. Mantel, N., and Haenszel, W. (1959): Statistical aspects of the analysis of data from retrospective studies of disease. *J. Natl. Cancer Inst.*, 22:719–748.

CHAPTER 8

Combination Chemotherapy

The early development of cancer chemotherapy was spurred on by dramatic responses to the few available single agents, most notably nitrogen mustard and methotrexate, in certain sensitive tumor types such as choriocarcinoma and acute leukemia (1–3). Relatively early on it became clear that the therapeutic potential of existing cytotoxic agents was limited. Administration of single drugs only rarely resulted in the attainment of durable complete remissions. Thus, the existence of primary or acquired drug resistance loomed as a major obstacle to the cure of disseminated neoplasia.

In the late 1950s, investigators began exploring combinations of cytotoxic agents in the clinic. This approach resulted in the eventual development of curative treatments for a number of disseminated cancers, including acute leukemias, lymphomas, and germ cell tumors (4–6). The increased effectiveness of combination chemotherapy gave additional rationale to the integration of chemotherapy into combined modality approaches and thus opened the way to the broad investigation of chemotherapy as an adjuvant to surgery or radiotherapy. At present, combination chemotherapy is at the core of state-of-the-art approaches to many neoplasms, and the further development of combinations of agents, as new active compounds are discovered, is one of the central challenges of clinical oncology.

The fundamental aim of combination chemotherapy is to produce a greater degree of cell kill than is obtained with single-agent treatment. For a combination to be truly useful clinically, it should constitute better therapy than alternative approaches; that is, it should yield higher remission rates, more durable remissions, increased survival, or better quality of life. For this to occur, the enhanced killing must be selective; enhancement of drug effect must be significantly greater for tumor cells than for normal host cells. If not, one simply sees enhanced toxicity to all cells and no net therapeutic gain.

The various rationales for the construction of particular combinations are generally either empirical or mechanistic in nature. By empirical we mean that two or more drugs are combined because of the individual activities of the constituent agents. The hypothesis here is that combinations of individually active agents will have substantially greater therapeutic activity than the component agents used singly. Alternatively, one may combine agents because of a particular mechanistic hypothesis relating to the biochemical or pharmacologic properties of the drugs when used together. These two classes of rationales are not mutually exclusive, and a given combination might be motivated by both kinds of considerations. This distinction is useful in ways that we shall return to later.

A brief word about terminology. In describing clinical results obtained with combination chemotherapy, it is best to stick to a description of the results themselves and avoid terms such as "synergistic" or "additive." In the experimental chemotherapy of transplantable murine tumors, where optimal doses can be defined and where controlled experiments to dissect the effects of alterations in a combination regimen are feasible, these terms have a precise meaning and are therefore useful; in clinical oncology, however, they have never been defined unambiguously (7). Quantitatively imprecise notions of synergism, such as "a greater response rate than would be expected from combining the component drugs" or "a greater than additive therapeutic effect," do not provide a usable operational definition of clinical synergism at all. These terms will not, therefore, appear anywhere in this chapter in connection with clinical results. A further discussion of some pertinent differences between laboratory models and clinical cancer is given in Ref. 7.

SCIENTIFIC CONSIDERATIONS

We shall begin by considering certain general properties of many effective drug combinations. For many years students of oncology have been taught that effective drug combinations tend to result when agents with the following properties are combined: (a) individually active against the tumor in question; (b) differing mechanisms of action, so that different biochemical events in the cell can be attacked simultaneously and so that the combination will be able to circumvent mechanisms of cellular resistance that apply to some, but not all, of the constituent agents; and (c) nonoverlapping toxicities, so that each agent can be given at or near its full single-agent dose. These lessons, with some redirection of emphasis, are as reasonable now as in the past and are discussed in further detail below.

Activity of Individual Agents

Experience suggests that agents without significant antitumor activity in their own right contribute little other than toxicity to combinations. The corollary is that the effectiveness of combination chemotherapy is generally proportional to the activity of the individual building blocks from which the combination is constructed (7).

This is not to say that relatively inactive agents can *never* have a place in combination treatment. For example, the attempt to modulate the antitumor effect of cytotoxic agents through the use of agents that have themselves no cytotoxic action is a subject of considerable current interest (8,9). Such experiments, however, are generally based on very specific mechanistic considerations. When combining agents without specific hypotheses concerning drug interaction, therefore, it seems wise to emphasize the use of known active drugs.

Non-cross-resistance of Individual Agents

The agents to be combined should be at least partially non-cross-resistant with each other. Before discussing this point further, let us define some terms. In the clinical situation, resistance implies that the dose of drug necessary to kill tumor cannot be delivered without unacceptably severe toxicity to the host. By contrast, sensitivity is present if antineoplastic effects occur at doses causing, at most, reversible toxicity (10). If the tumor cell population shows no sensitivity to the treatment on first exposure, we call the resistance "primary." If, on the other hand, the tumor initially regresses completely and then recurs despite continuation of treatment, the resistance may be termed "secondary" or "acquired."

Some instances of acquired resistance can be convincingly shown to have a genetic basis; resistance to methotrexate, for example, is sometimes due to amplification of the gene for dihydrofolate reductase. These amplified genes can be visualized as homogeneously staining regions of chromosomes (11). In the absence of a specific marker for resistance, however, a firm genetic basis for resistance may be extremely difficult to demonstrate clinically.

Any statement about clinical resistance to a drug must always be made with reference to a particular dose and schedule. A tumor that progresses during administration of an agent is resistant to that particular dose and schedule, but may subsequently respond to a higher dose or to more frequent administration. Moreover, a patient who has been in complete response and then relapses after discontinuation of therapy may respond to a second administration of the same regimen. Although not all the tumor was killed during the initial course(s) of treatment, one cannot presume clinical resistance of the recurrent tumor.

When induction of resistance to drug A also confers resistance to drug B, then A and B are said to be cross-resistant. In the clinic, one may conclude that agent B is at least partially non-cross-resistant to A if the administration of B produces responses in patients who are clearly resistant to full therapeutic doses of A. If patients have not been treated with full doses of A, either alone or in combination, then a subsequent response to B does *not* imply lack of cross-resistance, since complete clinical resistance to A has not been clearly demonstrated prior to exposure to B.

Partial non-cross-resistance is desirable among the components of a combination. If one built a combination out of three agents that exhibited complete overlap in activity (i.e., were completely cross-resistant), each agent would be capable of killing only the same subpopulation of (sensitive) cells. Thus, the combination of these agents would be no better therapy than the best of the three agents used singly. This is not to say that the coadministration of cross-resistant agents has no possible place in cancer therapy, for one could imagine two cross-resistant drugs with strikingly different pharmacological properties (e.g., one lipophilic and the other hydrophilic) being given in combination to attack tumor in systemic and central nervous system sanctuaries simultaneously.

In general, however, the use of non-cross-resistant agents in combination would seem to offer the greatest probability of improved efficacy. Agents are often thought to be non-cross-resistant if they have differing mechanisms of action or come from different chemical classes. The MOPP regimen for Hodgkin's disease, cytarabine + daunorubicin for acute nonlymphocytic leukemia, vincristine + prednisone + asparaginase for acute lymphoblastic leukemia, or vinblastine + bleomycin + cisplatin for testicular cancer are all curative regimens that were constructed partly on this basis.

For many diseases, the cross-resistance patterns of the existing active agents have not been worked out completely or rigorously, so decisions about what agents to bring together in combination must often be made on the basis of incomplete evidence. Evidence of lack of cross-resistance in *in vitro* cell culture systems may be of some assistance here, although the extent to which such data can be extrapolated to the clinic is problematic.

In trying to anticipate what agents might be cross-resistant, two important points should be kept in mind. First, chemical similarities between agents do not always imply cross-resistance. Different alkylating agents, for example, appear to lack cross-resistance, and combinations of them seem to be more active than single ones in laboratory models. Such combinations are currently under investigation in high dose in the clinic (12).

Second, chemical *differences* in structure, even profound ones, do not necessarily imply *lack* of cross-resistance. Recent work on the biology of drug resistance has revealed that the expression of certain multidrug resistance genes yields broad-spectrum resistance to natural products from a variety of chemical classes (13). Thus, cross-resistance bears no simple relation either to biochemical mechanism of action or to chemical structure. Although studies in cell culture systems or in *in vivo* murine tumor models may provide useful information, the demonstration of the extent of clinical cross-resistance (or lack of it) must ultimately come from clinical trials.

In addition, cells may have multiple mechanisms of resistance to particular drugs, and the ''multidrug resistance'' phenotype may not always reflect cross-resistance patterns in the primary treatment situation. For example, although anthracyclines and vincristine may share an acquired resistance phenotype, doxorubicin can still be shown to improve the effect of vincristine + prednisone in the control of primary acute lymphatic leukemia (14).

Nonoverlapping Toxicities

The major obstacle to administering full single-agent doses in the context of combinations is the existence of overlapping toxicities among many chemotherapeutic agents. For example, of the several agents commonly used against breast cancer, we have the spectrum of potential dose-limiting toxicities at conventional doses shown in Table 8.1.

This extensively overlapping pattern makes considerable caution necessary in the formation of combinations, since one might anticipate enhanced toxicity to bone marrow and mucosa with simultaneous administration. It may thus be necessary to

TABLE 8.1. *Toxic side effects of agents commonly used in breast cancer*

	Bone marrow	Mucosa	Myocardium	Neurologic
Alkylators	+			
Methotrexate	+	+		
5-fluorouracil	+	+		
Vincristine	±			+
Doxorubicin	+	+	+	

reduce the doses of the individual agents or increase the interval between doses. Either of these options has the effect of reducing the dose administered per unit time below that which has been shown to be effective. To minimize this problem, it is advisable, wherever possible, to employ agents with minimal overlap in toxicity patterns or to utilize pharmacologic protection (15,16). The lack of substantial overlap in toxicity for the agents employed in the MOPP combination for Hodgkin's disease allowed each agent to be given in nearly full dose and undoubtedly accounts in part for the effectiveness of this regimen.

So far, we have focused on the properties of the agents that make them ideal for incorporation into combinations. We now consider some of the important details involved in actually putting combinations together. In addition to selection of the component parts, we must establish the dose and schedule of each element of the combination.

DRUG SELECTION

If the disease in question has more than two or three active agents, the investigator must first decide which ones to include in the combination. Clearly, if one is working from some mechanistic hypothesis, then the hypothesis will dictate the choice. If, however, one wishes to combine agents empirically, the number of possible choices may be quite large, and one may have no compelling reason for favoring one alternative over any of the others. Returning to breast cancer, we have about six agents with response rates ranging from 20 to 40%; these drugs have incompletely overlapping toxicities and at least partial non-cross-resistance. Obviously, a very large number of combinations of from two to six agents is possible, and indeed, a quick look at the breast cancer literature would suggest that many of them have been tested clinically!

The central dilemma here is as follows. To maximize initial cell kill and suppress the emergence of resistance, thus minimizing the possibility of failure, one would ideally like to use all available non-cross-resistant agents, each in its maximum tolerated dose. Unless the toxicities are completely nonoverlapping, the greater the number of agents given together the more dose reduction must occur for each agent within the combination, to avoid intolerable toxicity from overlapping side effects.

It is therefore possible to end up with a combination of many drugs each given at an ineffective level.

One must also decide how the activities of the individual drugs should determine their priority for inclusion in a combination. If four candidate drugs have response rates ranging from 20 to 45%, how does one determine whether the inclusion of the drug with a 20% response rate is advisable? Omitting it may permit more intensive administration of the more active agents, but including it may be beneficial if the 20% agent has an important degree of non-cross-resistance with the others.

There are no general theoretical solutions to these very basic dilemmas, and the results of empirically based clinical studies provide little guidance. In breast cancer a variety of combinations of from two to five agents seem to produce about the same response rates and survival results, although the small number of direct comparative studies limits the strength of this conclusion. In ovarian cancer, for which several active agents currently exist, the best results with existing two-drug combinations are probably as good as results with more complex regimens (17). In the leukemias and lymphomas, where the number of active agents is greater, current research trends tend to emphasize the use of complex combinations involving eight or more drugs; for at least some of these diseases the evidence suggests that the more complex regimens yield better end results than the simpler ones (18,19,35).

DOSE SELECTION

Having decided what agents are to be included, one must decide how to give them. The simplest and most obvious answer is to attempt to administer each component according to the dose and schedule that appears optimal from existing single agent data, i.e., the dose schedule that yields the highest response rate of the agent when it is used singly. As previously noted, this approach is possible only when toxicities are essentially nonoverlapping. In addition, the frequency of myelosuppression and gastrointestinal mucosal toxicity among available cytotoxics has limited the number of such examples available in clinical chemotherapy (e.g., vincristine + prednisone, vinblastine + bleomycin + cisplatin, and streptozotocin + 5-fluorouracil). Thus, when a drug is placed into combination, full single-agent dosing is often simply not possible.

What is the effect of less than full dosing? The balance of evidence in the clinic favors the view that doses of drug should be as high as possible (7). Full-dose versus half-dose maintenance therapy produced more long-term remissions in a randomized study in acute leukemia (20). Current studies with very high doses of chemotherapy requiring bone marrow transplantation for support have yielded much higher response rates than one might expect from conventional doses of the same agents (12). Retrospective analysis of therapy for Hodgkin's disease suggests that longer remissions were associated with the administration of higher doses of drugs (21).

Recently, Hryniuk and Bush (22) compared the dose of drug per unit time (dose intensity) delivered in a number of different regimens for metastatic breast cancer.

Their analysis shows that clinical effectiveness is quantitatively related to the average dose intensity of treatment. The definition of dose intensity in this manner is rather different from previous ways of formulating dose-related hypotheses, in that the parameter of interest is the normalized dose over a certain treatment time period, rather than the size of an individual dose per se. As Hryniuk and Bush have pointed out, regimens that are apparently "low dose" (such as continuous weekly CMFVP) may have a higher relative dose intensity (because more drug is actually delivered over an entire treatment cycle) than CMFVP regimens featuring intermittent delivery of higher individual doses. This type of analysis has been extended to the breast adjuvant setting (23) with similar conclusions.

But even if one accepts the notion that combination chemotherapy should be given as vigorously as possible, we still have to decide how to match the doses of the individual agents in the combination. For example, consider a two-drug combination such as cyclophosphamide and doxorubicin. These agents have been most commonly administered by intravenous bolus once every 3 weeks or so. The acute dose-limiting toxicity of each is bone marrow suppression; thus, these agents are not normally given together without some reduction of the dose of each from the full single-agent dose. But how should the doses be reduced when the drugs are combined? Equivalently vigorous regimens of these two drugs could be achieved by employing an infinite number of different dose ratios. Each of these combinations, however, might have significantly different therapeutic characteristics. This is so for three reasons: (a) cyclophosphamide and doxorubicin have different degrees of activity against particular cancers; (b) their dose–response curves may well have different slopes; and (c) any interaction between two agents at the cellular level may depend on both dose and dose ratio.

In the absence of a firm scientific basis for choosing optimal dose ratios, clinicians have tended to approach the process empirically. Doses of the two agents may be selected on the basis of what the investigator estimates will yield tolerable toxicity; in establishing the dose ratio, one may give greater weight to the agent that is the more active for the disease in question; in other words, the more active agent will be given at a greater proportion of its single agent maximum tolerated dose than the less active agent. It should be remembered, of course, that criteria for defining a maximum tolerated dose change with time; more severe degrees of myelosuppression may be accepted now that a broader spectrum of antibiotics is available for infection control, than when the initial clinical trials with an agent were performed.

It should be clear that the complexities of dose-ratio selection, serious enough for a two-drug combination, become formidable for combinations of three or more agents. Our present inability to place dose-ratio selection on a firm scientific footing has uncertain consequences. With respect to the example of doxorubicin and cyclophosphamide given previously, it is admittedly not known whether the effectiveness of this two-drug combination is in fact highly dependent on dose ratio. Given the differences in activity from agent to agent, however, and the rather steep dose–response curves for many cytotoxic agents when used singly, there is no reason to assume that dose ratio should *not* make a difference in the clinic.

SCHEDULE SELECTION

As noted in the previous section, if one is selecting drugs on an empirical basis by their individual activity, one might most reasonably select the particular schedule that has been used with good effect in Phase II trials of the agent. In general, this should probably be the schedule that permits delivery of the agent at its maximal dose intensity.

If, however, the combination is being constructed according to mechanistic hypotheses, there may be additional considerations. Hayes et al. (24) used a cell-cycle based rationale to deliver a schedule of 8 days of oral cyclophosphamide at low dose (150 mg/m^2/day) followed by doxorubicin on day 8. Repeated biopsies of tumor in marrow showed that the cyclophosphamide increased the percentage of cells in S-phase by day 8, when doxorubicin was given. A higher percentage of patients with neuroblastoma achieved remission with this schedule than with other schedules of the same two agents, even in much higher doses.

Another widely studied example of considerable current interest is the interaction of methotrexate and 5-fluorouracil. A few years ago, based on their work in the laboratory, Cadman et al. (25) postulated that the effectiveness of these two drugs ought to depend on the temporal sequence in which they are administered. Studies in murine tumor models seemed indeed to show that when methotrexate preceded 5-fluorouracil, the combination was more efficacious than when the two drugs were given simultaneously or in the reverse sequence. The postulated mechanism of this effect, for which laboratory data *in vitro* provided support, was that exposure of tumor cells to methotrexate raised intracellular PRPP levels, which then increased the extent of activation of 5-fluorouracil to 5FdUMP and thus enhanced the cytotoxicity of a given dose of 5-fluorouracil. In the laboratory studies that motivated the clinical trials, not only the sequence but also the time interval between the administration of the two agents appeared to be an important determinant of the cytotoxic effect. Trials to test complex mechanistic hypotheses such as this are methodologically demanding, and we shall return to this issue later.

OPTIMAL DURATION OF THERAPY

How long should a treatment be carried on? Most investigators would probably agree that patients failing to respond to combination chemotherapy ought to have their treatment changed as soon as failure has been established. But what about the responders? Most of the very early studies in leukemia (e.g., VAMP, BIKE, POMP) gave therapy of limited duration (up to 15 months) and showed that although complete remissions were achieved, few patients were cured (26). It was therefore assumed that several years' duration of treatment was required in this tumor.

By contrast, for MOPP-treated patients with Hodgkin's disease, maintenance therapy for more than two courses after achievement of complete response does not prolong remission (21). For other highly sensitive tumors such as testicular cancer, it also appears that a relatively short duration of therapy is effective (27). For our purposes here, the main point is that determining the optimal duration of therapy requires systematic study for each disease, and perhaps even for each effective induction regimen.

In principle, therapy ought to continue until the point at which either all tumor has been eradicated or no further tumor cell killing is taking place. In the former case, therapy should be stopped altogether; in the latter, it should be changed to a regimen that will kill residual cells that are resistant to the initial treatment approach. Unfortunately, for patients in complete remission whose tumor is no longer measurable, the observer simply cannot tell when either of these points has been reached. The decision on how long to schedule therapy for responders must therefore be made somewhat arbitrarily.

The question of how long patients with complete responses should be treated cannot be divorced from the nature of the regimen used to induce the complete response in the first place. Complete response is a rather rough measure of treatment effect, and given the coarse diagnostic techniques currently in use, cell kill of only 2–3 logs will generally suffice to produce a complete response. It stands to reason, then, that all complete responses are not the same; the composition, intensity, and duration of the induction regimen itself ought to be major determinants of the quality of the complete response (i.e., how many logs of cell kill it actually represents) and of its potential durability.

When developing a new regimen, a termination time for therapy should be specified in the protocol, which might stipulate that treatment should continue for some fixed time period or for some arbitrary period beyond the point at which complete response is achieved. If a new combination results in a relatively high complete response rate, it might be reasonable to specify that the same combination be used again in patients who relapse, in order to see whether sensitivity to the initial regimen persists. If it does, then failure was not due to the acquisition of cellular resistance but to insufficient treatment intensity during initial therapy; perhaps doses were not high or frequent enough or treatment was not carried out for a sufficient number of cycles. This finding might then suggest a strategy involving different schedules or a search for sanctuary sites.

Certain experiences with salvage therapy have made it clear that failure to kill only the drug-resistant subpopulation is not the entire reason for the failure to cure with a particular combination. Patients receiving cyclophosphamide methotrexate + 5-fluorouracil (CMF) as adjuvant therapy for breast cancer who then relapse after 12 months and are retreated with CMF have response rates not very different from patients never previously exposed to cytotoxic agents (28). Patients with acute lymphatic leukemia who relapse after a year or more off therapy can have excellent responses to the drugs initially used in their treatment (26). In both cases, therefore, the entire sensitive cell population was not killed during initial therapy. As already noted, this may mean that the initial treatment was not given with sufficient intensity or that pharmacologic sanctuary sites may exist. Perhaps also the nondividing cell subpopulation may be relatively protected from the cidal effects of chemotherapy, in which case longer treatment periods may be more important than increasing the number of agents.

For patients in partial response, initial therapy has reduced tumor bulk significantly but incompletely. In the past, the general tendency has been to continue treatment until there is evidence of tumor regrowth, and this is still probably the most commonly adopted procedure. It is an understandable practice in many clinical contexts, particularly when alternative effective therapy is not available; clinicians reason that the treatment has helped the patient and that there is no point in stopping it until it has been shown to be ineffective in halting further tumor growth. Continuation also allows one to estimate the duration of partial response, which may be important in deciding the relative merits of competing treatments.

On the other hand, the continued administration of a drug combination that is causing no further evidence of antitumor effect beyond the initial shrinkage may be difficult to defend rigorously. Even if no alternative therapy is available, continuation of the initial regimen would be justifiable only in one of two hypothesized situations: (a) Clinical measurements are misleading and significant tumor cell killing is in progress. In some clinical contexts, such as the germ cell tumors, radiographs may give a misleading picture of the patient's response status, which can sometimes be established only by biopsy. (b) Drug-sensitive cells within the tumor mass, not yet completely eliminated by the therapy, continue to produce daughter cells that the continued therapy eliminates. Continuing treatment is a better way of controlling this sensitive subpopulation than stopping therapy and reintroducing it when evidence of progression occurs.

The question of whether continued treatment is more effective for partial responders than cessation of therapy and reintroduction of treatment upon progression has not often been studied. Such trials are readily designed; patients in stable partial response are randomized to either discontinue therapy and restart at the time of disease progression, or to continue therapy until disease progression. The endpoints would be survival, total time in remission, and quality of life. This question is the lesser priority, of course, than the development of more effective therapy that will increase the cure rate, but it certainly has relevance for the practical management of cancer patients for whom curative therapy is lacking.

ROLE OF THEORETICAL MODELS

As is apparent from the empirical nature of the previous discussion, we currently lack a comprehensive theory of combination chemotherapy. Such a theory would provide us with the solution to the fundamental problem at hand: what is the optimal strategy for combining the active agents for a particular cancer, given certain information about the therapeutic and toxicological characteristics of the drugs? In the absence of such a theory, though, the construction of theoretical models of the killing of tumor cells by cytotoxic drugs has been a productive method of generating testable therapeutic hypotheses.

Log-Kill Model

Originating from the observations of Skipper et al. (29) in mouse model systems, particularly the exponentially growing L1210 leukemia, the log-kill model postulated that the killing of tumor cells by drugs was a first-order process; that is, each dose of treatment resulted in the death of a fixed fraction (not a fixed number) of the remaining viable cells in the population. This assumption was the basis of much of the early support behind the concept that dose was a critical variable in the success of treatment. For if each treatment cycle results in the death of a fixed fraction of cells, and if the aim of therapy is to reduce the body burden of tumor to zero, it follows that the fractional reduction of tumor burden with each cycle should be maximized by increasing the intensity of therapy to the limits of tolerance.

Norton–Simon Model

The growth of most human tumors is more nearly approximated by a Gompertzian function than an exponential one, with the growth fraction decreasing as tumor size increases. Since the effectiveness of many chemotherapeutic agents is probably a function of a tumor's growth fraction, Norton and Simon reasoned that the cell kill achievable with a course of treatment might vary with changes in tumor size. More specifically, the intensity of treatment that suffices to cause regression of large tumors may not be sufficient to eradicate the remaining subclinical tumor in patients in clinical complete remission or in patients who are without evidence of gross disease following surgical extirpation of the primary tumor (30). This model led to the hypothesis that intensification of treatment after initial induction might lead to an increase in the effectiveness of chemotherapy. It is of interest that Mayer et al. (31) had drawn somewhat similar conclusions for acute leukemia on more empirical grounds some years before the Norton–Simon hypothesis had been developed. A recent review of the subsequent clinical studies that bear on the validity of the Norton–Simon hypothesis (32) has concluded that intensification may well have merit as a therapeutic strategy in some clinical circumstances. It also notes, correctly, that this conclusion does not establish rigorously the validity of the underlying kinetically based hypothesis, because the clinical trials that utilized intensification have often been designed such that other possible mechanisms of resistance are also circumvented.

Goldie–Coldman Model

Goldie and Coldman have adapted the somatic mutation theory to model the development of biochemical resistance to drugs as an acquired, heritable property of tumor cells (33). Assuming that mutations to drug resistance are random mutational events, the theory considers the impact of various therapeutic strategies on minimizing the probability that subpopulations of tumor cells resistant to multiple agents will evolve from a tumor that has no multiply resistant cells at the start. This formulation predicts that optimal therapy should consist of the maximal number of active drugs, given as early after diagnosis as possible, with the maximum dose intensities that are practical. This theory is consistent with a large volume of experimental data and with the results of some clinical trials (34). Trials designed specifically with the predictions of the somatic mutation theory in mind have been mounted too recently to permit definitive conclusions.

A well-constructed model, consistent with laboratory or clinical observations, is an important source of testable hypotheses, and it is in that light that the examples given above should be viewed. Although any given theoretical model may have its own committed partisans, the various models pertaining to chemotherapy should probably be viewed as potentially complementary rather than competitive. The Norton–Simon model addresses resistance that arises on a kinetic basis, while the orientation of Goldie–Coldman is genetic. Insofar as both formulations are consistent with much experimental and some clinical data, it seems likely that they both represent different aspects of a larger truth.

PRACTICAL ISSUES IN CLINICAL TRIALS METHODOLOGY

The development of many effective combinations over the past 25 years should not obscure the fact that this area is full of potential traps. We have already alluded to many dilemmas in the previous discussion and now turn to practical suggestions for dealing with some of them. Before we do, however, we should acknowledge explicitly that the development of effective combinations still remains one of the most intuitive areas in oncology. Combining drugs into effective regimens remains as much an art as a science, and there is rarely only one correct way to deal with any of the problems we discuss here. For simplicity we begin with the problems posed by combining two drugs.

Establishing a Maximum Tolerated Dose

You have decided to explore the combination of drugs A and B. Previous trials have established the maximum tolerated doses, the dose-limiting toxicities, and the response rates and durations for each drug. Where to begin?

In trying to anticipate the toxicities of drug combinations, one should pay attention to possible pharmacological interactions between the individual agents. If, for example, cisplatin produces renal functional impairment, the toxicity of bleomycin, which is excreted by the kidneys, may be greatly accentuated if the two drugs are given together. Although most toxicities of combinations can be anticipated, one should be prepared for surprises. In a recent clinical trial evaluating combinations of alkylating agents in high dose, the addition of melphalan to the combination of cisplatin, BCNU, and cyclophosphamide produced unacceptable degrees of nephrotoxicity, this despite the fact that melphalan alone is not notably toxic to the kidneys, nor was the three-drug combination to which it was added (12). Careful monitoring for interactions will be taken as a given in further discussion.

Now, assume first that the dose-limiting toxicities of the two agents are completely nonoverlapping. As noted previously, it is likely, though not certain, that the dose-limiting toxicities of AB will be the sum of the separate toxicities of A and B. It is likely, but again not certain, that you will be able to administer A and B each at its maximum tolerated dose in the combination. Because of the uncertainty about this, and the possible adverse impact on patient safety if you run into unanticipated interactions, it seems prudent to do what amounts to a Phase I evaluation of the two drugs in combination. One relatively efficient way to proceed is to fix the dose of one of the agents (say A) at or near its maximum tolerated dose, and combine with it B at 50–60% of the maximum tolerated dose of B. Three patients are treated with AB at this dose; if toxicity permits, the dose of B is successively escalated, with 3 patients per level, until the maximum tolerated dose of B in the context of the combination AB is reached. At that point, it is probably appropriate to treat about 6–8 patients, rather than 3, simply to be sure that the maximum tolerated dose of the combination is securely defined, before broader (perhaps multicenter) testing of AB is undertaken. A Phase I trial of this type should require no more than 15–20 patients.

Now assume that the toxicities of A and B are at least partially overlapping. The procedure is basically the same as just outlined but there are some important differences in detail. First, it is less obvious where to fix the dose of A initially. You strongly suspect before the trial starts that you are not going to be able to give full doses of both drugs together. Thus, the higher you set the initial dose of A, the less room you will have to escalate B before the overlapping toxicities produce the dose-limiting toxicity of the combination. Second, the presence of overlapping toxicities means that, at least in theory, you have to be very vigilant about significantly enhanced toxicity from A and B together to the target organ(s). Finally, one must take the time course of the appearance and resolution of toxicities into account in the design of the combination. For example, the known patterns of toxicity for cyclophosphamide and doxorubicin when used singly make it perfectly reasonable to expect that these agents could be given in combination once every 3 weeks. By contrast, in trying to combine methyl-CCNU and doxorubicin, the fact that methyl-CCNU expresses its dose-limiting myelosuppression 4–5 weeks following a dose seriously limits your ability to recycle doxorubicin in full dose once every three weeks.

For these reasons the initial dose of A, the entry dose of B, and the escalation scheme for B must be done a little more cautiously than in the case of nonoverlapping toxicities. Starting doses might well be a little more conservative and the escalation steps a bit narrower. In both cases, however, this procedure establishes the maximum tolerated dose for the combination without guesswork and reduces the need for dose adjustments after a combination is entered into Phases II or III. It is an efficient way of assessing the feasibility of AB with respect to toxicity. The advantages of establishing with reasonable rigor a maximum tolerated dose for the combination in this way, prior to Phase II or III testing, would seem to outweigh the modest inconvenience of a formal dose-finding phase.

Study of Efficacy

Having shown that A and B can be given together with tolerable and reproducible toxicity, and having defined a combination of the two that seems suitable for further study, what is the next step? The most obvious possibility, and logistically the easiest, is probably a Phase II study of AB in the disease of interest. Such a trial yields information about the response rate and response duration, as well as further information about toxicity. If AB produces wonderful results, unprecedented for the disease in question (e.g., MOPP in Hodgkin's disease in 1969), or conversely if the regimen produces few or no responses or intolerable toxicity (which should not happen, of course, if a careful Phase I trial has been done beforehand), then the results of such a Phase II evaluation may be truly informative.

Recall, however, that A and B have been combined because each is active. Such combinations may be expected to produce at least some responses. In practice, it is often very difficult to decide from an uncontrolled Phase II trial of relatively few patients whether the results are promising or not. The size of most pilot studies (20–30 patients) is too small to provide reasonably precise estimates of the true response rate. Despite the imprecision of such studies, many are performed and reported (7). Unfortunately, promising response rates in such studies are often found to be overestimates when measured against results in subsequent controlled trials. A previously cited review of the head and neck cancer literature (35) documented that the average response rate for experimental regimens was 45% in uncontrolled studies and only 29% in subsequent controlled trials of the same regimens. In half the randomized studies, methotrexate alone produced a higher response rate than the combination to which it was compared.

An alternative to the pilot Phase II study is to go directly to a Phase III comparison of AB with a pertinent control treatment; this may be A or B or some other drug or combination, depending on the specific circumstances. The sample size requirements for such a study may be quite large if relatively small differences are of interest and if the study is designed as a classical Phase III comparison. On the other hand, other statistical designs make this approach more attractive. Ellenberg and Eisenberger (35) have proposed a design in which a comparative trial is initiated, but the data are examined after a fixed number of patients have been entered. If the number of responses to experimental therapy B is the same or fewer than the number of responses to standard therapy A, then the trial is terminated and B is discarded. Otherwise, the trial proceeds to the second stage, and the remaining patients are entered according to the fixed sample size design. This procedure differs from other early stopping procedures in two important ways. First, it is concerned only with a difference in one direction: B is of interest only if it is better than A. Second, it allows early stopping if the two arms do not differ by more than a specified amount. This design results in a potential reduction in the required number of patients since it permits stopping the trial if the results determine that the new treatment is unlikely to be more than a certain specified amount better than the standard.

Another possibility is to perform a randomized Phase II study of AB and the control; the trial can be planned so that an analysis following the projected accrual results in either (a) termination of the study if the results are judged not promising; or (b) continuation of accrual and conversion of the study into a formal Phase III comparison with appropriate sample sizes if this appears justified by the results.

Either of these options is likely to be more productive than an uncontrolled Phase II evaluation in a limited number of patients. Although it might be argued that the Phase II trial provides valuable information about whether a subsequent comparative trial is really justified or not, such uncontrolled studies would seem to have a relatively high probability of giving either an inconclusive answer or the wrong answer, simply on grounds of small sample size. And if the sample size is increased to provide tighter confidence intervals around the estimates of response rate (or other parameters of interest), then the required number of patients may be little different from those necessary for the randomized designs just presented.

More Than Two Drugs

For a number of malignancies, many different active agents are available. As noted previously in our comments about breast cancer, the number of possible two-, three-, four-, and five-drug combinations that one can form from the six or seven active drugs is very large. For the hematological malignancies, the number of active drugs is much greater yet. Under such circumstances investigators have often elected to combine several agents at once; the resulting regimens may turn out, therefore, to be quite complex. The hypotheses guiding the construction of such combinations may have a kinetic or biochemical basis; they may represent attempts to apply theoretical models or strategies worked out in murine tumor systems; or they may simply be empirical attempts to use many active agents in as vigorous a manner as possible. The common denominator underlying most of them, however, is the conviction that a significant treatment advance is most likely with the application of more, rather than fewer, agents.

This approach is to be contrasted with the stepwise construction of combinations, in which agents are added, one at a time, and the effects of each addition are systematically assessed in comparative trials (e.g., AB vs. A, then ABC vs. AB, etc.). This stepwise approach has been used in several important disease-oriented settings relating to the development of combined modality therapy, notably in breast cancer (36), Wilms' tumor (37), and Ewing's sarcoma (38).

These two different approaches each have advantages and disadvantages. The formation of complex combinations in a nonstepwise manner has provided us with some of the most successful examples of therapy for disseminated cancer: MOPP for Hodgkin's disease (4), similar regimens for the non-Hodgkin's lymphomas (17) and germ cell tumors (5), and any number of multidrug combinations for acute leukemia. When such regimens result in striking improvements in complete remission rates and survival, they provide support for the underlying hypothesis and tend to vindicate use of the general approach in other diseases as well.

On the other hand, the common use of the nonstepwise approach has certain implications that we should acknowledge. The most obvious is that it does not yield information about the contribution of a specific agent to the overall effect, both therapeutic and toxic, of a regimen. Now why should we care about this at all? Concern with this issue strikes some as scholastic nitpicking. If combination ABC is effective, why should we care about the individual contributions of A, B, and C? The chief reason is that, from a purely medical point of view, if drug C is irrelevant to the therapeutic effect of ABC (i.e., if AB is just as effective as ABC), it makes little sense to use ABC. The continued use of C in this context serves only to increase the toxicity of the regimen and perhaps also its financial cost. The presence of an ineffective drug in the regimen also tends to limit further innovation with that regimen, simply because the ineffective agent continues to express its toxic effects on normal tissues and this, in turn, limits further additions to the regimen or further attempts to increase treatment intensity.

Obviously, if De Vita and his collaborators (5) had chosen to build MOPP up in sequential steps of two-, three-, and four-drug regimens, they could in the process have defined the roles of the constituent agents. At the time, however, they were much more interested in testing the hypothesis that combinations of active agents, each given at or near the full single-agent dose, would be curative. A stepwise approach would have taken much longer to get to the same point, though admittedly it would have yielded information along the way that was not obtainable from the testing of the four-drug combination as a unit.

A major problem with investigating the role of individual components after the effectiveness of the combination has been established is that once a drug combination has been shown to be effective therapy, clinicians are reluctant to tamper with it. They become nervous at the prospect that deleting components of the full regimen may compromise its effectiveness. In addition, such trials, to be done properly, require large numbers of patients. In a recent trial, 214 patients were studied to demonstrate that vinblastine 0.3 mg/kg/cycle was as effective as 0.4 in nonseminomatous testicular cancer (39). These large numbers are required because one has to insure that small but medically significant differences *will* be detected. If inadequate accrual results in failure to identify such small differences as really significant, then it is conceivable that "nonsignificant" small differences in sequential trials might cumulate and eventually a worse therapy could become standard. Shuster (40) has likened this phenomenon to the following parable:

> When a King reached his thirtieth birthday, he commanded his son, then 6 years old, to report to him every day whether or not the King's appearance had changed from the previous day. Every day for 15 years, the son examined his father carefully and reported that there was no change. The King at 45 believed he had the identical

appearance that he had had at 30. At 21, the King's son married and left the palace. The King approached his second son to take on the daily inspection. The second son said, "It will be my honor, old father."

A further implication of not knowing the contribution of the individual components is that the interpretation of certain kinds of subsequent trials with the same combination may be very difficult. This is particularly true of studies in which other agents are substituted for components of the original combination [see Chapter 6, example 5 (ABC vs. AXC)]. For example, some investigators have attempted to modify MOPP by substituting other drugs (nitrosoureas, vinblastine) for the components of MOPP, in the hope of producing a less toxic combination with at least equal effectiveness. As we have discussed in Chapter 6, such an approach may yield ambiguous information. If the role of X in the combination ABX is undefined, then the finding that ABY is just as good as ABX but less toxic may mean either that Y should be substituted for X or that they are both irrelevant to the activity of their respective combinations. Of course, if ABY is better than ABX, then something of positive value has been learned.

Another quite practical consequence of a nonstepwise approach results from the current requirements of the Food and Drug Administration (FDA) concerning the licensing of investigational agents for commercial distribution. In brief, the FDA requires that new agents be shown to be safe and effective before it will authorize marketing of the agent by pharmaceutical companies. Such a demonstration is best accomplished by controlled trials involving either direct comparison to a valid control (A vs. X) or stepwise addition to control and comparison with it (AX vs. A). When such data are lacking, the FDA is loathe to approve new drugs unless the available clinical data overwhelmingly suggest efficacy. The absence of such studies keeps potentially useful agents in investigational status for a long time, making them relatively difficult for physicians to obtain. Over the past decade drug sponsors have had this experience with a number of investigational agents or formulations whose efficacy is widely credited in the oncology community; these currently include high-dose methotrexate, teniposide, and ifosfamide.

The lesson, therefore, is that both approaches are needed. They are complementary rather than competitive, with each offering information that the other does not. When the number of active agents is very limited, stepwise development is much easier to implement (e.g., gastrointestinal cancers, hypernephroma, melanoma). Conversely, where there are several active agents (hematological malignancies) this approach may be difficult or impossible to implement productively. The choice between these approaches in particular clinical settings will depend on the availability of compelling hypotheses, the number of available agents, and the state of existing therapy for the disease in question.

Importance of Hypothesis Verification

Clinical trials based on biological hypotheses are of particular interest since the results of such trials, if they are properly designed and conducted, may tell us something of fundamental importance in addition to whether a treatment works or not. As we become more knowledgable about the biology of neoplastic disease, we can expect that clinical trials will relate increasingly to mechanistic hypotheses of one kind or another. In this context, it will become increasingly important to attempt to verify the validity of the underlying hypotheses in parallel with the clinical trial itself.

Consider again the case of sequenced methotrexate and 5-fluorouracil discussed earlier in this chapter. This hypothesis and the associated preclinical findings generated much interest among oncologists, who then mounted many studies in various tumor types. The great majority of these trials, however, were small pilot studies without controls; it thus proved very difficult to say with any assurance whether any particular methotrexate–fluorouracil sequence was more effective than the simultaneous use of the two agents (or, for that matter, better than either agent used singly). In addition, it has proved very difficult to verify in the clinic the significance of the underlying biochemical hypothesis; such verification requires biochemical studies in parallel with a suitable clinical trial with the aim of measuring intracellular PRPP levels and extent of 5-fluorouracil activation, and comparison of these results with what would have been achieved with 5-fluorouracil alone. Such studies are by no means simple; if they were, they would have been done with considerable dispatch.

Now a skeptic might argue that this is all quite unnecessary; after all, what you really care about is developing a better therapy, and even if a particular hypothesis is not consistent with the clinical data, all that really matters is that the new treatment be shown clinically to be an advance. The truth, however, is that if one has both the data on clinical efficacy and the laboratory correlates, then one has a much firmer basis for further investigation. If the clinical effect is positive and parallel laboratory studies are able to establish that the postulated interaction is indeed present, then this argues for the clinical relevance of the hypothesis and may suggest further productive avenues of research. On the other hand, if the new treatment is shown to be effective but one can find no evidence for the postulated interaction, or the interaction is seen, but no enhanced clinical benefit occurs, then the particular hypothesis is probably irrelevant. Finally, if neither clinical enhancement nor the laboratory correlate is noted, then the hypothesis has not been tested adequately and a revised clinical experiment should be implemented, perhaps by alternating the dose and schedule of the agents in question.

The moral is simple: whenever possible, clinical trials based on mechanistic hypotheses should, in addition to providing firm clinical data, attempt correlative studies that test the validity of the hypothesis. Small pilot studies to demonstrate that the biochemical effects occur can precede larger clinical studies and this may be the most efficient design. We do not mean to imply that rigorous laboratory correlation is always possible; sometimes the technology to collect the specimens or to perform the required assays is not available. We also acknowledge that, even when such studies are possible, they are almost never simple. Nevertheless, for the reasons outlined above, the rewards from such an approach would seem well worth the effort.

Dose Ratios

We alluded earlier to the potential importance of dose ratios in determining the efficacy of a regimen. This question is logistically very difficult to study in the clinic. The standard clinical trials approach would be a large comparative trial comparing the dose ratios of interest. For adequate statistical power such trials would have to accrue hundreds of patients. A potential alternative that would not require such large sample sizes is afforded by the technique of response surface methodology (41). In this procedure one varies independently the doses of the two agents, thereby forming a two-dimensional grid of dose combinations (Fig. 8.1). Clinical responses occurring at each point on the grid are noted; the totality of response rates occurring over the entire grid forms a mathematical surface whose maxima and minima can be modeled over the particular dose combinations of the two agents. We are then interested in locating the maximum of the response surface, which constitutes the solution to the problem. The technique is in principle generalizable to any number of drugs and also to defining optimal treatment intervals within a regimen. Although in use for many years in industrial settings, application of response surface methodology to clinical trials is still very new; currently the Mid-Atlantic Oncology Program is conducting the first clinical trial utilizing this methodology to define an optimal CMF-type regimen in metastatic breast cancer. It is not yet clear whether some of the practical problems connected with this approach will permit its widespread use, but the technique would seem at this point to have impressive potential to contribute to the optimization of combination therapy design.

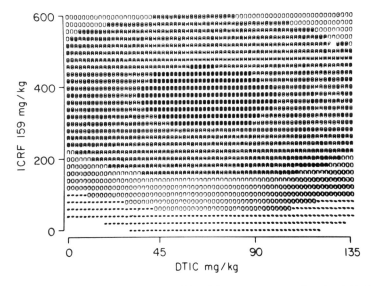

FIG. 8.1. Response surface methodology. Plot of dose–response surface in which the darker shadings indicate regions of improved treatment, i.e., longer survival. (Reprinted from Ref. 41).

REFERENCES

1. Goodman, L. S., Wintrobe, M. M., Dameshek, W., et al. (1946): Nitrogen mustard therapy: Use of methyl bis (B-chlorethyl) amino hydrochloride for Hodgkin's disease, lymphosarcoma, leukemia, and certain allied and miscellaneous disorders. *J.A.M.A.*, 32:126–132.
2. Li, M. C., Hertz, R., and Spencer, D. B. (1956): Effect of methotrexate upon choriocarcinoma and chorioadenoma. *Proc. Soc. Exp. Biol. Med.*, 93:361–366.
3. Farber, S., Diamond, L. K., Mercer, R. D., et al. (1948): Temporary remissions in acute leukemia in children produced by folic antagonist 4-amethopteroylglutamic acid (aminopterin). *N. Engl. J. Med.*, 238:787–793.
4. Frei, E., and Freireich, E. J. (1965): Progress and perspectives in the chemotherapy of acute leukemia. *Adv. Chemother.*, 2:269–298.
5. DeVita, V., Serpick, A., and Carbone, P. P. (1970): Combination chemotherapy in the treatment of advanced Hodgkin's disease. *Ann. Intern. Med.*, 73:881–895.
6. Einhorn, L. H. (1981): Testicular cancer as a model for a curable neoplasm: The Richard and Hilda Rosenthal Foundation Award lecture. *Cancer Res.*, 41:3275–3280.
7. Wittes, R. E., and Goldin, A. (1986): Unresolved issues in combination chemotherapy. *Cancer Treat. Rep.*, 70:105–125.
8. Leyland-Jones, B., and O'Dwyer, P. J. (1986): Biochemical modulation. Application of laboratory models to the clinic. *Cancer Treat. Rep.*, 70:219–230.
9. Martin, D. S., Stolfi, R. L., Sawyer, R. C., and Young, C. W. (1985): Application of biochemical modulation with a therapeutically inactive modulating agent in clinical trials of cancer chemotherapy. *Cancer Treat. Rep.*, 69:421–423.
10. Osieka, R. (1984): Primary and acquired resistance to antineoplastic chemotherapy. A preclinical and clinical study. *Cancer*, 54:1168–1174.
11. Alt, F. W., Kellems, R. E., Bertino, J. R., and Schimke, R. T. (1978): Selective multiplication of dihydrofolate reductase genes in methotrexate-resistant variants of cultured murine cells. *J. Biol. Chem.*, 253:1357–1370.
12. Peters, W. P., Eder, J. P., Henner, W. D., et al. (1986): High-dose combination alkylating agents with autologous bone marrow support: A Phase I trial. *J. Clin. Oncol.*, 4:646–654.
13. Ling, V., Kartner, N., Sudo, T., et al. (1983): Multidrug-resistance phenotype in Chinese hamster ovary cells. *Cancer Treat. Rep.*, 67:869–874.
14. Hitchock-Bryan, S., Gelber, R., Cassady, J. R., and Sallan, S. E. (1986): The impact of induction anthracycline on long-term failure-free survival in childhood acute lymphoblastic leukemia. *Med. Pediatr. Oncol.*, 14:211–215.
15. Scheaf, W., Oklein, H., and Brock, N. (1980): Controlled studies with an antidote against the urotoxicity of oxazophorines. *Cancer Treat. Rep.*, 63:501–505.
16. Howell, S. B., Pfeifle, C. E., Wung, W. E., and Olshen, R. A. (1983): Intraperitoneal cisdiammine dichloroplatinum with systemic thiosulphate protection. *Cancer Res.*, 43:1426–1431.
17. Young, R. C., Knapp, R. C., Fuks, Z., and Disaia, P. J. (1985): Cancer of the ovary. In: *Cancer: Principles and Practice of Oncology*, edited by V. T. DeVita, Jr., S. Hellman, and S. A. Rosenberg, pp. 1083–1118, 2nd ed. Lippincott, Philadelphia.
18. Sullivan, M. P., Boyett, J., Pullen, J., et al. (1985): Pediatric Oncology Group experience with modified LSA$_2$-L$_2$ therapy in 107 children with non-Hodgkin's lymphoma (Burkitt's lymphoma excluded). *Cancer*, 55:323–336.
19. Klimo, P., and Connors, J. M. (1985): MACOP-B chemotherapy for the treatment of diffuse large-cell lymphoma. *Ann. Intern. Med.*, 102:596–602.
20. Pinkel, D., Hernandez, K., Borella, L., et al. (1971): Drug dosage and remission duration in childhood lymphatic leukemia. *Cancer*, 27:247–256.
21. Longo, D. L., Young, R. C., Wesley, M., et al. (1986): Twenty years of MOPP therapy for Hodgkin's disease. *J. Clin. Oncol.*, 4:1295–1306.
22. Hryniuk, W., and Bush, H. (1984): The importance of dose intensity in chemotherapy of metastatic breast cancer. *J. Clin. Oncol.*, 2:1281–1288.
23. Hryniuk, W. M., Levine, M. N., and Levin, L. (1986): Analysis of dose intensity for chemotherapy in early (stage II) and advanced breast cancer. *Natl. Cancer Inst. Monogr.*, 1:87–94.
24. Hayes, F. A., Green, A. A., and Mauer, A. A. (1977): Correlation of cell kinetic and clinical response to chemotherapy in disseminated neuroblastoma. *Cancer Res.*, 37:3766–3770.

25. Cadman, E., Davis, L., and Heimer, R. (1979): Enhanced 5-fluorouracil nucleotide formation following methotrexate: Biochemical explanation for drug synergism. *Science*, 205:1135–1137.
26. Leventhal, B. G., Levine, A. S., Graw, R. G., Jr., et al. (1975): Long-term second remissions in acute lymphatic leukemia. *Cancer*, 35:1136–1140.
27. Vugrin, D., Whitmore, W. F., and Golbey, R. B. (1983): VAB-6 combination chemotherapy without maintenance in treatment of disseminated cancer of the testis. *Cancer*, 51:211–215.
28. Bonadonna, G., Valagussa, P., Rossi, A., et al. (1985): Ten year experience with CMF based adjuvant chemotherapy in resectable breast cancer. *Breast Cancer Res. Treat.*, 5:95–115.
29. Skipper, H. E., Schabel, F. M., Jr., and Wilcox, W. S. (1964): Experimental evaluation of potential anticancer agents. XIII. On the criteria and kinetics associated with "curability" of experimental leukemia. *Cancer Chemother. Rep.*, 35:1–111.
30. Norton, L., and Simon, R. (1977): Tumor size, sensitivity to therapy, and design of treatment schedules. *Cancer Treat. Rep.*, 61:1307–1317.
31. Mayer, R. J., Weinstein, H. J., Coral, F. S., et al. (1982): The role of intensive postinduction chemotherapy in the management of acute myelogenous leukemia. *Cancer Treat. Rep.*, 66:1455–1462.
32. Norton, L., and Simon, R. (1986): The Norton–Simon hypothesis revisited. *Cancer Treat. Rep.*, 70:163–169.
33. Coldman, A. J., and Goldie, J. H. (1985): Role of mathematical modeling in protocol formulation in cancer chemotherapy. *Cancer Treat. Rep.*, 69:1041–1046.
34. Santoro, A., Bonadonna, G., Bonfante, V., and Valagussa, P. (1982): Alternating drug combinations in the treatment of advanced Hodgkin's disease. *N. Engl. J. Med.*, 306:770–775.
35. Ellenberg, S. S., and Eisenberger, M. A. (1985): An efficient design for Phase III studies of combination chemotherapies. *Cancer Treat. Rep.*, 69:1147–1152.
36. Fisher, B., Redmond, C., Fisher, E. R., and Wolmark, N. (1986): Systematic adjuvant therapy in treatment of primary operable breast cancer: National Surgical Adjuvant Breast and Bowel Project experience. *Natl. Cancer Inst. Monogr.*, 1:35–43.
37. D'Angio, G. J., Evans, A. E., Breslow, N., et al. (1976): The treatment of Wilms' tumor: Results of the National Wilms' Tumor Study. *Cancer*, 38:633–646.
38. Nesbit, M. E., Jr., Perez, C. A., Tefft, M., et al. (1981): Multimodal therapy for the management of primary, nonmetastatic Ewing's sarcoma of bone: An Intergroup study. *Natl. Cancer Inst. Monogr.*, 56:255–262.
39. Stoter, G., Sleyfer, D. T., tenBokkel Huinink, W. W., et al. (1986): High-dose vs. low-dose vinblastine in cisplatin–vinblastine–bleomycin combination chemotherapy of non-seminomatous testicular cancer: A randomized study of the EORTC genitourinary tract cancer cooperative group. *J. Clin. Oncol.*, 4:1199–1206.
40. Shuster, J. J., Krischer, J. P., and Boyett, J. M. (1985): Ethical issues in cooperative cancer therapy trials from a statistical viewpoint. II. Specific issues. *Am. J. Pediatr. Hematol. Oncol.*, 7:64–70.
41. Carter, W. H., Jr. (1985): Response surface methodology and the design of clinical trials for the evaluation of cancer chemotherapy. *Cancer Treat. Rep.*, 69:1049–1052.

CHAPTER 9

Combined Modality Therapy

The idea that two or more modalities employed together might be more effective therapy than a single modality follows naturally from observations in the clinic and the laboratory. At most primary sites, surgery cures a high proportion of patients with low-stage disease. Even for localized disease, however, the effectiveness of surgery is limited by technical considerations; vital normal structures must be left in place, and sophisticated techniques of reconstruction are all too often incapable of ameliorating the devastating cosmetic effects of radical resection. More fundamentally, however, the surgeon cannot resect what he cannot see, and the tendency of many cancers to spread microscopically beyond the bounds of feasible resection poses an insuperable challenge to even the most skilled operator.

Like surgery, radiotherapy can cure an appreciable fraction of patients with relatively low-stage cancer. Unlike surgery, however, radiotherapy can, in an anatomically conservative fashion, rather effectively sterilize large areas affected with microscopic spread of tumor. On the other hand, large tumor masses that can be resected by a skilled surgeon often respond only incompletely to even full courses of radiation.

For many years, the complementary effects of the two local modalities has suggested to investigators that their use in combination might be more fruitful than the use of either one singly. The development of high-energy radiation sources made the delivery of tumoricidal doses of radiation with tolerable toxicity more practical and stimulated interest in exploring combinations of surgery and radiotherapy. A very large number of reports in the clinical literature testifies to the long-standing interest in such approaches for many solid tumors.

In principle, surgery and radiotherapy can control cancer only in the local areas where they have been applied. For this reason, most attempts to combine them have been for the treatment of cancers where local control looms as a significant clinical problem, such as locally advanced carcinomas of the head and neck, rectum, bladder, breast, and brain. Some studies have also shown the value of radiation at the time of primary diagnosis to sites of common micrometastatic deposits of tumor such as the lung in Ewing's sarcoma (1) or the brain in small cell lung cancer (2).

Systemic chemotherapy has the immense theoretical advantage of controlling disease anywhere in the body. Unhappily, however, the treatment of many disseminated cancers with existing cytotoxic agents has proved to be less than uniformly effective. With the exception of a number of relatively uncommon tumors, complete responses are unusual and long-term control or cure rates are low.

The earliest notions about surgical adjuvant chemotherapy were based on the assumption that chemotherapy might be used to destroy malignant cells released into the circulation at the time of surgical ablation of the primary tumor (3). We know now that a large percentage of patients already have metastatic disease at the time of detection of the primary tumor. Laboratory models employing a wide spectrum of histological tumor types transplanted into a number of different strains of mice, showed generally that the use of chemotherapy and surgery in concert produced more cures than either modality used singly (4). Experiments of this kind provided strong motivation to clinicians to integrate chemotherapy into combined modality approaches for the treatment of human cancer.

Several success stories in the clinic show the impact of combined modality therapy on the eventual cure of cancer patients. Perhaps the best example is afforded by Wilms' tumor of the kidney. The survival rate was only 15% from 1914 to 1930, when surgical techniques were imperfect. It climbed to 33% from 1931 to 1939 when operative methods improved and to 47% from 1940 to 1947 when post-operative radiation was added to treatment (5,6). Then, in 1967, Cancer and Leukemia Group B (7) reported a 2-year survival rate of 89% for patients given actinomycin D in the postoperative period, as opposed to 50% for those not given chemotherapy. Subsequently, the National Wilms' Tumor Study Group (NWTS) was organized and a systematic refinement of multimodality therapy for this disease has continued.

Several factors have contributed to this enviable success story. In the first place, the majority of patients present with surgically resectable gross disease; 64% of patients in the NWTS 2 study had all detectable tumor removed at the time of initial surgery. In the second place, this tumor is sensitive to the effects of both radiation and chemotherapy, so that it is possible to devise effective treatment regimens for residual disease. In fact, current studies in the resectable forms of this disease are aimed at reducing therapy until the minimal curative regimen is defined. Thus, refinements in the use of each modality have resulted in consistent, significant improvement in therapy over a 40–50-year period. The Wilms' model is a particularly gratifying one. The integration of chemotherapy into combined modality approaches to treatment has also produced medically significant improvements in the therapy of a number of other cancers such as rhabdomyosarcoma, Ewing's sarcoma, osteosarcoma, breast cancer, and carcinomas of the colon, rectum, and anus. Admittedly, the more common and resistant epithelial tumors of adulthood are still very far from the excellent survivals achieved in several of the pediatric tumors.

DEFINITIONS

The term *combined modality therapy* (CMT) refers to the integration of two or more cancerocidal modalities into a planned treatment course. We emphasize that there is nothing haphazard about this integration; its details must be planned with minute care. The patient who has failed surgery and is then treated with radiotherapy as salvage on a ''let's hope for the best'' basis has not received CMT as the term is generally understood today.

Because surgery was the first effective means of treating cancer, many clinicians (particularly surgeons!) have viewed it as the fundamental therapeutic maneuver to which the more recently developed ones have been added in a helping, or adjuvant, capacity. Thus, one commonly refers to the use of adjuvant radiotherapy after the surgical resection of a rectal cancer, or to adjuvant chemotherapy after resection of a Stage II breast cancer. It should be clear, however, that because of the complementary effects of the different therapeutic modalities, the labeling of one modality as adjuvant to another is somewhat arbitrary. The term is, however, firmly established in current usage. We shall, therefore, refer to a modality as *adjuvant* in a particular context if it is the one that is added to the treatment with the more established cure rate. In this sense, surgery is an adjuvant to chemotherapy when resection follows chemotherapeutic induction of remission in limited-disease small cell lung cancer or in testicular cancer with bulky retroperitoneal disease. Radiotherapy may be adjuvant to chemotherapy in the setting of advanced-stage Hodgkin's disease. The term ''neoadjuvant,'' used by some to designate chemotherapy given prior to surgery, will not be used here.

The use of therapy to treat micrometastatic disease in certain sanctuary sites, such as intrathecal chemotherapy or radiation to the central nervous system in acute leukemia and other disease, has commonly been referred to as ''prophylaxis.'' This is something of a misnomer, since one is really treating disease that is already present but not yet clinically apparent. Although a more accurate designation would be ''treatment of micrometastic disease,'' the term ''prophylaxis'' is probably with us for good.

GOALS AND ENDPOINTS

The principal goal of CMT is to increase the effectiveness of treatment over what can be obtained from single-modality therapy. The primary endpoint of interest is survival. The most compelling evidence of the effectiveness of CMT (or of any therapy for fatal disease) is a significant shift to the right of the survival curve and an increase in the tail of the survival curve (cure rate). As noted already in Chapter 3, in studies that utilize survival as a major endpoint, it is often relevant to distinguish between total mortality (death from all causes) and cancer-related mortality (death from cancer and its treatment). In populations that have very high rates of competing causes of death, an effect on total mortality may be very difficult to demonstrate. Women diagnosed with node-negative breast cancer in the 65–69-year age group will have one non-cancer-related death for every breast cancer death. Thus, any trial will require very large numbers of patients for adequate statistical power (8). Patients with lung or head and neck cancers tend to be older males with a rather high prevalence of alcohol and/or tobacco abuse; thus, the rates of death from ischemic heart disease, chronic lung and liver disease, and second primary cancers are appreciable and may obscure all but the largest differences in cancer treatment trials.

It seems to us that a close look at survival calculated in both ways is the most reasonable course. The analysis by all causes of death will be most useful for indicating whether the therapy should be given very broadly across the population at large, outside the clinical trials setting. The cancer-related survival curves may also be useful for this purpose, though perhaps their greater utility is to indicate whether the CMT is having an effect on the natural history of the malignancy in a favorable direction. This analysis may then point to productive directions for future trials.

Disease- or recurrence-free survival is often used as a surrogate measure of survival (see Chapter 2). One important way of looking at disease-free survival is in terms of control rates at the primary site. This is a particularly important endpoint in trials of combined local therapy, since it may not be reasonable to expect any kind of local therapy, no matter how effective, to improve survival if the major factor determining survival is the occurrence of distant metastases. The most one can reasonably expect from optimal local therapy is uniformly good control (i.e., continuous complete remission) at the primary site. This line of reasoning seems valid if the distant metastases that ultimately kill the patient have occurred before the start of local therapy. If not, of course, the way the primary is treated might well have an effect on the rate of formation of metastases and subsequent survival.

It follows, therefore, that CMT might well induce an apparent improvement in local control without an impact on overall survival. Results like this have been seen in a number of trials. A study by the European Organization for Research on Treatment of Cancer (EORTC) of preoperative radiation therapy in resectable rectal carcinoma, yielded a 5-year survival of 65% in both groups, while the 5-year local recurrence-free survival was 85% in the combined treatment group versus 65% in the group treated with surgery alone (9). Such data clearly emphasize the need for better systemic therapy. They also point out the importance of assessing quality of life, which may be heavily influenced by patterns of relapse in patients with rectal carcinoma (see Chapter 3). For the most part, quality of life endpoints have not been central to the design of most CMT trials; they are, however, important in an overall assessment of the value of any treatment innovation.

The balance of toxicities of alternative modes of treatment becomes particularly important in clinical settings where an appreciable fraction of patients are long survivors. In such situations the surfacing of medically important chronic toxicities can have a significant impact on the overall judgment about whether a therapy is worth generalizing to the population at large. This is particularly so if the beneficial effect of treatment upon survival is only modest. In the setting of adjuvant chemotherapy, the importance of serious adverse toxicities is of especial concern because the techniques for patient selection onto these trials cannot generally insure that all patients entering on treatment actually have the residual disease that they are presumed to have. We shall return to this point later on.

HYPOTHESES AND THE DESIGN OF REGIMENS

The design of CMT regimens shares certain formal similarities with the construction of drug combinations (see Chapter 8): (a) Generally, the inclusion of a given modality in CMT for a given tumor makes sense only if the modality has demonstrable activity when used singly against that tumor. If, for example, there is no known chemotherapy that will affect the growth of measurable disease on a particular cancer type, it does not make sense to devise an adjuvant trial of chemotherapy for that cancer.

(b) The non-cross-resistant properties of CMT is one of its most agreeable features. The resectability of bulk disease bears no direct relationship to the tumor's resistance to drugs or radiation. The relationship between resistance to radiation and to drugs is considerably more complicated. Generally, the two have appeared to be roughly correlated: tumor types that exhibit significant resistance (or sensitivity) to radiation tend also to be relatively refractory (or sensitive) to chemotherapy. Recent studies have also suggested that certain mechanisms of induction of resistance to radiation, such as hypoxia (10), may also induce resistance to drugs. Despite these limitations, however, combining modalities presents another avenue of attacking a tumor that cannot be extinguished by any one modality alone.

(c) The combination of modalities at their full single-modality treatment levels may be limited by overlapping toxicity. Obviously, the effects of surgery on the host differ qualitatively from that of chemotherapy and radiotherapy, but the relationship is there nonetheless: the side effects of each modality place limits on the overall design of CMT regimens, and to the extent that treatment intensity must be reduced, the contribution of the attenuated modality to the overall antitumor effect will decrease in parallel.

Following is a discussion of the ways in which the three modalities can be combined.

Surgery and Radiation

As noted previously, the use of the local modalities in combination exploits their complementary abilities to eliminate bulk and microscopic disease within the treatment volume. Which modality should be given first is still a matter of some controversy. The use of preoperative radiotherapy was originally motivated by the supposition that at least partial sterilization of the tumor prior to resection would prevent dissemination of tumor cells at the time of surgical manipulation and, by reducing the tumor's size and its adherence to surrounding structures, would aid in the resection itself. However, neither radiation nor chemotherapy would be given, except in most unusual circumstances, without an initial biopsy that yields a tissue diagnosis of cancer. In this sense, then, almost no radiotherapy is preoperative.

Radiotherapy prior to definitive surgery may still be favored sometimes. One such situation is in the patient with bilateral retinoblastoma. This diagnosis is often made on direct examination without biopsy. Radiotherapy is frequently administered as initial therapy in an attempt to save at least partial vision in one or both eyes and enucleation is performed only if disease progresses to the point where it appears that useful vision cannot be retained. It should be emphasized that this is a highly radiosensitive tumor, and that even when it progresses, disease usually remains confined to the globe for a long time.

The maximum tolerated dose of preoperative radiation is limited not only by the usual limits of normal tissue tolerance but also by the obvious requirement for good wound healing within the treatment volume; without this, the surgical complication rate may well exceed acceptable limits. This is not so much of a problem with the reverse sequence, since postoperative radiotherapy is generally not started for 1–2 weeks until wound healing has already begun. It should also be obvious that the postoperative use of radiotherapy does not interfere with full surgical or pathologic staging of the primary tumor and its regional nodes. In addition, with postoperative therapy the prior removal of relatively resistant bulk tumor mass leaves only sub-clinical disease for the radiation to deal with.

Local Therapy Followed by Chemotherapy

This is the treatment sequence that has been most completely studied in laboratory models of CMT, and it has been explored clinically in numerous trials in many tumor types, including breast, large bowel, lung, melanoma, and the soft-tissue sarcomas. In theory it has the advantage that the body burden of tumor is minimal at the time of exposure to drugs, because all bulk disease, which may serve as a nidus for the generation of resistant cell populations, has been removed. On the other hand, this sequence often imposes a very considerable delay between diagnosis and the institution of the chemotherapy (11). In most trials, this time interval is at least a few weeks; in the case of some tumors, where the local treatment itself is complex or multistaged (as in head and neck cancer), it can be for several months. Since such delays may be deleterious to outcome, the sooner the treatment can be started the better. The crucial role of timing in the effectiveness of CMT has been consistently emphasized by the animal models of adjuvant chemotherapy (11).

Chemotherapy Followed by Local Therapy

The use of chemotherapy immediately upon diagnosis has been explored inten-sively in several tumor types. One of the early rationales for this approach was quite similar to that of preoperative radiation: tumor shrinkage induced by chemo-therapy might make local control easier to achieve with subsequent surgery or radiation. Accordingly, initial chemotherapy has received much attention in tumor types for which local control is a significant problem (head and neck, esophagus) or for which other issues in local treatment are of central importance (limb salvage in osteosarcoma). In beginning chemotherapy shortly after diagnosis, this sequence also introduces systemic treatment of disseminated disease at the earliest possible time; this feature explains its appeal for tumors where the development of distant metastases limits survival (breast, osteosarcoma). It also offers a means of possibly scaling down the scope of radical surgery; if the addition of initial chemotherapy increases local control rates and/or survival compared with local therapy alone, one might inquire whether radical or disfiguring surgery could be replaced by operations that are anatomically more conservative. One should not, of course, assume that this can be done unless data from a formal clinical trial have confimed that no loss in efficacy results. Another theoretical advantage is that the response to initial chemotherapy can be assessed in the surgical specimen and therapy changed in the postoperative period if the patient does not appear to be responding. This approach has yielded promising results in osteosarcoma (12), although the hypothesis has not been tested in a controlled fashion.

On the other hand, this approach has at least three potential liabilities. The use of chemotherapy as first treatment, when tumor bulk is maximal, may serve to select out resistant subpopulations from the primary tumor. This liability is only theoretical at present, but it cannot be discounted entirely; formal comparison of preoperative and postoperative chemotherapy scheduling are unavailable for any tumor type, although such a study is currently underway in the Pediatric Oncology Group in osteosarcoma. Second, the delay of surgery or radiotherapy while several cycles of chemotherapy are being administered might prejudice outcome if non-response to chemotherapy permits the progression of local disease to a state of unresectability. Although this is a significant theoretical risk, it seems not to have occurred with any frequency in the trials reported to date, probably because the whole approach is generally only utilized when very active chemotherapy regimens are available. Finally, in the opposite situation, if chemotherapy results in striking regression of tumor, either physicians or patients may feel encouraged to refuse surgery, in the hope that chemotherapy has "gotten it all." In one uncontrolled study where amputation was not performed after excellent local responses to intra-arterial cisplatin in osteosarcoma, there was a disappointingly high rate of local recurrence (3 of 3 patients) (13). Patient refusal of planned surgery has, in fact, occurred in at least one institution's experience with this approach (14).

Simultaneous Radiation and Chemotherapy

The use of drugs and radiation simultaneously has potentially attractive features. Since many anticancer agents act as radiosensitizers, the simultaneous delivery of drugs and radiation may increase the killing effect of radiotherapy within the treatment volume. In addition, to the extent that full therapeutic doses of cytotoxic agents are used early in the treatment plan, the regimen will also provide systemic treatment of disease outside areas of locoregional spread. Unfortunately, the radio-sensitization properties of most anticancer agents are not very selective for tumor, and many trials have documented significant enhancement of radiation toxicity to normal tissues within the treatment volume without a real increase in useful therapeutic effect.

Alternating Chemotherapy and Radiotherapy

In a series of studies in an animal model, Looney and Hopkins (15) have shown that radiation and chemotherapy are best integrated by alternating them in sequence. Animals that are not cured either with full-course radiation or chemotherapy, or with the combination of full-course radiation followed by chemotherapy, may be cured if the radiotherapy is broken up into segments between which the chemotherapy is interposed. The mechanism for the dependence of effect on sequencing of modalities is not completely clear, but may relate to the enhanced dose intensity of each of the two modalities when given in alternating fashion. This kind of sequencing has been utilized in the clinic with reasonable results (summarized in Ref. 15), though the uncontrolled studies done so far have not established that this approach is superior to more conventional sequencing.

Combined Modality Therapy for Pharmacologic Sanctuaries

Combined modality therapy may be the best way to approach tumor that has metastasized to "privileged sites." The realization that the central nervous system served as a pharmacologic sanctuary for leukemia cells, led to direct treatment of the central nervous system with radiation, an approach that represented a major advance on the road to cure for acute lymphatic leukemia (16).

The series of clinical dose-finding experiments that were performed before an active regimen was discovered took about 5 years and involved two negative trials at 500 and 1200 cGy before the effective dose of 2400 cGy was identified (see Fig. 9.1). This series of experiments is thought provoking for anyone interested in

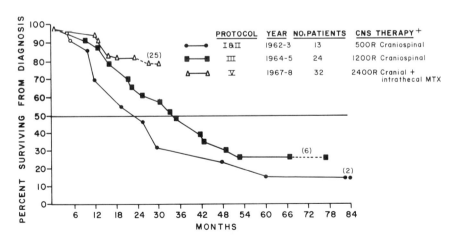

FIG. 9.1. Therapy of childhood leukemia. Summary of a series of experiments used in finding the proper dose for cranial radiation for treatment of clinically inapparent disease in acute leukemia. (Redrawn from Ref. 16.)

clinical research, since it shows how careful investigation of dose and schedule may turn a negative experiment into a major breakthrough if the underlying hypothesis is correct.

Since cranial radiation was later found to produce undesirable central nervous system toxicity, the current method of treating clinically inapparent central nervous system disease in acute leukemia is intrathecal chemotherapy (17). Toxic interactions between agents given by various routes have to be considered in developing a tolerable combination treatment regimen of this sort. A fraction of the methotrexate given intrathecally leaks into the systemic circulation and may result in mucositis, but it results in less overall myelosuppression than craniospinal radiation because of the large bulk of marrow included in the radiotherapy field (18).

SELECTION OF PATIENTS

The target population for a study of CMT must be defined very carefully. We shall use the case of adjuvant chemotherapy to illustrate some of the key issues. Drug regimen ABC, with significant activity against advanced disease of a particular tumor type, is to be tested in the postoperative adjuvant setting. How does one select a suitable patient population for study? The job is to define a patient group whose *prognosis* after standard therapy (in this case, surgery alone) is such that the *potential benefit* of adjuvant therapy justifies the *estimated risks* of treatment. Following is a discussion of how these three factors can be dealt with in practice.

Prognosis

As a general rule, the patients selected for most adjuvant trials do not do well after local therapy alone. This relatively poor prognosis, coupled with the possibility of therapeutic improvement, is what justifies entering them on a therapeutic experiment in the first place. The prognosis should be defined by criteria that are established and reproducible. These might be the number of positive regional nodes, the degree of tumor differentiation, tumor size, or other measurable characteristics. In breast cancer, the relative importance of a number of such factors has been assessed systematically in patients treated with surgery alone; the principal factor is the number of lymph nodes with metastatic involvement (0, 1–3, or 4 +) (19) (Table 9.1). One can see that the prognosis for treatment failure ranges from 13% for those with no positive nodes to 59% for those with 4 or more nodes.

How poor should the prognosis be to justify entry onto the trial? This depends largely on the complexity and toxicity of ABC. Generally, for new treatments without a previous track record in the adjuvant setting, the more potentially toxic and intensive the regimen the poorer the baseline prognosis should be for patients to justify their entry in the study. It is obvious from Table 9.1 that one would feel

TABLE 9.1. *Prognostic importance of nodal status in patients with breast cancer*

No. positive nodes	No. patients ($N = 614$)	% Treatment failure	
		10 yr	5 yr
0	279	20	13
1–3	160	47	39
4+	175	71	69
4–6	65	59	
7–12	55	69	
13+	55	87	

Reprinted from Ref. 19.

more justified in using "experimental" therapy in patients with 4 or more positive nodes than in those with no positive nodes. As a next step, if a relatively toxic treatment has shown evidence of effectiveness in a poor-prognosis group, one may have strong motivation to study its effect in patients with a much better underlying prognosis. On the other hand, if ABC is an essentially nontoxic therapy that can be given to outpatients by mouth with minimal expense and inconvenience, then one might contemplate initially entering patients with a rather good prognosis, provided that there is no reason to think that the treatment is associated with adverse long-term consequences or a worsening of the clinical course. This latter consideration (i.e., the possibility of tumor stimulation in some patients) was a cause of concern among some oncologists in the 1970s in connection with the use of hormones as adjuvants in Stage I breast cancer.

If patients with an extremely poor prognosis are selected for adjuvant trials, their disease may be so advanced that therapy has no chance to accomplish much. In the present example, if breast cancer patients with very extensive axillary involvement (e.g., more than 10 or 12 positive nodes) are selected for study, they may include a high percentage of patients with occult *macro*metastatic disease. It is possible that this constitutes an unfair test of an hypothesis that relates the greatly enhanced effectiveness of chemotherapy to metastases that are at most of *micro*scopic size.

Selecting patients with a suitably poor prognosis has another, purely statistical aspect of great practical importance. The sample size necessary for a trial to detect a given difference of interest depends most importantly on the number of adverse events (in this example, recurrence or death) occurring in the study population. If a trial is composed of a very favorable patient population, for which event rates are low, a very much larger sample size will be required than if prognosis were less good. Although the decision about entry of a given class of patients should be made on medical grounds, the statistical consequences have to be planned very carefully in advance, to assure that such trials are indeed practicable. The statistical issues of comparative studies are discussed more extensively in Chapter 7.

Potential Benefit

Clinical investigators do not generally initiate therapeutic studies unless they anticipate at least some possibility of benefit, but estimating the likely magnitude of this benefit in advance is usually not possible. If the test regimen is a modification of one for which adjuvant data are already available, then intelligent guesses can be made of the likely range of a therapeutic effect. In addition to helping decide on suitable study populations, such estimates are also extremely useful in performing realistic sample size calculations that should precede any comparative trial (see Chapter 6).

Generally, one tends to regard an adjuvant study with more or less enthusiasm in proportion to the activity of the test regimen in advanced disease: the higher the response rate in advanced cancer, the more reasonable it is to anticipate that the regimen will be an effective surgical adjuvant. In fact, it is generally difficult to justify testing as an adjuvant a regimen that had *not* shown activity in advanced disease. For regimens of low activity, however, response rate in advanced disease is not a good predictor of adjuvant efficacy; as shown in Table 9.2 (11), although the activities of 5-fluorouracil in colon cancer, dacarbazine in melanoma, and melphalan in breast cancer are in the same range, the first two have produced no statistically significant benefit as adjuvants in individual adjuvant trials.

Once therapy for advanced disease becomes extremely effective, however, there is an interesting twist. The experience in testicular cancer (20) and Hodgkin's disease (21) (Fig. 9.2) suggests that the use of combination chemotherapy as an adjuvant to surgery or radiotherapy, respectively, may have no greater impact upon overall survival than careful observation and use of the same combination following clinically evident relapse. In other words, in disease for which extremely effective systemic treatment exists, with high complete response rates and cures in advanced disease, a policy of observing patients after local therapy and treating with chemo-

TABLE 9.2. *Relation between response rate in advanced disease and efficacy as postoperative adjuvant*

Disease	Regimen	Response rate	Results of adjuvant trials
Breast	L-PAM	20–25%	Positive
	CMFVP	40–60%	Positive
	CMF		Positive
Melanoma	DTIC	9–30%	Negative
Colorectal	FU	12–20%	Negative
	Methyl-CCMU		Negative
	FU		

Reprinted from Ref. 11.

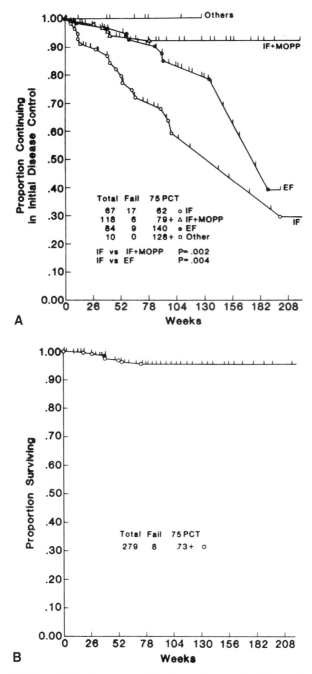

FIG. 9.2. Relatively high salvage rate with chemotherapy after failure of local treatment with radiotherapy results in a marked difference in disease-free survival (**A**) but no difference in overall survival (**B**) in this early analysis of the intergroup Hodgkin's disease study. (Data from Ref. 21.)

therapy only those who actually relapse may be just as effective as treating all patients with the same regimen as an adjuvant. Effects like this are impossible to predict in advance, and cannot be confidently extrapolated from one tumor type to another. They do serve to remind us, however, that trying to figure out "potential benefit" using information other than that obtained from adjuvant trials themselves is likely to be difficult at best.

Similar considerations may apply also to combinations of surgery and radiation. For tumor types such as larynx cancer, in which failures to radiation alone can often be salvaged by surgery, the development of CMT strategies are much less important than they would be if failure to initial treatment were tantamount to a death sentence. In situations where salvage therapy can be quite effective, therefore, the risks of employing two or more modalities in combination must be carefully weighed against the relatively small improvements that may accrue with the use of CMT compared with the judicious use of the modalities sequentially, as needed.

Estimated Risks

Proper concern with risks of a new intervention is an essential feature of any good clinical experiment. Oncologists are accustomed to a greater level of risk in therapy than physicians treating most other disorders. The obvious justification is the lethality of most cancers in the absence of effective treatment, and the unfortunate fact that we do not yet have treatment that is devoid of annoying, and sometimes very nasty, side effects.

Although CMT is no different from other treatment innovations in respect to the need for careful risk assessment, some features of CMT warrant particular emphasis. The manner in which patients are selected for adjuvant chemotherapy trials means that the physician is necessarily treating some individuals for whom local therapy alone is curative. For these patients, the chemotherapy is totally superfluous and stands to contribute only risk. The problem is that we have no way to exclude these patients from the trial in advance. Our inability to do this haunts the design of virtually all adjuvant trials and explains in part why the toxicity of adjuvant regimens often seems to generate so much more discussion than the use of equivalently toxic regimens in the setting of more advanced disease. The toxic death of a patient on an adjuvant study, who may already have been cured by local therapy and who may be on study simply because our crude diagnostic tests give us no valid way of excluding him, is an appalling prospect. It also explains, in part, the enthusiasm of most physicians for the development of increasingly sensitive diagnostic techniques and increasingly discriminating prognostic factor analyses. A less dramatic but very important practical issue in this context is that patients on adjuvant trials, having no evidence of or symptoms from their cancer, would generally be fully functional except for treatment-related morbidity. Since most adults have jobs to hold down and families to care for, any inability to perform normal daily functions may have significant immediate consequences, not the least of which may be the loss of medical insurance with the loss of a job.

For these reasons, oncologists have often displayed a real reluctance to deliver adjuvant regimens at full tolerated dose (11). Failure to do this may surely be one reason why the integration of chemotherapy into CMT has not shown more striking results in many trials. The greater sensitivity of most childhood solid tumors and the ability of children to tolerate, in general, greater degrees of drug-induced toxicity have led to a greater success rate in the adjuvant therapy of pediatric solid tumors. This in turn leads pediatric oncologists to be much more inclined to use a maximally vigorous approach to therapy. When a child is diagnosed as having cancer, as long as the chance for cure seems reasonable, everything else in the child's life can take second place to treatment. Thus, the evidence for success may depend on the willingness to administer full-dose therapy, and the willingness to administer full-dose therapy may depend on the evidence for success.

When treating advanced metastatic solid tumors, oncologists and patients do not often have to contend with the long-term effects of the treatment, since many of these diseases are fatal within weeks or months. In the adjuvant setting, however, a proportion of patients will become long survivors, even if the chemotherapy is not particularly effective. We still have yet to learn what full doses of anthracyclines do to cardiac function 20–30 years later, or what cisplatin does to renal function as cured patients age. The chronic effects of all the modalities, therefore, become important potential consequences of therapy. Late effects of cytotoxic drugs or radiation on various organ systems, particularly when these two modalities are given in a combined approach, are of particular concern. In the setting of Hodgkin's disease, for example, some have claimed that there may be more leukemogenesis and sterility after MOPP than after ABVD (22). If the two regimens were equally effective, this might be a reason for choosing the latter as primary treatment. There may also be more sterility and second cancers in patients treated with CMT (radiation and chemotherapy) than in those patients treated with either modality alone (23). The time distribution of the appearance of secondary leukemias and solid tumors is still being worked out, with the median incubation period of the latter apparently longer than that of the former (24).

Although concern with these issues is appropriate, it must never turn into a preoccupation that impedes further innovation. Chronic and long-term effects of treatment must, where possible, enter into the risk/benefit assessment in the planning stage of any clinical trial. The late effects that actually occur in the trial must be carefully quantitated and characterized. They are an important part of the determination of the overall value of a new treatment. But our willingness and enthusiasm for exploring treatment innovations must not be paralyzed by vague fears of what late effects *may* occur to the cured patient many years after cure of the cancer.

CURRENT ISSUES

The last 15–20 years of clinical trials have established the role of CMT in a number of different tumors. In children, the treatment of the majority of malignancies is with multimodal therapy. In adults, research into optimal ways of combining modalities continues, although a relative paucity of effective agents for the treatment of several very common tumors has hindered rapid progress. Since CMT strategies are likely to be effective in proportion to the effectiveness of their constituents, the further development of adjuvant chemotherapy depends in an important way on the discovery of more effective individual agents and drug combinations than we now possess. It should be emphasized that it is not only the development of new drugs that will improve CMT, but the continued refinement and improvement in radiotherapeutic and surgical techniques as well. Radiolabeled antibodies might allow one to target radiotherapy and deliver a dose locally that was previously impossible to give. In addition, it is conceivable that improvement in systemic therapy would lead one to reexplore the need for better local therapy in a particular disease. In Ewing's sarcoma, where amputation was abandoned long ago, some surgeons continue to feel that patients whose primary tumor is resected do better than those who do not have definitive surgery (25). The difficulty with this specific argument is that patients with primary disease in "expendable" bones such as fibulae and ribs tend to do better than those with primary disease in sites such as the pelvis, whether they are operated on or not. The effect of surgery has not been studied in a randomized controlled fashion in these operable sites. The point, however, is that improvement in therapy with one modality may lead one to try to develop improvements in another modality.

We shall now consider briefly a variety of issues that are of current concern in the design, execution, and reporting of CMT trials. Integration of biological response modifiers into CMT is discussed in Chapter 10.

DESIGN OF REGIMENS

Adjuvant chemotherapy studies generally employ regimens that have appeared most active against the same tumor in advanced stages. In the absence of other ways of deciding what regimens ought to be effective against micrometastatic disease, this has seemed the procedure most likely to yield positive results. For the most part the doses and schedules used in the adjuvant setting have paralleled those for advanced disease. Although some theoretical modeling has suggested that the sensitivity of tumor may actually decrease as the body burden of tumor is reduced following induction therapy (26), these considerations have not influenced the design of most adjuvant trials. As noted before, a concern with quality of life has probably induced many physicians to attenuate doses in the adjuvant setting (11). Because the therapeutic objective here is increasing the cure rate, however, the chemotherapy in CMT regimens ought to be delivered at full therapeutic doses. If anything, even more attention should be paid to maintaining the intensity of treatment in this setting than in the advanced disease situation, where the chances of curing many solid tumors with available chemotherapeutic agents may well be remote. The duration of treatment should also be considered. In an initial study Bonadonna et al. (27)

showed that CMF given monthly for 12 cycles improved disease-free survival after surgery in node-positive breast cancer patients. In a later study 6 cycles were found to be as effective as 12 cycles and patients receiving only 6 cycles were more likely to receive full-dose therapy. Of course, when 12 cycles are given there are more opportunities for dose reduction, but it may also be that physicians are more willing to give full dose if they know the course will be relatively short.

In designing CMT regimens, physicians must anticipate interactions between modalities. The delivery of radiotherapy and chemotherapy in close temporal proximity may impede our ability to deliver the full dose of one modality or the other in many clinical situations (15). Sometimes deletion of one of the chemotherapeutic agents makes full dosing possible with the remaining drugs, but this can hardly be termed full-dose therapy (28). In other cases, simultaneous treatment schemes have had to be abandoned in favor of other strategies.

The clinical experience giving chemotherapy in very close association with surgery (perioperative treatment or treatment within a day or two of operation) is very limited. Despite the fact that animal models all stress the importance of timing in determining effectiveness, most clinicians have been reluctant to give cytotoxic treatment within hours or days of surgery, probably for fear of increasing the complication rate. One study (29) in breast cancer of cyclophosphamide (5 mg/kg/day i.v. for 6 days) versus no chemotherapy, where randomization was done by telephone from the operating room and the first injection was given immediately after closure of the surgical wound, showed significant benefit and no interference with normal healing of the surgical wound. Early results of another breast cancer adjuvant study using CMF in the immediate postoperative period documented some increase in the local infection rate and increased trouble with wound healing compared with conventional scheduling (30).

For combinations of surgery and radiotherapy, the governing principle has usually been to give them in as close a temporal relationship as possible. Postoperative radiotherapy is generally started as soon as wound healing is well enough along not to be jeopardized by radiation. Certain retrospective analyses have documented an increased recurrence rate in patients who experienced a significant delay in the onset of radiation (31). Such data support the importance of minimizing the interval between resection and subsequent radiotherapy. For preoperative radiation schedules, the interval between radiation and surgery is often a function of radiation dose. For relatively low doses of radiotherapy, surgery may follow within a few days without an unacceptable complication rate; for higher doses of radiotherapy, however, a longer delay is mandatory to allow local radiation reactions to subside before operation.

An interesting contrast between radiation and chemotherapy is in the matter of dose, when either modality is combined with surgery. As noted previously there is no evidence at all that the chemotherapy dose may be less in the adjuvant than in the advanced disease setting. By contrast, radiotherapists have known for years that the radiation dose required to sterilize micrometastatic disease is significantly less than that required to cause complete and permanent disappearance of bulk tumor masses. Accordingly, the doses routinely employed in postoperative radiation schedules are generally less than those needed when radiotherapy is used alone against bulk tumor masses (32).

SUBGROUP-SPECIFIC EFFECTS

The realization that all patients with a particular disease do not respond the same to treatment carries obvious implications for medical decision making. For example, the demonstration that a particular adjuvant therapy has a beneficial effect of a certain magnitude on a population of patients with Stage II breast cancer does *not* mean that the size of this effect is the same for the receptor-positive and receptor-negative patients, or for those with 1–3 and ≥ 4 positive nodes. Thus, physicians naturally want to examine the results of their clinical experiment within various patient groups defined by relevant clinical parameters. Usually, as in the breast cancer example just mentioned, these parameters are the ones suspected of influencing the effect of treatment or the disease's natural history. The laws of probability, however, make it likely that, if we analyze a sufficient number of subgroups in our patient population, we shall eventually find a difference that approaches conventional levels of statistical significance, even if the true results are not different (see Chapter 7).

This leads to one of the most vexing and common problems in large clinical trials: how seriously should one take a result that alleges subgroup-specific effects? There are no simple answers to this question that apply to all clinical situations, but a few general comments are in order. First of all, allegations of subgroup-specific differences are more plausible if they have been replicated in an independent trial of similar design. Second, they are more believable if they are associated with some reasonable biologic rationale. The fact that estrogen-receptor positive patients seem to have a greater therapeutic effect from adjuvant tamoxifen than receptor-negative patients is inherently more plausible than the claim that, for example, patients with lesions of the left breast did better on tamoxifen than those with lesions resected from the right.

The third point, closely related to the second, is that subgroup differences are more convincing if they have been postulated at the start of the trial, are part of the therapeutic hypothesis, and have been a basis for the trial's stratification. A corollary to this point is that one should be very wary of subset differences that have turned up in the course of exploratory analyses of the data at the end of the trial. When such differences in subgroups turn up, they may be useful in generating hypotheses for future studies but they should rarely be taken as definitive.

LONG-TERM FOLLOW-UP AND REPORTING OF RESULTS

As already noted, many studies of CMT are concerned with endpoints that take a long time to generate. How long clearly depends on the particular cancer being studied, but even for very aggressive neoplasms that kill relatively quickly, one should be wary of drawing early conclusions. Patients with small cell lung cancer limited to the primary complex have median survival of about 12 months. The large majority of treatment trials have been reported at relatively early time points in the evolution of the data. Although this practice permits the delineation of response rates, acute toxicities, and actuarial projections of disease-free and total survival, a final analysis of survival is possible only after most of the deaths in the population have occurred. Early reporting also does not allow a reasonably complete description of some of the important late effects of CMT. Although these have sometimes been reported later as part of the total institutional experience across several individual protocols (27), it is quite uncommon to see full final reports of individual trials in the literature.

For a disease such as breast cancer, where the natural history of the illness extends over more than a decade, a full understanding of the impact of treatment may well require follow-up for the duration of life of the study subjects (and the investigators!). At the very least, when the time course of the illness extends over such long periods, it would seem prudent to continue active follow-up for at least the length of time required for the survival curve of an untreated population of patients with the disease to become parallel to that of the general age-matched population without the disease.

Meanwhile, as we wait for study results to mature, what is a reasonable policy for the publication and dissemination of interim results? A look back at the experience with the interim analyses of one influential breast cancer adjuvant study is of interest. Updates of this trial, which compared postoperative CMF to observation alone, have been presented almost yearly during the first decade of follow-up. Particularly during the early years (33–35), conclusions about the major endpoints were very unstable (Table 9.3) and had to be revised substantially with each further year of follow-up. In this situation, as each new analysis was performed at close to yearly intervals, the effect of the chemotherapy was seen to be less durable. This was without any change in the patient population being studied.

Sometimes the differences in outcome with repeat analysis can be even more striking, particularly if new information has accrued about the patients. A recent report from the Southwest Oncology Group of a review of an ovarian cancer study originally published in 1979, showed a marked decrease in the response rate and median survival in the 1985 report compared with the original (36) (Table 9.4). The differences resulted from a review of the pathology with exclusion of 88 of the original 200 registered patients. These patients failed to meet strict pathologic criteria for a diagnosis of ovarian cancer of the epithelial type on review and had fared better overall than those patients who did meet the diagnostic criteria. The authors felt that this high number of pathology exclusions was unusual and occurred because this was the first study the group had performed that required pathologic review. The bulk of pathologic material was reviewed years after patient registration. Nevertheless, despite the fact that there may be an explanation for the change in the data, and even if the new report may be somewhat embarrassing, it is important that final analyses be published.

TABLE 9.3. *First three reports of the Milan studies of breast adjuvant chemotherapy with CMF: Comparison of results*

	First report (33)		Second report (34)		Third report (35)	
	Control	CMF	Control	CMF	Control	CMF
Total	179	207	179	207	179	207
Mean follow-up	14 mos.		21 mos.		40 mos.	
Data projected to:	27 mos.		36 mos.		48 mos	
Recurrence rate						
Overall	24%	5.3%	45.7%	26.3%	52.7%	34.4%
By nodes						
1–3	22.9%	3.6%	37.9%	19.1%	—	—
≥ 4	40.7%	8.8%	64.9%	41.5%	67.6%	51.0%
By menopausal status						
pre	24.3%	5.2%	47.6%	14.7%	59.2%	25.0%
post	23.7%	5.3%	40.1%	36.2%	47.6%	43.8%
Dead of disease	6%	0.48%	21.4%	10.4%	29.4%	17%
Relapses after successful completion of 1 year of therapy	None		Many		Many	

TABLE 9.4. *Preliminary, interim, and final results of study SWOG No. 7706 for ovarian cancer*[a]

Date of report[b]	Number of patients enrolled	Number of patients evaluable	% CR + PR[c]	Median survival (mos.)
1979 (17)				
FHAP	54	29	48	12+
FHP	111	74	31	14
1980 (18)				
FHAP	56	48[d]	31	12
FHP	114	106[d]	25	13
1985 current report				
FHAP	69	38[a]	26	8
FHP	131	74[a]	26	7

[a]Histology was retrospectively reviewed leading to the exclusion of a number of patients who failed to meet the criteria for ovarian cancer of the epithelial type and who fared better than the group as a whole. This resulted in an apparent decrease in response rate and survival.
[b]FHP = 5-FU, hexamethylmelamine, cisplatin; FHAP = FHP + doxorubicin.
[c]CR, complete response; PR, partial response.
[d]Includes fully and partially evaluable patients.

Reprinted from Ref. 36.

REFERENCES

1. Nesbit, M. E., Jr., Perez, C. A., Tefft, M., et al. (1972): Multimodal therapy for the management of primary, nonmetastatic Ewing's sarcoma of bone: An intergroup study. *Natl. Cancer Inst. Monogr.*, 56:255–262.
2. Bleehen, N. H., Bunn, P. A., Cox, J. D., et al. (1983): Role of radiation therapy in small cell anaplastic carcinoma of the lung. *Cancer Treat. Rep.*, 67:11–20.
3. Karrer, I., Humphreys, S. R., and Goldin, A. (1967): An experimental model for studying factors which influence metastasis of malignant tumors. *Int. J. Cancer*, 2:213–223.
4. Griswold, D. P., Jr. (1986): Body burden of cancer in relationship to therapeutic outcome: Consideration of preclinical evidence. *Cancer Treat. Rep.*, 70:81–86.
5. Belasco, J. B., Chatten, J., and D'Angio, G. J. (1984): Wilms' tumor. In: *Clinical Pediatric Oncology*, edited by W. W. Sutow, D. J. Fernbach, and T. J. Vietti, pp. 588–621, 3rd ed. Mosby, St. Louis.
6. D'Angio, G. J. (1985): Oncology seen through the prism of Wilms tumor. *Med. Pediatr. Oncol.*, 13:53–58.
7. Burgert, E. O., Jr., and Glidewell, O. (1967): Dactinomycin in Wilms' tumor. *J.A.M.A.*, 199:464–468.
8. Zelen, M., and Gelman, R. (1986): Assessment of adjuvant trials in breast cancer. *Natl. Cancer Inst. Monogr.*, 1:11–17.
9. Gerard, A., Berrod, J. L., Fene, F., et al. (1985): Interim analysis of a Phase III study on preoperative radiation therapy in resectable rectal carcinoma. Trial of the gastrointestinal tract cancer cooperative group of the European Organization for Research on Treatment of Cancer (EORTC). *Cancer*, 55:2373–2379.
10. Rice, G. C., Hoy, C., and Schimke, R. T. (1986): Transient hypoxia enhances the frequency of dihydrofolate reductase gene amplification in Chinese hamster ovary cells. *Proc. Natl. Acad. Sci. USA*, 83:5978–5982.
11. Wittes, R. E. (1986): Adjuvant chemotherapy—Clinical trials and laboratory models. *Cancer Treat. Rep.*, 70:87–103.
12. Rosen, G., Caparros, B., Huvos, A. G., et al. (1982): Neoadjuvant (preoperative) chemotherapy for osteogenic sarcoma: Selection of postoperative adjuvant chemotherapy based upon the response of the primary tumor to neo-adjuvant chemotherapy. *Cancer* 49:1221–1230.
13. Jaffe, N., Murray, J., Wallace, S., et al. (1986): Limb salvage (LS) utilizing preoperative intra-arterial cis-diamminedichloroplatinum-II (P-IA-CDP), local en bloc resection and endoprosthetic replacement in pediatric osteosarcoma. *Proc. A.S.C.O.*, 5:204.
14. Weaver, A., Flemming, S., Kish, J., et al. (1982): Cis-platinum and 5-fluorouracil as induction therapy for advanced head and neck cancer *Am. J. Surg.*, 144:445 448.
15. Looney, W. B., and Hopkins, H. A. (1986): Alternation of chemotherapy and radiotherapy in cancer management. Results in experimental solid tumor systems and their relationship to clinical studies. *Cancer Treat. Rep.*, 70:141–162.
16. Aur, R. J. A., Simone, J., Hustu, O., et al. (1971): Central nervous system therapy and combination chemotherapy in childhood lymphocytic leukemia. *Blood*, 37:272–281.
17. Freeman, A. I., Weinberg, V., Brecher, M. L., et al. (1983): Comparison of intermediate-dose methotrexate with cranial irradiation for the post-induction treatment of acute lymphocytic leukemia in children. *N. Engl. J. Med.*, 308:477–484.
18. Aur, R. J. A., Hustu, H. O., Versoza, M. S., et al. (1973): Comparison of two methods of preventing central nervous system leukemia. *Blood*, 42:349–357.
19. Fisher, E. R. (1986): Prognostic and therapeutic significance of pathological features of breast cancer. *Natl. Cancer Inst. Monogr.*, 1:29–34.
20. Williams, S., Muggia, F., Einhorn, L., et al. (for the Testicular Cancer Interstudy Group) (1986): Resected stage II testicular cancer: Immediate adjuvant chemotherapy versus observation. *Proc. A.S.C.O.*, 5:98.
21. Sullivan, M. P., Fuller, L. M., Chen, T., et al. (1982): Intergroup Hodgkin's disease in children study of stages I and II: A preliminary report. *Cancer Treat. Rep.*, 66:937–947.
22. Valagussa, P., Santoro, A., Fossati-Bellanti, F. G., et al. (1986): Second acute leukemia and other malignancies following treatment for Hodgkin's disease. *J. Clin. Oncol.*, 4:830–837.
23. Coleman, C. N. (1986): Secondary malignancy after treatment of Hodgkin's disease. An evolving picture. *J. Clin. Oncol.*, 4:821–824.

24. Blayney, D. W., Longo, D. L., Young, R. C., et al. (1987): Decreasing risk of leukemia with prolonged follow-up after chemotherapy and radiotherapy for Hodgkin's disease. *N. Engl. J. Med.*, 316:710–714.

25. Wilkins, R. M., Pritchard, D. J., Burgert, E. O., Jr., and Unni, K. (1986): Ewing's sarcoma of bone: Experience with 140 patients. *Cancer*, 58:2551–2555.

26. Norton, L., and Simon, R. (1986): The Norton–Simon hypothesis revisited. *Cancer Treat. Rep.*, 70:163–170.

27. Bonadonna, G., Valagussa, P., Tancini, G., et al. (1986): Current status of Milan adjuvant chemotherapy trials for node-positive and node-negative breast cancer. *Natl. Cancer Inst. Monogr.*, 1:45–49.

28. Glick, J. H, Danoff, B., Haller, D., et al. (1983): Integration of adjuvant chemotherapy with definitive radiotherapy for primary breast cancer. In: *Adjuvant Therapy of Cancer, IV*, edited by S. E. Salmon and S. E. Jones, pp 291–300, Grune and Stratton, New York.

29. Nissen-Meyer, R., Host, H., Kjellgren, K., et al. (1986): Treatment of node-negative breast cancer patients with short course of chemotherapy immediately after surgery. *Natl. Cancer Inst. Monogr.*, 1:125–128.

30. Ludwig Breast Cancer Study Group (1983): Toxic effects of early adjuvant chemotherapy for breast cancer. *Lancet*, 2:542–544.

31. Vikram, B., Strong, E. W., Shah, J., and Spiro, R. H.(1980): Elective postoperative radiation therapy in stages III and IV epidermoid carcinoma of the head and neck. *Am. J. Surg.*, 140:580–584.

32. Hellman, S. A. (1985): Principles of radiation therapy. In: *Cancer: Principles and Practice of Oncology*, edited by V. T. DeVita, Jr., S. Hellman, and S. A. Rosenberg, pp. 227–255, 2nd ed. Lippincott, Philadelphia.

33. Bonadonna, G., Brusamolino, E., Valagussa, P., et al. (1976): Combination chemotherapy as an adjuvant treatment in operable breast cancer. *N. Engl. J. Med.*, 294:405–410.

34. Bonadonna, G., Rossi, A., Valagussa, P., et al. (1977): The CMF program for operable breast cancer with positive exillary nodes. Updated analysis on the disease-free interval, site of relapse and drug tolerance. *Cancer*, 39:2904–2915.

35. Bonadonna, G., Valagussa, P., Rossi, A., et al. (1978): Are surgical adjuvant trials altering the course of breast cancer? *Semin. Oncol.*, 5:450–464.

36. Laufman, L. R., Green, J. B., Alberts, D. S, et al. (1986): Chemotherapy of drug-resistant ovarian cancer: A Southwest Oncology Group Study. *J. Clin. Oncol.*, 4:1374–1379.

CHAPTER 10

Biologic Response Modifiers

Previous chapters have discussed the study of therapies that are directly cytotoxic to tumor cells. Because these therapies are toxic to normal cells as well, investigators have strong motivation to develop approaches having a much greater degree of selectivity. The exquisite specificity of the immune system has long made it a potentially attractive mediator of selective antitumor effects. Only within the past few years, however, has the vast increase in biological knowledge and in our technical capabilities for producing clinical reagents made the beginnings of a rational approach to this problem feasible.

In this chapter we shall deal with some of the issues in clinical trials posed by the development of approaches that are not themselves directly cytotoxic. We shall see that many of the paradigms used for the evaluations of cytotoxic treatments cannot be applied to this area without substantial modification. Because a systematic approach to the assessment of noncytotoxic approaches is still so new, many of the questions discussed in this chapter currently lack satisfactory answers.

The area of biological response modification is one of the fastest moving in all clinical cancer research. For that reason, and because the thrust of this book is the methodology of clinical cancer research, we have chosen to keep this discussion rather general. A more detailed treatment of many of the specific issues connected with individual classes of biologicals is not necessary for our purposes and would run the risk of becoming outdated very quickly.

DEFINITION OF TERMS

Medicines of biological origin have played an important role in therapeutics for a long time. Plants and microorganisms have served as the source of many of our most active pharmacologic agents, including several widely used cytotoxic compounds such as daunorubicin, bleomycin, and mitomycin C. When the term "biological" is used in oncology, however, it generally refers rather loosely to whole cells or cell fractions (bacterial or mammalian) or to defined products of mammalian cells. Eventually, of course, the DNA sequences coding for a defined product may be identified and transferred to a prokaryotic organism for large-scale production of pure material.

By contrast, the term "biologic response modifier" (BRM) refers to agents or approaches that modify the host's biological response to tumor cells with resultant therapeutic effects (1). It should be clear from these definitions that a given biological may or may not be a BRM. Conversely, biologic response modification may be produced by chemicals not of biologic origin. In common usage, however, the terms BRM and biological are often employed synonymously.

The rational clinical development of agents that are presumed to exert an antitumor effect by modifying host responses depends in an obvious way on our understanding of the underlying mechanism of these responses, how they are modified by the agent of interest, and how this modification may be monitored. It goes without saying that the present state of our knowledge of many fundamental processes in tumor biology—antitumor effects of the immune system, differentiation, and metastasis, to name three potentially exploitable areas—is still rather primitive. The fact that many biologicals are presumed to act through incompletely understood host mechanisms rather than via direct tumor cell killing leads to several complex problems in performing interpretable clinical trials. These problems must be faced squarely in conceptualizing and performing trials, but they should not be cause for despair. After all, a number of effective pharmacologic agents for the treatment of cancer emerged as useful before their mechanism of action was understood. In fact, clinical correlations with successful antitumor therapy may well help us eventually to understand some of the basic underlying mechanisms for selective cell kill by the immune system.

PROBLEMS IN THE STUDY OF BRMS

Pleiotropism

It was hoped for some time that as the agents under investigation went from relatively crude microbial agents [e.g., *Bacillus Calmette Guérin* (BCG) or *Corynebacterium parvum*] to chemically defined, purified, even homogeneous substances, only one function or action in the host would be observed. Many molecules, however, tend to be pleiotropic in their effects on the immune system or on other host functions. As an example, some of the known functions of interferon (IFN)-alpha include cytostasis, increased expression of certain cell surface antigens, increased levels of certain enzymes, and augmentation of NK cell numbers (2). Under such circumstances it may be difficult or impossible to define "the" mechanism of action.

Standardization

For many BRMs, units are expressed in terms of a particular biologic activity. As noted above, this activity may not be the only one expressed by the agent, nor in fact even be most important for control of tumor growth. With IFN, units are expressed as the amount of decrease in viral plaque formation in tissue culture. One might anticipate that a recombinant material would be easier to standardize than a natural product. One IFN preparation currently in clinical trial (human lymphoblastoid IFN) is that material produced in human lymphoid tissue culture in response to infection with Sendai virus; this material consists of at least 12 distinct subtypes of IFN-alpha (3). By contrast, IFN-alpha produced by recombinant DNA technology is a homogeneous molecular species. Transfering genetic information to a bacterium, however, does not necessarily assure that the resulting protein will be identical to that made by the human cell. Bacteria cannot glycosylate proteins, for example, and many of these substances as synthesized in mammalian cells are, in fact, glycoproteins. The lack of glycosylation of the recombinant protein might make it appreciably different from the natural product in terms of biodistribution or functional activities.

Once a biologic activity has been accepted as the standard, it is important that it be assayed reproducibly. Herberman (4) describes the evaluation of 12 different interleukin-2 (IL-2) preparations, 6 natural and 6 recombinant, which were referred to the Biologic Response Modifiers Program of the National Cancer Institute (NCI) for evaluation. When the preparations were all compared to a BRMP standard preparation for their activity in promoting growth of T-cell lines, there was in some cases a 100-fold or more difference between the companies' stated units of activity and the BRMP reference units actually measured. This type of painstaking standardization should be required of any agent before the start of clinical trials.

Species Specificity

The complexity of assaying these materials and developing relevant *in vivo* preclinical models is materially increased by the fact that a variety of potentially useful BRMs do not cross the species barrier. An agent might have potent effects, either directly on human tumor cells or indirectly via patients' effector mechanisms, but be entirely ineffective in rodents. For such BRMs (e.g., most human IFNs and monoclonal antibodies against human tumors), it has been necessary to rely on *in vitro* preclinical assessments and on studies of human tumor xenografts in nude mice rather than on the usual preclinical screening that is performed for chemical compounds. Needless to say, the nude mouse is hardly an adequate animal model for studying the effects of BRMs that require the mediation of an intact immune system.

DESIGN OF TRIALS

Selection of Appropriate Dose

Determination of the optimal dose for clinical study is a particularly vexing problem for BRMs. The dilemma may be posed as follows. We have a substance that is presumed to exert an antitumor effect by modifying some aspect of the host's response to the tumor. Preclinical work may have revealed not one but several effects of this substance on, say, various regulatory or effector limbs of the immune system. Perhaps, as with IFN-alpha, there may even be evidence of a direct anti-proliferative effect against tumor cells. What kind of clinical trial(s) is adequate to establish the optimal dose under such complex circumstances?

Before going any further we need to consider the term ''optimal.'' Optimal with respect to what? Since we are interested in killing or arresting the growth of cancer cells, the optimal antitumor dose would seem to be most relevant clinically. With agents that are directly cytotoxic to tumor cells, we usually assume the maximum tolerated dose is also the optimal dose. This does not seem to be a reasonable assumption for BRMs, simply because there is no reason whatsoever to suppose that the maximum tolerated dose is the optimal dose for modifying the biological responses that are hypothesized to be relevant to tumor killing. In fact, preclinical data for at least some BRMs suggest a bell-shaped relation between BRM activity and dose (5). In addition, whether the optimal BRM dose and the optimal antitumor dose are identical ought theoretically to depend on the correctness of the therapeutic hypothesis, i.e., that the particular biologic response we are attempting to optimize is decisively related to tumor cell killing. In early studies of immunotherapy with tumor cell vaccines in soft tissue sarcoma (6), and with allogeneic cells and BCG in acute myelogenous leukemia (7), high titers of cytotoxic antibodies were produced in the patients, in the one case against tumor cell lines in tissue culture and in the other case against HL-A antigens on the immunizing cells. Although one might suppose that production of an antibody that is cytotoxic *in vitro* would be a desired endpoint, there was no evidence of a beneficial clinical effect.

Thus there are two optimal doses of interest in trials of BRMs: the optimal antitumor dose (OAD) and the optimal BRM dose (OBRMD). The relation between these will depend most importantly on which biologic resonse one is attempting to optimize and the relation, if any, between this response and the observed antitumor effect. The implication, of course, is that in the course of early clinical trials of BRMs, one must monitor not only antitumor response, toxicity, and pharmacoki-netics, but also the biological parameters one is trying to influence.

This is all much easier said than done. The reader will appreciate that the de-termination of ''optimality'' in medicine is a very rigorous task usually involving large comparative trials. In the present context, where testing of several dosage levels might be theoretically pertinent, the trials would become quickly impractical. No suprise, then, that the clinical data currently available do not yet rigorously clarify the existence of an optimal dose separate from the maximum tolerated dose of any particular modulating agent for either antitumor or BRM activity. With IFN-alpha, for example, highly sensitive malignancies such as hairy cell leukemia have responded well to low doses (e.g., 2 MU/m^2 daily or 3 times/week), and, therefore, higher doses have not commonly been explored (8,9). In less sensitive tumors, however, when dose–response studies have been done, higher doses have been associated with greater antitumor activity. In a randomized trial in renal cell carcinoma, for example, 20 MU/m^2 yielded 12/41 responses compared with 0/15 at 2 MU/m^2 (10). This result was confirmed in a smaller randomized trial with partially purified leukocyte IFN (11). Similar results have also been observed in a sequential trial in Kaposi's sarcoma where a greater proportion of responses (38%) was seen at the higher dose (36 $\times$ 10^6 U) than at a lower dose (3% at 3 $\times$ 10^6) (12).

One interpretation of these findings might be that the antitumor effect in each of these situations is not the same. Tumor control could represent the direct sensitivity of one or all of the target cells to IFN, or it could represent the fact that the host mechanism required to control renal cell carcinoma and/or Kaposi's sarcoma is different from that required to control hairy cell leukemia. It is obvious that our lack of understanding of the basic mechanisms underlying the effects inhibits our ability to interpret the results. But trials comparing several dose levels of a BRM and including a negative control probably represent the only present approach to clarifying these issues, even if the studies are difficult to perform.

Selection of Ideal Dose Schedule

An immune response, when stimulated, normally does not continue indefinitely, nor is the response to the second exposure to an antigen the same as that to the first exposure. In the same way, repeated administration of a BRM may produce a different response than single administration does. Repeated daily administration of IFN-alpha results in decrease rather than augmentation of NK activity (13). Under such circumstances, therefore, one might conclude that an intermittent dose schedule may be more effective. However, to the extent that tachyphylaxis to the toxic effects of the agent also occurs, a chronic dosage schedule might be better tolerated than an intermittent one. Symptoms of fever, rigors, and nausea during the first week of regular IFN-alpha administration may be more frequent and more severe than symptoms with the same dose during the eighth week. Thus, if an intermittent schedule is elected, an escalating dose schedule may be required in order to reach an effective dose (12).

Delivery of Active Material to Tumor Site

With most agents, including cytotoxic drugs, the choice of an optimal route is governed by such matters as the pharmacological behavior of the drug, bioavailability, relative toxicities, and convenience. These considerations should not be overlooked in the study of biologicals. For example, the subcutaneous injection of IFN-alpha leads to prolonged serum levels while little or no circulating IFN is detected after subcutaneous or intramuscular injection of IFN-beta (14). With biological agents, however, there are some additional considerations. In early studies with crude infectious material such as BCG, there was concern that the use of the intravenous route might produce systemic infection. Even with killed bacteria there is always the potential problem of anaphylaxis with repeated injections of foreign proteins. In addition, efficacy (defined as complete disappearance of tumor) was seen only in situations associated with direct contact between tumor cells and adjuvant. Early studies by Morton et al. (15) showed that regression of intradermal melanoma lesions often occurred when they were directly injected with BCG. Only about 10% of patients showed regression of uninjected nodules, however, and responses were unlikely to occur if disease had spread beyond the skin. Regional treatment of intrapulmonary disease (e.g., by intrapleural injection in patients with Stage I carcinoma of the lung) was also the subject of a promising early report (16), but a later randomized study of 400 patients did not confirm this result (17).

Several trials of intradermally injected BCG in acute leukemia were performed in the 1970s, presumably with the rationale that the activated cells circulating after local contact in the skin would destroy tumor cells. These studies followed the provocative observation by Mathe et al. (18), suggesting benefit to adjuvant therapy with BCG and allogeneic leukemia cells. Attempts in other controlled studies to reproduce this result (19,20) were not successful, however, and there have been no unambiguously successful reports of systemic immunotherapy with BCG in other human cancers.

A number of BRMs can be administered systemically, but some of these molecules are labile, have a short half-life in the circulation, and do not distribute evenly throughout the body. After intravenous administration, IL-2 has a serum half-life of only a few minutes and may not accumulate in sufficient levels in the lymphoid organs or at sites of tumor growth where it probably mediates its effects. In an attempt to overcome these problems, Rosenberg and his colleagues (21,22) have performed multiple leukophereses on patients to collect large quantities of autologous killer cells that can then be expanded in number by *in vitro* incubation with IL-2 and reinfused into the patient; IL-2 is then administered systemically in high dose to support *in vivo* growth of the killer cells. This approach was demonstrated in animal models to be more successful than the administration of IL-2 alone in high doses, although IL-2 alone did have some antitumor effect. This therapy is clearly capable of inducing a significant antitumor effect although at the price of significant acute toxicity (21). Continuing investigation of this approach is directed toward increasing its antitumor activity while, if possible, decreasing the associated toxicity (22).

The problem of an inadequate supply of activated cells at the local tumor site to accomplish tumor destruction has been a major mechanical difficulty with immune modulation. In an attempt to use an *in vivo* rather than *in vitro* expansion of an activated cell population and still retain direct contact between activated immune cells and tumor cells, Fidler (23) treated animals with intravenously administered liposomes containing muramyl dipeptide or other diffusible macrophage activators. The majority of the liposomes (80–90%) are taken up by the reticuloendothelial cells in the liver, spleen, lymph nodes, and bone marrow and by circulating monocytes. By exploiting this localization pattern, liposome-encapsulated materials can be targeted to macrophages *in vivo* and activated at the site (e.g., the lungs), where the metastatic tumor deposits are occurring. This approach is undergoing Phase I testing at the present time.

Evaluation of Immune Modulation

In trials with immunomodulators, attempts to measure putatively relevant effects on the immune response are essential. Effector functions such as activity of cytotoxic T cells, NK cells, and macrophages; assays for general immune competence including the quantitation and typing of lymphocyte subpopulations and their *in vitro* proliferative responses; and studies of other specific functions such as the production of lymphokines may all be needed to evaluate a single product.

The selection of assays to include in a particular trial is often problematical. First of all, many of these assays are technically difficult to reproduce. There appears to be substantial spontaneous fluctuation in reactivity in the control assays over a period of time. This fluctuation can occur in target cell sensitivity as well as in effector cell activity. For many assays, the best approach to "normalizing" data has been the collection and cryopreservation of large quantities of cells by leukophoresis from normal donors (24). This allows the investigator to thaw aliquots from several normal donors each day an experiment is performed. On the other hand, certain cell functions survive cryopreservation better than others. Monocyte-mediated cytotoxicity, for example, is well preserved, but NK activity is much less reliably reproduced when cells are processed in this fashion.

There is also an intrinsic fluctuation in immunological reactivity of each donor, and presumably of each cancer patient that is independent of the administration of the BRM. The interpretation of changes in immune response in the course of treatment must take these spontaneous variations into account. One way of doing this is the establishment of a normal range for each patient of the activity in a critical assay by analysis of multiple baseline determinations (e.g., of NK cell activity prior to interferon administration) (24), which can then be compared with multiple posttreatment assays.

At least in part for these reasons, the serial monitoring of immune status in many trials has been less than satisfying. In the early studies of IFN-alpha, levels of circulating NK cells appeared to respond quite variably, often falling rather than rising. As a result, investigators turned to other more reproducible measures of IFN effect, such as the level of $2'5'$ oligoadenylate synthetase (OAS) induced in peripheral blood mononuclear cells. In patients with juvenile laryngeal papillomatosis, OAS levels correlate well with response to IFN therapy (25). In patients with epidemic Kaposi's sarcoma and HIV infection, where immune function is grossly abnormal at the start of therapy, often with high spontaneous levels of IFN and OAS, correlation has not been so good (26).

Importance of Host Factors

In addition to the intrinsic variation in assays, there may be a wide variation in the baseline condition of the host response one is trying to modify. In preclinical testing of BRMs, the effect of the agent may be different in tumor-bearing from that in nontumor-bearing mice. In particular, in animal models immunotherapy has been most effective in a situation of minimal tumor burden (27). Many of the most striking experiments have involved prophylaxis with the agent administered some time prior to or with tumor cell administration, rather than after the tumor is already established. This is hardly a realistic model for the treatment of established cancer.

In the clinic also, tumor burden may be a major determinant of success with immunomodulating therapy. Previously treated patients with advanced disease and large tumor burdens may have different immunological responses to modulators than those who are less ill (28). A randomized trial of short-term levamisole treatment was undertaken in a cancer population unresponsive to dinitrochlorobenzene (DNCB) to determine whether this agent increased delayed hypersensitivity. During DNCB challenge, 50 of 100 patients received levamisole (150 mg daily × 3); the other 50 were challenged but not given the drug. The conversion rate to DNCB positivity was 20% (10/50) for those treated with levamisole and 12% (6/50) for controls. Although this difference is obviously not significant, there was a significant inverse relationship in the total population between extent of disease and the incidence of conversion to a DNCB reactive state. Thus, in this trial, the tumor burden rather than the immunomodulator appeared to be the significant variable with respect to immune reactivity (29).

The reasons why large tumor burdens depress the response to challenge with new antigens are not entirely clear. It has been known for years that patients with advanced stages of Hodgkin's disease (30) or malignant melanoma (31) have a higher prevalence of depressed delayed hypersensitivity than patients with less advanced disease. Thus, as tumor burden increases, the ability of the immune system to mount cellular responses against new exogenous antigens decreases. It may also be that the immune system may be capable of destroying only a certain load of tumor, and that body burdens greater than a certain level cannot be eliminated by endogenous host defense mechanisms alone, even if these mechanisms can be effectively stimulated.

Enhancement of Tumor Growth

From a theoretical point of view, one might conceivably stimulate a desirable and an undesirable effect simultaneously. Yu et al. (32) have demonstrated the simultaneous presence of cytotoxic and inhibitor lymphocytes against tumor cells in the blood of osteosarcoma patients receiving chemotherapy. The concept of enhancement of tumor growth by antibody and by cells has been shown in animal model systems (33). It is not clear whether a similar phenomenon occurs clinically. Enhancement of tumor growth is in principle very difficult to detect in the absence of suitable controls, and most trials of biologicals in humans have been uncontrolled or have revealed no evidence for enhancement. One controlled trial of levamisole in lung cancer revealed a higher mortality in the postoperative period among those patients receiving levamisole when compared with controls; this resulted in a significantly shorter survival in the levamisole group. No immunologic explanation for this result was apparent (34). Because immune enhancement of tumor growth can be regularly demonstrated in model systems, however, it is particularly important to design clinical immunotherapy trials such that a deleterious result can be detected if it occurs. This means, in essence, that an appropriate control should be included whenever possible.

ANTIBODY THERAPY

Clinical Uses of Antibodies

Antibodies against components of tumor cells have a number of obvious potential applications in treatment. First, they might be directly cytotoxic to cells, with or without the mediation of complement. They might also serve as an opsonin for cell-mediated cytotoxicity. By complexing with growth factors or growth-factor receptors on the tumor cell surface, they might interfere with critical steps in a tumor's growth. Much current research is focusing on the coupling of monoclonal antibodies to cytotoxic drugs, bacterial toxins, or radionuclides as a way of routing the toxic moieties directly to tumor and increasing selectivity. Monoclonal antibodies to human carcinoma-associated antigens are now being reported with increasing frequency (35). Carcinoma-associated antigens detected by these antibodies may be expressed on only a subpopulation of cells from a single tumor type or may be more "public," i.e., more widely expressed and be found on more than one tumor type or even on some normal adult cell populations. Clearly, such tumor-related properties as heterogeneity of antigen expression in different patients or even from cell to cell within the same patient will have a major impact on the usefulness of highly specific antibodies.

Some monoclonal antibodies have been used clinically for diagnosis. For example, a murine monoclonal antibody has been produced against DU-PAN 2, a high molecular-weight surface glycoprotein of a pancreatic ductal adenocarcinoma cell line (36). Elevated levels of this antigen were detected in the serum in 31/33 patients with adenocarcinoma of the pancreas; 5/6 patients whose lesions were surgically resectable showed return to normal within 1 to 3 weeks after surgery. With tumor progression, DU-PAN 2 levels increased in all patients an average of 2 months before evidence of progressive disease by clinical parameters. Thus, serial DU-PAN 2 determinations appeared to be a sensitive monitor of disease progression in pancreatic cancer, but did not allow quantitation of tumor burden.

Radiolabeled antibodies can be used to localize tumors by scanning techniques. Studies have recently been initiated in patients using intraperitoneal administration of [131]I B 72.3 monoclonal antibody to detect intraabdominal colorectal cancer metastases (37). Note, however, that antibodies that are active *in vitro* may not be useful *in vivo*. A particular monoclonal antibody raised against breast tumor antigens turned out to be unsuccessful for imaging because of the antibody's relatively high affinity for granulocytes (38). The ability to image a tumor with a given antibody may prove to be a useful technique for selecting patients who are likely to benefit from therapeutic doses of the same antibody, given either alone or conjugated to a toxin or a radionuclide.

Therapeutic Uses of Antibody

As with any systemic agent, an antibody's pharmacokinetic properties, as well as its degree of access to tumor in various locations, will be major determinants of its therapeutic potential. Several other considerations that are peculiar to antibody therapy should also be considered in the design of clinical trials.

Nature of the Antibody

Most monoclonal antibodies produced to date are of murine origin. They will therefore be recognized as foreign proteins by the human host, which, in turn, may react immunologically against them. Allergic reactions will therefore be significant obstacles to murine monoclonal antibody administration unless effective measures are taken to contain them. These may include pharmacologic attempts to block the generation of an allergic response. Some investigators have employed the sequential use of radiolabeled immunoglobulins from a variety of species (goat, rabbit, etc.) in the same patient (39).

Thus far, the majority of monoclonal antibodies in clinical trial have been of IgG type. Some *in vitro* evidence suggests that for antibodies with a given specificity, the isotype may have a significant influence on the ability of the antibody to elicit antibody–target cell interactions. In attempting to dissect the factors in the immune response responsible for lysis of human target cells, Johnson et al. (40) discovered that only antibodies in the IgG_{2a} subclass and macrophages activated by thioglycolate (as opposed to BCG) appeared to be active in ADCC (antibody-dependent complement cytotoxicity) tumor lysis. For this reason they administered an IgG_{2a} monoclonal antibody (17-1A) raised against human colon carcinoma cells to patients with gastrointestinal adenocarcinoma both alone (41) and after incubation with autologous leukocyte preparations (42). The clinical results from these particular trials were disappointing; however, our ability to engineer isotype variants with identical specificities may be an important tool for seeing to it that antibodies brought to clinical trial are optimal.

Nature of the Antigen

Many carcinoma-associated antigens are stable components of the cell membrane and are not internalized, capped, or shed when complexed with antibody. However, the tendency of some antigens to disappear from the cell surface in the presence of antibody (antigenic modulation) is a potential obstacle to treatment. In *in vivo* studies with the infusion of anti cALLa antibody in patients with acute leukemia, Nadler et al. (43) found that antigen-positive cells disappeared after a very short period of exposure to antibody but reappeared in the patients' circulation within hours of cessation of infusion. Proper scheduling of antibody administration might well circumvent this obstacle. In addition, the internalization of antigen–antibody complexes from the tumor cell surface may be of actual advantage to the therapist if the antibody is armed with a toxin or a cytotoxic agent that exerts its lethal effects intracellularly.

Dose

Most of the Phase I trials done to date have not pursued a systematic approach to the delineation of a maximum tolerated dose. It is difficult to know whether the maximum tolerated dose is indeed an approximation of what ought to be the optimal dose. Presumably what one wants to do with antibody therapy is coat a certain critical number (or percentage) of accessible tumor-associated antigens with the reagent. Since the dose-limiting toxicities of a foreign protein bear no necessary relation to its therapeutic mechanism of action, the assumption that the maximum tolerated dose ought to be defined and used in further study seems more tenuous than it is with conventional cytotoxic drugs.

What other approaches to defining the proper dose are available? Available techniques for assessing the binding of antigen by antibody in tumor tissue (44) might permit titration of dose to a more tumor-specific endpoint. For an antibody that fixes complement, the rate of utilization of circulating complement might be an indirect measure of when the optimal dose had been reached.

Nevertheless, if more rational alternatives are not available, it still seems advisable to define and use the maximum tolerated dose in the conventional manner. Interesting data from at least one preliminary evaluation of monoclonal antibody R24 in patients with melanoma suggests that tumor cells growing in the face of therapy still bear the target antigen (44). This suggests that access of antibody (or perhaps some host component) to the tumor tissue may be a significant obstacle to successful treatment. Delivering the maximum dose is a reasonable way to attempt to overcome problems of access. Thus, if the maximum tolerated dose is not used in subsequent Phase II studies, the absence of activity may simply reflect insufficient dosing, rather than intrinsic inactivity of the antibody per se. The best strategy, of course, will be to assess dose–response relationships systematically as part of the comprehensive clinical evaluation of the active antibody.

Schedule

If, as with other systemically administered agents, the aim is to select a schedule that will provide the maximum tolerated concentration over the treatment period, we still face with antibody therapy a few constraints that do not exist with other kinds of agents. Insofar as modulation is an obstacle to successful therapy, we should aim for short repeated treatment courses, timed according to the disappearance and reappearance of antigen, so that any cells protected by modulation might be reexposed to the antibody. As noted previously, however, repeated courses of a foreign protein may be impossible because of allergic reactions. Such schedules may also elicit the formation of specific antibody that may neutralize the antitumor effect of the administered antibody. One approach may be to give sequential courses of antibodies from different animal sources. A completely satisfactory solution to this latter problem may have to await wider availability of chimeric or human monoclonal antibodies.

Presence of Circulating Antigen

Significant quantities of circulating antigen might tie up antibody as complexes and prevent the antibody's access to tumor. Variable levels of circulating antigen from patient to patient might well be a source of variability in the maximum tolerated dose in individual patients, as well as in the antitumor results achieved. Plasmapheresis prior to antibody administration (45), as well as high initial doses of antibody have been proposed as a way of circumventing this obstacle to successful treatment.

Patient Selection

Since the aim of medical intervention in any clinical trial is patient benefit, even in early trials that seek to define tolerable doses for later study, it makes sense to limit accrual to antibody studies to those patients having tumors with the requisite antigenic targets. Ideally, screening patients for such trials would involve testing of antibody reactivity with a sample of each patient's tumor before study entry. Alternatively, such screening might involve the demonstration by radionuclide scanning that radiolabeled antibodies are selectively taken up by the patient's tumor. In practice, however, some antibodies in clinical use appear to have such broad reactivity with certain histological types that testing of each patient may not be necessary; the R24 antibody, for example, appears to react with a very high proportion of melanomas thus far tested (46). On the basis of such information, it may be possible to select patients of a given primary site on histological type alone. The reader should note the contrast with most cytotoxic drug studies, where selection of patients by tumor type does not occur until Phase II.

Immunotoxins and Radiolabeled Antibodies

The chemical coupling of a highly specific antibody to a toxin or radionuclide is a very appealing therapeutic approach. Preclinical studies in murine models have shown the feasibility of this approach, and much effort is currently directed toward the development of active conjugates. Toxins of interest include a number of chemotherapeutic agents (methotrexate, vinca alkaloids) and nonspecific cellular poisons (ricin, ricin A chain). The chemistry involved in the synthesis of active conjugates is generally very complex; the trick is to link the toxin to the antibody without destroying the specificity or pharmacologic behavior of the antibody.

The current status of work with radiolabeled antibodies has been summarized in a recent symposium (47). Promising preliminary results have been reported at a variety of sites, including liver and ovary. In general the dose-limiting toxicity of the approach appears related to the radiation rather than the antibody.

Antiidiotype Therapy

Most human B lymphocytic malignancies are thought to be derived from a single original transformed B cell. This implies that the cells of the tumor uniformly express an immunoglobulin molecule that is unique for each tumor. Antibodies in this situation can be made that are truly tumor specific, i.e., that are directed toward these unique (idiotypic) structures in the variable region of the immunoglobulin molecule. Eleven patients were treated with antibodies having such specificity (45), with 1 durable complete response and 5 objective remissions that were "clinically significant." Therapy was complicated if there was circulating idiotypic protein, since the concentration of mouse antibody required to achieve tumor penetration under these circumstances was increased. Another complication in this study was that 5/11 patients developed an immune response to mouse immunoglobulin and once this occurred further therapy was ineffective.

MATURATIONAL AGENTS

For a long time clinicians have recognized that certain malignant tumors may undergo histological maturation to an apparently more differentiated phenotype. Embryonal carcinoma of germ cell origin undergoes evaluation to mature teratoma (48); neuroblastoma sometimes forms ganglioneuroma. Although these changes may evolve spontaneously, most of the reported cases have occurred in the context of therapy, usually with cytotoxic drug combinations. The clinical significance of this phenomenon appears to be that evolution of a histologically malignant tumor to a more mature, benign-appearing phenotype carries with it a favorable prognosis for improved survival (48).

New techniques in molecular biology have recently permitted the extension of these observations to acute leukemia. Studies of premature chromosome condensation have documented identical karyotypic abnormalities (e.g., minute chromosomes, hyperdiploidy) in pretreatment malignant marrow samples and mature peripheral blood granulocytes obtained after treatment (49,50). After conventional dose cytarabine, Fearon and colleagues (51) found that morphologic differentiation of malignant tissue had occurred. White cells from 3/13 patients whose bone marrow appeared to be in remission were derived from a single clone and probably represented maturation of the patients' original leukemic line. Thus, the existence of differentiation in human cancer may be a more general phenomenon than was formerly suspected. It should be emphasized, however, that neither the clinical nor the laboratory observations to date prove conclusively that therapy has in fact induced maturation. It remains possible that the appearance of mature, histologically "benign" tissue at sites previously involved with malignant tumor is due to selective killing of the more malignant appearing elements. At the present state of our knowledge there is no way to distinguish with certainty between these possibilities.

In principle, one can assess the appearance of increased degrees of differentiation by looking for morphological evidence of maturation or for the new production of differentiated gene products by tumors. For example, the production of mucin, keratin, or melanin by tumors not previously producing those substances might be evidence of maturation in the appropriate clinical context.

In the case of germ cell tumors, neuroblastoma, and leukemia mentioned above, the aim of therapy has been to produce a cytotoxic effect, and any maturation that may have occurred was an unintentional by-product. More recently, however, as the process of differentiation has become the focus of intensive laboratory investigation, interest in differentiation itself as a therapeutic goal has quickened. A large variety of chemical structures can be shown to induce differentiation of a number of premalignant or malignant cell lines *in vitro*. These include the retinoids (vitamin A and its synthetic analogs) derivatives of vitamin D, cyclic adenosine monophosphate and its nucleoside analogs, a number of cytotoxic agents, and certain small, polar–planar molecules such as dimethylsulfoxide (52).

In *in vivo* models, however, or as noted above in the clinic, it may be operationally difficult to distinguish between cytotoxicity and differentiation. For example, the use of low doses of cytarabine in patients with acute leukemia and with myelodysplastic syndromes was based on the hypothesis that differentiation could be induced without significant cytotoxicity and all the undesirable and dangerous effects on normal tissue that accompany cell killing. The significant myelosuppressive effects that often result from treatment with low-dose cytarabine, however, suggest that significant cytotoxicity is present and the relative importance of cytotoxicity and maturation in the therapeutic effect of low-dose cytarabine therapy is at present uncertain (53).

With purposeful attempts at maturational therapy in their infancy, what are the implications for clinical trials? It would seem, first of all, that the usual clinical endpoints of response may need to be reassessed. These trials should logically involve some assessment of whether maturation has actually occurred with therapy. The usual endpoint of tumor shrinkage, universally employed when cytotoxicity and cell death are the goals of therapy, may be misleading in the context of maturational studies, where a change in cell phenotype is what is sought. As is well known in the therapy of germ cell tumors, the *absence* of significant tumor shrinkage is still compatible with apparently total histological maturation from an undifferentiated embryonal carcinoma to fully mature teratoma. One might think that the induction of differentiation ought at least to result in cessation of further tumor growth. This may be true in most cases, if the effect occurs within a cell division or two of the start of therapy. On the other hand, experience with the germ cell tumors has, in fact, revealed that apparent enlargement of tumor masses can also occur with effective therapy if the treatment results in the formation of cystic masses as part of the mature teratoma (48).

There would seem to be no good substitute, therefore, for measuring differentiation directly if it is the intended goal of therapy. Feasible approaches for doing this, however, are not simple. As noted above, molecular biological techniques that can establish the monoclonality of the differentiated cells after therapy and the pretreatment tumor population are probably the least ambiguous way to show that maturation has occurred. In cases where certain phenotypic changes accompanying differentiation of normal cell lineages are well characterized (such as orderly changes in the expression of cell surface antigens or in cytoplasmic enzyme activities), it may be possible to follow the evolution of parallel events in the tumor cell population longitudinally with therapy. Doing so obviously requires the performance of serial biopsies as treatment proceeds. Also, if there is heterogeneity in phenotypic expression within the same patient at any given point in time, the interpretation of any observed changes over time may be difficult, unless they are very dramatic. Despite the difficulties, however, it seems clear that the use of endpoints that reflect the differentiation process directly is indispensible for the rational development of this whole approach.

As with cytotoxic agents, knowledge of an agent's cellular pharmacology and pharmacokinetics provides a useful guide to clinical development. If one knows that a certain concentration of a differentiator is required *in vitro* to produce differentiation in cell lines and that this concentration must be sustained for a minimum time period, it would seem logical to design the clinical trials in such a way as to achieve the putatively effective serum levels for the required duration. The clinical testing of hexamethylene bisacetamide (HMBA), a polar–planar compound currently in development as a differentiator, is being guided by such considerations (54). The concentration and exposure-time requirements for differentiation of cell lines *in vitro* have been used to guide dose and duration of infusion in the early clinical trials done to date.

Since trials involving this approach are currently in early stages, it may be premature to worry about the ultimate end of such treatment. If patients with testicular tumors that show conversion to a mature phenotype have a very good prognosis, then it is not idle to suppose that the same result may occur with more refractory neoplasms. On the other hand, it is not known whether any differentiation that may accompany therapy will be terminal or, instead, whether malignant cells having a mature phenotype will retain the ability to dedifferentiate to a more malignant phenotype. If histologically mature cells retain the same chromosomal markers as their malignant ancestors, why should we expect them to remain well-behaved in the absence of the agent that presumably forced the differentiation? The answers to these questions are unknown, but will be of great importance in determining important characteristics of the treatment such as the duration of therapy. It should need no emphasis that although the endpoints of the early clinical trials of maturational agents are the occurrence of differentiation, the ultimate value of the treatment will be expressed in terms of survival and quality of life.

COMBINATION THERAPY WITH BRMS AND OTHER MODALITIES

Many clinical trials groups are investigating the effects of BRMs, particularly cloned biologic products, including IFN-gamma, IL-2, and tumor necrosis factor, either alone or in combination with each other as adjuvants to local therapy or integrated into combinations with chemotherapy. There are many positive reasons for combining BRM and other therapies. Since BRMs are most active in model systems when tumor burden is low, it might be important to decrease initial tumor load with another modality first. In addition, BRMs might sensitize the tumor cell to the effect of the other modality. Human IFN-beta has sensitized bronchogenic carcinoma cells *in vitro* to radiation cytotoxicity presumably via interfering with enzymes important for radiation repair (55). In addition, one BRM might enhance the effect of another. IFN through its effects on cell surface may enhance the expression of tumor-associated antigens (56) and increase the total number of receptors for another agent such as tumor necrosis factor (57).

The recent availability of molecularly cloned hematopoietic colony stimulating factors (CSF) for both granulocyte (G-CSF) and the granulocyte-macrophage (GM-CSF) lineages (58) has dramatically increased the possibilities for successful combined therapy. The CSFs are capable of rapidly inducing large increases in the numbers of circulating blood elements in their respective series. Although one can easily imagine many potential uses of such BRMs, two obvious questions concerning combinations of the CSFs and cytotoxic drugs stand out: (a) Does the coadministration of CSF with an effective but myelotoxic chemotherapy regimen obviate the myelotoxicity of the regimen? and (b) Does the coadministration of CSF and a partially effective chemotherapy regimen permit delivery of higher doses of the regimen with a resulting increase in the effectiveness of the chemotherapy?

These questions can only be answered definitively by controlled trials. To answer question (a), one first identifies an effective but myelosuppressive regimen in a particular disease. Then one works out in a preliminary Phase I pilot the dose and schedule of CSF that, in association with the particular chemotherapy reigmen, keeps the circulating blood counts above some desired level. Then the randomized trial (chemotherapy versus chemotherapy + CSF) may proceed. The key endpoints are relative blood counts and, more importantly, some direct measures of patient morbidity (number of infections, hospitalizations, toxic deaths, etc.).

Question (b) requires a somewhat different approach. After defining a suitable chemotherapy-disease combination in which the administration of chemotherapy is limited by bone marrow tolerance, one performs a Phase I study of chemotherapy and CSF in which the chemotherapy is escalated to the limits of tolerance in the presence of CSF. This Phase I pilot is rather complicated, since it is likely that higher doses of CSF may permit more chemotherapy to be given. Thus, the Phase I pilot would probably have to include provisions for escalating both the CSF and the chemotherapy. In any case, once the new maximum tolerated dose of the chemotherapy has been defined in the presence of CSF, the randomized trial (chemotherapy versus chemotherapy + CSF, with each treatment arm at its maximum tolerated dose) may then proceed. The key endpoints of this trial are remission rates and durations, survival, and quality of life.

An immune response stimulated in other ways by BRMs might also allow patients to tolerate more cytotoxic therapy than an unstimulated immune system. On the other hand, some experiments in animal models demonstrate that the administration of a cytotoxic agent that is also immunosuppressive, can ablate a potentially useful immune response. In one preclinical study, cyclophosphamide administered to a tumor at a critical point in the immune reaction produced temporary regression, but eventually the neoplasms grew and destroyed all the treated animals, while some of the controls that received no chemotherapy eventually achieved complete immune-mediated regression of their tumor (59). It would seem prudent therefore, to consider the use of the two obvious controls when evaluating combinations of cytotoxic agent A and immunomodulator B, to help assess these potential interactions.

The combination of antibodies with other therapies has already been discussed. The concept of combining growth factors or maturational agents with chemotherapy is intriguing. A number of chemotherapeutic agents act most particularly on cells in the S-phase and a growth factor that could stimulate a greater fraction of cells to become sensitive to a DNA synthesis inhibitor might be very useful, although the potential dangers of stimulating tumor growth seem obvious.

Despite initial hopes to the contrary it is amply clear by now that BRM administration often results in significant toxicity. For this reason, the successful integration of BRMs with other modalities still depends on our ability to construct active yet tolerable regimens from agents with nonoverlapping dose-limiting effects.

CONCLUSIONS

The complexity associated with the evaluation of each BRM, some of which is discussed above, prevents screening large numbers of potential BRMs as has been done with cytotoxics. The Biologic Response Modifiers Program of the NCI has conducted a preclinical evaluation of the effects of 10–20 compounds per year with study of the effects of multiple doses on various components of the immune system as well as on aspects of tumor growth. This contrasts with approximately 10,000 potential cytotoxic agents screened per year in transplantable murine tumors (60).

As one considers the difficulties in assessing the therapeutic activity of BRMs, one becomes particularly conscious of our heavy reliance on preclinical models for such important issues in cytotoxic drug development as selection of an appropriate starting dose and schedule. But, in addition, we also rely heavily on the *clinical cytotoxic* properties of chemotherapeutic agents to decide what doses and schedules are feasible for further study and how drugs should be combined with each other. With BRMs these familiar guideposts may be either absent or irrelevant, and new paradigms are clearly necessary. This chapter has outlined some of the important issues, almost all of which are currently unresolved. With our increasing ability to clone almost any kind of biological molecule or produce monoclonal antibodies with a wide variety of specificities, the next few years will challenge the ingenuity of clinical investigators in an unprecedented fashion.

REFERENCES

1. Mihich, E., and Fefer, A. (1983): Biological response modifiers: Subcommittee report. *Natl. Cancer Inst. Monogr.*, 63:251.
2. Fish, E. N., Banerjee, K., and Stebbing, N. (1983): Human leukocyte interferon subtypes have different antiproliferative and antiviral activities on human cells. *Biochem. Biophys. Res. Commun.*, 112:537–546.
3. Finter, N. B., and Fantes, K. H. (1980): The purity and safety of interferon prepared for clinical use: The case of lymphoblastoid interferon. In: *Interferon, Vol. II*, edited by I. Gresser, pp. 65–80. Academic Press, London.
4. Herberman, R. B. (1985): Design of clinical trials with biological response modifiers. *Cancer Treat. Rep.*, 69:1161–1164.
5. Bast, R. C., Jr., Zbar, B., Borsos, T., and Rapp, H. J. (1974): BCG and cancer, part I. *N. Engl. J. Med.*, 290:1413–1419.
6. Morton, D. L., Holmes, E. C., Eilber, F. R., and Wood, W. C. (1971): Immunological aspects of neoplasia: A rational basis for immunotherapy. *Ann. Intern. Med.*, 74:587–604.
7. Baehner, R. L., Bernstein, I. D., Sather, H., et al. (1979): Improved remission induction rate with D-ZAPO but unimproved remission duration with addition of immunotherapy to chemotherapy in previously untreated children with ANLL. *Med. Pediatr. Oncol.*, 7:127–139.
8. Quesada, J. R., Reuben, J., Manning, J. T., et al. (1984): Alpha interferon for induction of remission in hairy cell leukemia. *N. Engl. J. Med.*, 310:15–18.
9. Golomb, H. M., Jacobs, A., Fefer, A., et al. (1986): Alpha-2 interferon therapy of hairy-cell leukemia: A multicenter study of 64 patients. *J. Clin. Oncol.*, 4:900–905.
10. Kirkwood, J. M., Harris, J. E., Vera, R., et al. (1985): A randomized study of low and high doses of leukocyte A interferon in metastatic renal cell carcinoma. The American Cancer Society Collaborative Trial. *Cancer Res.*, 45:863–871.
11. Quesada, J. R., Rios, A., Swanson, D., et al. (1985): Antitumor activity of recombinant derived interferon alpha in metastatic renal cell carcinoma. *J. Clin. Oncol.*, 3:1522–1528.
12. Real, F. X., Oettgen, H. F., and Krown, S. E. (1986): Kaposi's sarcoma and the acquired immunodeficiency syndrome: Treatment with high and low doses of recombinant leukocyte A interferon. *J. Clin. Oncol.*, 4:544–551.
13. Maluish, A. E., and Herberman, R. B. (1985): Assessment of biological responses: What to measure and when. *Cancer Treat. Rep.*, 69:1165–1169.
14. Gobel, U., Arnold, W., Wahn, V., et al. (1981): Comparison of human fibroblast and leukocyte interferon in the treatment of severe laryngeal papillomatosis in children. *Eur. J. Pediatr.*, 137:175–176.
15. Morton, D. L., Eilber, F. R., Holmes, E. C., et al. (1974): BCG immunotherapy of malignant melanoma. *Ann. Surg.*, 180:635–643.
16. McKneally, M. F., Maver, C., Lininger, L., et al. (1981): Four year follow-up on the Albany experience with intrapleural BCG in lung cancer. *J. Thorac. Cardiovasc. Surg.*, 81:485–492.
17. Mountain, C. F., and Gail, M. H. (1981): Surgical adjuvant intrapleural BCG treatment for Stage I non-small cell lung cancer. *J. Thorac. Cardiovasc. Surg.*, 82:649–657.

18. Mathe, G., Amiel, J. L., Schwarzenberg, L., et al. (1969): Active immunotherapy for acute lymphoblastic leukaemia. *Lancet*, i:697–699.
19. Heyn, R. M., Joo, P., Karon, M., et al. (1975): BCG in the treatment of acute lymphocytic leukemia. *Blood*, 46:431–442.
20. British Medical Research Council, Leukaemia Committee and Working Party on Leukaemia in Childhood (1971): Treatment of acute lymphoblastic leukaemia: Comparison of immunotherapy (BCG), intermittent methotrexate, and no therapy after a five month intensive cytotoxic regimen (Concord trial). *Br. Med. J.*, 4:189–194.
21. Rosenberg, S. A., Lotze, M. T., Muul, L. M., et al. (1985): Observations on the systemic administration of autologous lymphokine-activated killer cells and recombinant interleukin-2 to patients with metastatic cancer. *N. Engl. J. Med.*, 313:1485–1492.
22. Rosenberg, S. A., Lotze, M. T., Muul, L. M., et al. (1987): A progress report on the treatment of 137 patients with advanced cancer using lymphokine-activated killer cells and interleukin-2 or high dose interleukein-2 alone. *N. Engl. J. Med.*, 316:889–897.
23. Fidler, I. J. (1985): Macrophages and metastasis—a biological approach to cancer therapy: Presidential address. *Cancer Res.*, 45:4714–4726.
24. Maluish, A. E., Ortaldo, J. R., Sherwin, S. A., et al. (1983): Changes in immune function in patients receiving natural leukocyte interferon. *J. Biol. Response Mod.*, 2:418–427.
25. Lodemann, E., Kornhuber, B., Gerein, V., and von Ilberg, C. (1984): (2'-5') Oligo (A) synthetase as a monitor of interferon action in juvenile laryngeal papillomatosis. *J. Interferon Res.*, 4:283–290.
26. Preble, O. T., Rook, A. H., Steis, R., et al. (1985): Interferon induced 2'-5' oligoadenylate synthetase during interferon-alpha therapy in homosexual men with Kaposi's sarcoma: Marked deficiency in biochemical response to interferon in patients with acquired immunodeficiency syndrome. *J. Infect. Dis.*, 152:457–465.
27. Bast, R. C., Jr. (1985): Principles of cancer biology: Tumor immunology. In: *Cancer: Principles and Practice of Oncology*, edited by V. T. DeVita, Jr., S. Hellman, and S. A. Rosenberg, pp. 125–150, 2nd ed. Lippincott, Philadelphia.
28. Bast, R. C., Zbar, B., Borsos, T., and Rapp, H. J. (1974): BCG and cancer, part 2. *N. Engl. J. Med.*, 290:1458–1469.
29. Hirshaut, Y., Pinsky, C. M., Frydecka, I., et al. (1980): Effect of short-term levamisole therapy on delayed hypersensitivity. *Cancer*, 45:362–366.
30. Brown, R. S., Haynes, H. A., Foley, H. J., et al. (1967): Hodgkin's disease. Immunological, clinical, and histologic features of 50 untreated patients. *Ann. Int. Med.*, 67:291–302.
31. Camacho, E. S., Pinsky, C. M., Braun, D. W., Jr., et al. (1981): DNCB reactivity and prognosis in 419 patients with malignant melanoma. *Cancer*, 47:2446–2450.
32. Yu, A., Watts, H, Iaffe, N., and Parkman, R. (1977): Concomitant presence of tumor specific cytotoxic and inhibitor lymphocytes in patients with osteogenic sarcoma. *N. Engl. J. Med.*, 297:121–127.
33. Prehn, R. T. (1972): The immune reaction as a stimulator of tumor growth. *Science*, 176:170–171.
34. Anthony, J. M., Mearns, A. J., Mason, M. K., et al. (1979): Levamisole and surgery in bronchial carcinoma patients: Increase in deaths from cardiorespiratory failure. *Thorax*, 34:4–12.
35. Schlom, J. (1986): Basic principles and applications of monoclonal antibodies in the management of carcinomas. *Cancer Res.*, 46:3225–3238.
36. Mahvi, D. M., Meyers, W. C., Bast, R. C., et al. (1985): Carcinoma of the pancreas: Therapeutic efficacy as defined by a serodiagnostic test utilizing a monoclonal antibody. *Ann. Surg.*, 202:440–445.
37. Carasquillo, J. A., Colcer, D., Sugarbaker, P., et al. (1986): Intraperitoneal infusion with I[131] B 72.3 monoclonal antibody in patients with peritoneal carcinomatosis from colon cancer. *Proc. 33rd Annu. Mtg. Soc. Nucl. Med. (abstr.)*.
38. Hayes, D. F., Zalutsky, M. R., Kaplan, W., et al. (1986): Pharmacokinetics of radiolabeled monoclonal antibody B6.2 in patients with metastatic breast cancer. *Cancer Res.*, 46:3157–3163.
39. Lenhard, R. E., Jr., Order, S. E., Spunberg, J. J., et al. (1985): Isotopic immunoglobulin: A new systemic therapy for advanced Hodgkin's disease. *J. Clin. Oncol.*, 3:1296–1300.
40. Johnson, W. J., Steplewski, Z., Koprowski, H., and Adams, D. O. (1985): Destructive interactions between murine macrophages, tumor cells, and antibodies of the IgG$_{2a}$ isotype. *Adv. Exp. Med. Biol.*, 184:75–80.

41. Sears, H. F., Herlyn, D., Steplewski, Z., and Koprowski, H. (1985): Phase II clinical trial of a murine monoclonal antibody cytotoxic for gastrointestinal adenocarcinoma. *Cancer Res.*, 45:5910–5913.

42. Sears, H. F., Herlyn, D., Steplewski, Z., and Koprowski, H. (1984): Effects of monoclonal antibody immunotherapy on patients with gastrointestinal adenocarcinoma. *J. Biol. Response Mod.*, 3:138–150.

43. Nadler, L. M., Ritz, J., Griffin, J. D., et al. (1981): Diagnosis and treatment of human leukemias and lymphomas utilizing monoclonal antibodies. *Prog. Hematol.*, 12:187–225.

44. Houghton, A. N., Mintzer, D., Corden-Cardo, E., et al. (1985): Mouse monoclonal IgG3 detecting GD3 ganglioside: A phase I trial in patients with malignant melanoma. *Proc. Natl. Acad. Sci. USA*, 82:1242–1246.

45. Meeker, T. C., Lowder, J., Maloney, D. G., et al. (1985): A clinical trial of anti-idiotype therapy for B cell malignancy. *Blood*, 65:1349–1363.

46. Real, R., Houghton, A., Urmacher, C., et al. (1982): Monoclonal antibodies detecting melanoma antigens in tissue sections. *Proc. A.A.C.R.*, 23:255.

47. *Natl. Cancer Inst. Monogr.* (1987): *In press.*

48. Wong, W. K., Wittes, R. E., Hajdu, S. I., et al. (1977): The evolution of mature teratoma from malignant testicular tumors. *Cancer*, 40:2987–2992.

49. Beran, M., Andersson, B. S., Ayyar, R., et al. (1985): Clinical response and mechanisms of action of low dose cytosine arabinoside (Ara-C) in myelodysplastic syndromes (MDS) and myelogenous leukemias (AML, CMML). *Proc. A.S.C.O.*, 4:678 (*abstr.*).

50. Hittelman, W. N., Hawkins, M., Doyle, S., and Beran, M. (1985): Direct cytogenic evidence of induced maturation of leukemic cells *in vivo. Proc. A.A.C.R.*, 26:181 (*abstr.*).

51. Fearon, E. R., Burke, P. J., Schiffer, C. A., et al. (1986): Differentiation of leukemia cells to polymorphonuclear leukocytes in patients with acute nonlymphocytic leukemia. *N. Engl. J. Med.*, 315:15–24.

52. Cheson, B. D., Jasperse, D. M., Chun, H. G., and Friedman, M. A. (1986): Differentiating agents in the treatment of human malignancies. *Cancer Treat. Rev.*, 13:129–145.

53. Cheson, B. D., and Simon, R. (1987): Low-dose Ara-C in acute non-lymphocytic leukemia and myelodysplastic syndromes: A review of 20 years experience. *Semin. Oncol.*, 14(*Suppl. 1*):126–133.

54. Chun, H. G., Leyland-Jones, B., Hoth, D., et al. (1986): Hexamethylene bisacetamide: A polar–planar compound entering clinical trials as a differentiating agent. *Cancer Treat. Rep.*, 70:991–996.

55. Gould, M. N., Kakria, R. C., Olson, S., and Borden, E. C. (1984): Radiosensitization of human bronchogenic carcinoma cells by interferon beta. *J. Interferon Res.*, 4:123–128.

56. Greiner, J. W., Horan Hand, P., Noguchi, P., et al. (1984): Enhanced expression of surface tumor associated antigens on human breast and colon tumor cells after recombinant leukocyte alpha interferon treatment. *Cancer Res.*, 44:3208–3214.

57. Aggarwal, B. B., Eessalu, T. E., and Hass, P. E. (1986): Characterization of receptors for human tumor necrosis factor and their regulation by α-interferon. *Nature*, 318:665–667.

58. Clark, S. C., and Kamen, R. (1987): The human hematopoeitic colony-stimulating factors. *Science*, 236:1229–1237.

59. Glynn, J. P., Halpern, B. G., and Fefer, A. (1969): An immunochemotherapeutic system for the treatment of a transplantable Moloney virus induced lymphoma in mice. *Cancer Res.*, 29:515–520.

60. Hawkins, M. J., Hoth, D. F., and Wittes, R. W. (1986): Clinical development of biological response modifiers: Comparison with cytotoxic drugs. *Semin. Oncol.*, 13:132–140.

CHAPTER 11

Elements of a Protocol

A protocol is the detailed written plan of a clinical experiment. The word protocol is derived from the Greek "proto-kollon" and originally referred to the first leaf glued to the front of a manuscript which contained notes as to the contents (1). In modern research usage it is the blueprint for an experiment. It is important to remember that a poorly designed protocol cannot be "rescued" to give important information after the fact. If diagnostic criteria have not been rigorously applied, we may not know exactly what kind or how much tumor patients had at the start of treatment. If treatment schedules were not clearly stated, then each patient may have been treated a different way. Although some information can perhaps be gleaned from retrospective analysis of a well-designed trial, the biostatistician should be consulted from the beginning to assure that the information required to answer the principal questions will, in fact, be collected appropriately.

The elements of a protocol are listed in Table 11.1.

TITLE PAGE AND TABLE OF CONTENTS

The title page should clearly identify the protocol as well as the chairman of the study and the coinvestigators with their subspecialty indicated if this is a multi-

TABLE 11.1. *Subject headings for a protocol*

1. Title page and table of contents
2. Aims or objectives of the study
3. Introduction and scientific background for the study
4. Patient eligibility
5. Treatment programs, including schematic diagram
6. Agent information
7. Procedures and treatment modifications in case of toxicity
8. Required clinical and laboratory data
9. Criteria for evaluating the effect of treatment
10. Criteria for removing the patient from study
11. Statistical considerations
12. References
13. Recording forms
14. Informed consent

modality study. The table of contents should be clear and detailed so investigators can refer quickly to a specific subsection (e.g. dose reduction for toxicity) once they are treating a patient on study, and will not have to waste time searching through a long document. Anything that increases the efficient use of the protocol will increase the accuracy with which it is applied and, in the long run, will increase the evaluability of all the patient entries.

AIMS OR OBJECTIVES OF THE STUDY

It is important to describe the study objectives quite specifically in the protocol. As has already been noted, a study should be designed in such a way that it asks a question that can be answered in quantitative terms. The study must ask questions for which a limited number of answers are logically acceptable. If a clinician wants to ''study the effect of drug X on cancer Y,'' he has not asked a critical question in the sense implied here, for almost anything observed is part of the ''study'' of the effect. A trial that asks only a diffuse question leads to diffuse answers. An example of a more specific way to ask the question would be: ''Does drug X given at the dose that has been determined to be the maximum tolerated dose in man lead to a complete plus partial response rate in disease Y of at least 20%?'' This is obviously a Phase II question, but all questions can be framed in specific fashion.

A protocol should not ask too many questions. Complex studies are often stopped well before all the questions have been answered and sometimes no question is answered adequately. The realities of patient numbers required dictate that most studies should be restricted to one major question. An example of a design that eventually proved to be too complex is the Pediatric Intergroup Hodgkin's study (2). This study was initially designed to compare disease-free and overall survival in patients with Stages I and II Hodgkin's disease randomized to receive either involved-field or extended-field radiation or radiation + MOPP. Patients were supposed to be followed until relapse and then, if they had received only radio-therapy, treated with MOPP to see whether salvage with late chemotherapy would give the same overall survival as early chemotherapy plus radiation. The data for initial disease-free interval were faithfully collected, but by the time the patients were relapsing, protocol discipline had waned, new chemotherapies such as ABVD had come along, and patients were not restaged and maintained on protocol in an evaluable fashion. Thus, the answer to this important question was not discovered with this study. It is conceivable that if only one radiation regimen had been selected, the answer might have been arrived at since fewer patients would have been required.

The question posed by the protocol should be designed in such a way that the next logical step is obvious despite the protocol outcome. If the protocol is com-parative, then either positive or negative results should be informative for patient management (3). Examples of such studies are given in Chapter 6 and include the comparison of radiotherapy with no maintenance after surgery in Stage IV gliomas and the comparison of total with partial mastectomy for patients with Stage I breast cancer. If either procedure is better than the other in terms of survival then that would serve as the basis for future therapy. If they are the same, then the least toxic or the least disfiguring would probably be selected. In the Phase II example given above, if sufficient patients had been studied to assure that the drug was not active at the 20% level, then the next step would presumably be to try another drug. If the drug is active, then perhaps it will be incorporated into Phase III studies of first-line therapy for patients with that disease.

BACKGROUND AND RATIONALE

The background section should contain both the preclinical and the clinical rationale for the trial. Thorough literature review should assure that the question has not already been answered, a risk which is most likely if a "good idea" has already undergone several negative trials. If the question involves an experimental drug the IND sponsor (see Chapter 3) may have important updated information and be aware of all current trials. Not all information is published, particularly negative results.

If there has already been extensive experimentation in the disease, tables summarizing the previous trials are often most helpful. If there is a previous protocol on whose findings this one is based, the rationale and sequence of ideas should be clear. If one arm from the previous study is to be considered the "standard" arm of this study, detailed results should be given, particularly if the study is not yet published, with a thoughtful justification for any changes in schedule. Chapter 6 discusses the reasons why it is important to include concurrent randomized control arms, even if this represents the repetition of an arm from a previous study.

Of course we all hope that the experiments we perform will be worthy of publication upon completion and a protocol should be written with that eventual aim in mind. The background and rationale should be written in such a way that they will serve as a good basis for the discussion section of an eventual peer reviewed manuscript. They should explain not only what is planned but *why*. This is the critical portion of the document which serves to educate those who are to use the protocol, so that they will be able to administer the therapy properly and also so that they can carry on rational discussions with the patient and family about the relative risks and benefits of participation.

PATIENT ELIGIBILITY

Specific criteria for patient eligibility differ for each type of protocol. These criteria must be carefully spelled out so that if an intervention is shown to be successful or unsuccessful, the medical and scientific community know to what population of patients the results are referable. It must be remembered that patients referred to a cancer center for study may not necessarily be representative of patients as a whole with the same diagnosis.

Examples of specific criteria that must be mentioned in the protocol are discussed below.

1. *Nature and quantity of disease.* Is histologic confirmation of the diagnosis required? If not, how will the diagnosis be proven? What stages of disease can be treated? What amount of disease should the patient have? Is it necessary that the patients have measurable disease, evaluable disease, or completely resected disease?

2. *Eligible subsets of patients.* What age? What performance status and expected survival? Reasons for the importance of this particular prognostic designation are discussed in Chapter 3. What other prognostic subgroups? A trial in acute leukemia, for example, might show very different results if all patients regardless of age or white count are included than it would if the trial were restricted to patients with white counts $< 10,000/mm^3$ at diagnosis who were over 2 and under 10.

3. *Eligibility of previously treated patients.* If previously treated patients are eligible, would treatment with a particular drug (e.g. an analog of the one under study) render them ineligible, or cause them to be stratified and randomized separately? Specific descriptions of the amount and nature of prior therapy allowed must be made.

If a particular prognostic feature has been shown to be extremely important in previous studies (e.g., stage), then entry should be restricted for this criterion or patients should be stratified for this factor to assure that adequate balance within treatment groups will occur. Some statisticians advise that the eligibility criteria be very broad, because subset analyses can always be performed later. This approach has the following deficiencies: (a) considerable effort and resources may be expended studying patients who may not be expected to benefit from or tolerate a new therapy; (b) misleading conclusions may result from multiple subset analyses; and (c) one must be careful to plan the study so that adequate numbers of patients within each major subset are available for subset analysis. On the other hand, if the eligibility criteria are broad and no subset analysis is performed, then a conclusion of no difference may result from a positive effect in one subset being cancelled out by a negative effect in another. Before deciding what your specific criteria are going to be, be sure that you have access to enough patients within the groups you have chosen to answer the question.

TREATMENT PROGRAM INCLUDING SCHEMATIC DIAGRAM

This section should start with a concise rephrasing of the question to be asked in the protocol. For example:

"This protocol is designed to compare 6 courses with 15 courses of chemotherapy after surgery for the effect on disease-free survival in tumor X. All patients will receive the same treatment for the first 6 courses. They will then be randomized, if still in remission, to receive no further therapy (Arm A) or 9 further courses of therapy (Arm B)."

A protocol should give a detailed statement of the regimen of treatment each group of patients is to receive. The doses should be given by unit (e.g., mg/m^2)

and, if the investigators wish to limit the total maximal permissible doses, these should be stated both for individual doses (e.g., 2 mg for vincristine), and for lifetime doses (e.g., 450 mg/m^2 daunorubicin in patients who do not receive mediastinal irradiation and 350 mg/m^2 in those who do).

The specific method of administering each drug and precautions to be taken must be spelled out in detail; for example, the amount of fluid needed before, during, and after each intravenous dose and why; the possible local toxicity at the injection site; relation of oral drug administration to meals. Any other agents that are to be given concurrently, (e.g., as antidotes to toxicity or to promote drug excretion) should be given with doses.

It is important to make clear how long the total time and amount of treatment should be. If in your overall plan you expect to give 15 courses of treatment at monthly intervals, you should also clearly decide whether, if a choice must be made, you want to treat for 15 months and then stop even if several doses of drug have had to be omitted or delayed because of established toxicity criteria or whether you want to get in 15 total courses of therapy no matter how long that takes. The answer to this question depends on your principal aim but it should be clear in your protocol. It is generally easier to prescribe a certain number of courses than it is to prescribe a certain minimum time.

The time intervals between treatments must also be clearly stated if the courses are intermittent. It is not enough to say "repeat treatment every 3–4 weeks." Does that mean there should be a 3-week interval between the last day of course 1 and the first day of course 2 or does it mean that course 2 should start 3 weeks from the first day of course 1? Making these intervals identical will result in more uniform behavior on the part of your coinvestigators and you will be better able to estimate the patients' tolerance for the treatment, since schedule changes will be done on the basis of stated toxicity criteria rather than at the investigators' whim or misinterpretation of your instructions.

Many protocols will employ different treatment regimens for different phases of the disease. For example, in leukemia, treatment is often divided into three phases: (a) *Induction*, i.e., that phase of treatment which goes on until there is no longer any visible disease; (b) *Consolidation*, a short phase of intensive treatment once remission has been achieved and; (c) *Maintenance*, where patients are treated for some arbitrarily defined period of time to attempt to eradicate the last tumor cell. The description of treatment for each phase should be clearly delineated.

Even if your study is not comparative and you think duration of therapy will be short for most patients, it is wise to put some limit on treatment. If this is a Phase II study, you must define what duration of treatment should be given before the patient is considered a failure and also how long treatment should be given if the patient should have a response. There is a general discussion of these issues in Chapter 8.

It is a good idea to give a schematic diagram of the study design showing the randomization(s) for the various groups of patients. In some of the big, multidisciplinary studies of single diseases such as Wilms' tumor and rhabdomyosarcoma these schemas can be extremely complex and extremely helpful. Whenever possible, specific drug doses should be included on the schema. Once a schema is made available, people may no longer look at the body of the protocol itself, so if a dose is to be adjusted, then that adjustment must be clearly indicated on the schema (see Table 11.2 for an example).

AGENT INFORMATION

General background information about each agent including physical and chemical descriptions similar to those in a package insert need to be given in one section of the protocol along with a description of how the drugs are formulated and by whom they are supplied. Important toxicities should be mentioned in this section as well as any drugs or solvents with which the agent is incompatible. Local toxicity of the agent should be described as well as systemic effects. If there are precautions that should be observed by the individuals administering or formulating the agent, those should be noted here as well. In general, the package inserts for commercially available drugs, or, if the drug is experimental, the clinical brochure from the IND sponsor will be the best sources of this information. The IND sponsor will, in addition, have a drug monitor for each experimental agent, with whom it is possible to speak directly. It is critical that the pharmacist have access to all the pertinent information about the agent and also about the record keeping that may be required before the study begins.

DOSAGE MODIFICATION AND PROCEDURES TO BE FOLLOWED IN EVENT OF TOXICITY

The first statement in this section should again be an overall description of the philosophy of dosage adjustment for toxicity. It should be clear whether it is more important to get in a total dose of drug, even if there will be delay between doses, or more important to give the drug on schedule even if it has to be given in reduced doses. Even though detailed instructions about how to adjust the dose for toxicity must also be given, this sort of overall summary will help all coinvestigators deal with situations that may not be completely covered in the toxicity guidelines. If the major thrust of the investigation is to achieve peak levels of a particular agent, then reduced doses should not be given on schedule if the patient's white count is too low, but rather the dose should be delayed until it is felt the full dose will be tolerated. For example, if the study is to evaluate the effect of 6-mercaptopurine given at high intravenous doses in order to achieve significant levels in the spinal fluid, the purpose will not be accomplished if the drug is given at 25% of the originally scheduled dose, even if the patient could "tolerate" that level (4). On the other hand, if the question involves a comparison of schedules, such as maintenance courses given every 4 weeks compared with every 8 weeks in acute leukemia (5), then obviously the drug should be given on schedule even if doses have to be reduced.

TABLE 11.2. Schema for multiinstitutional protocol of Hodgkin's disease showing time frame and doses with dose modifications for chemotherapy[a]

	MOPP/ABVD	MOPP/ABVD	MOPP/ABVD	MOPP/ABVD			
Approx. month	0 1	2 3[b]	4 5	6[b] 7	8	9[c]	

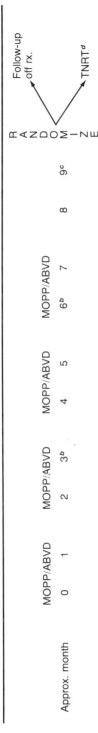

R
A
N
D
O
M → Follow-up off rx.
I
Z → TNRT[d]
E

Each 2-month cycle is as follows:

MOPP
Mustargen: 6 mg/m² i.v. push days 1,8
Oncovin: 1.5 mg/m² i.v. push days 1,8
Procarbazine: 100 mg/m² p.o. days 1–14
Prednisone: 40 mg/m² p.o. days 1–14

ABVD
Adriamycin: 25 mg/m² i.v. push days 29,43
Bleomycin: 10 mg/m² i.v. push days 29,43
Vinblastine: 6 mg/m² i.v. push days 29,43
Dacarbazine: 375 mg/m² i.v. push days 29,43

[a] See Appendix to protocol for chemotherapy dose modifications.
[b] Clinical restaging. Includes CT of chest.
[c] At 9 mos. patients are restaged. Those with suspected residual disease will have biopsy. If positive, patient is off study. If patient is felt to be disease free, randomized to no further treatment or TNRT to begin 6 weeks after end of chemotherapy.
[d] TNRT = 3 weeks—mantle (150 cGy/fraction × 14); 2 weeks—rest; 3 weeks—paraaortic nodes and spleen (150 cGy/fraction × 14)*; 2 weeks—rest; 3 weeks—pelvic field (150 cGy/fraction × 14). Withhold XRT for 1 week if APC ≤ 1000 uL and platelets ≤ 75,000 uL.
See Section 6.4 of protocol for additional regions to be treated at discretion of radiotherapist and section 6.5 for further discussion of dosage modification.

If the toxicities of the drug are already well known, then the dosage modifications should be spelled out in detail for each important one. When dealing with blood counts it should be clearly stated whether the modification is to be made on the basis of the nadir reached in the counts (in which case the patient will have had to have had blood counts drawn often enough to have some ideas of what the nadir was and when it occurred) or whether adjustments will be made only on the basis of the counts on the day the next dose of medication is scheduled to be given. Specific instructions should be given for other toxicities as well. For example, for an anthracycline, the level of change in the QT interval or ejection fraction that will be considered sufficiently severe to result in holding or reducing a dose should be stated. Vague phrases such as "monitor cardiac function closely" should be avoided. Imagine yourself as a house officer who knows nothing about oncology reading the instructions and write them accordingly. Standard toxicity criteria can be referred to. It is permissible to say: "The dose of drug should be reduced by 50% for the next course if Grade III–IV gastrointestinal toxicity was seen with the previous course." This then might represent dosage reduction for mucositis, nausea and vomiting, ileus, or diarrhea, but the reason for dosage modification should be precisely recorded. (These grades should obviously be defined elsewhere in the protocol.)

If the criteria for dosage adjustment will be different for each period during the protocol, be sure to indicate this. In leukemia, for example, low blood counts will not be considered a reason for stopping the initial course of induction therapy when they are most reasonably ascribed to disease infiltrating the marrow, although it might well be a reason for delaying therapy during maintenance.

Some protocols include an instruction to increase the dose of drug if a previous course has been well tolerated. If this is planned, the degree of toxicity that will permit dose escalation should be clearly noted, for example, "escalate dose by 10% if nadir granulocyte from previous course is above $1000/mm^3$ and no other dose-limiting toxicity was seen." If this is a combination drug study, it should be clear whether all drugs, or only one is to be escalated. In general, it seems most logical to escalate only one drug at a time.

This section should also include advice about what to do to alleviate symptoms if toxicity has occurred. Note, for example, that steroid eyedrops and premedication with systemic steroids are often helpful if a patient has developed a febrile reaction to cytosine arabinoside with conjunctivitis. If remedies that are known to be effective are recommended rather than left to the discretion of the individual physician administering the protocol, the patients will benefit and the treatment program will be more homogeneous.

Procedures to be followed to document the severity of toxicity should be outlined. How often should each test be done? If a specific symptom or sign appears, what workup should be done? If a patient has hematuria, is cystoscopy required to evaluate the degree of bladder involvement? If it is important that an expected toxicity be recorded (e.g., neuropathy or alopecia from vincristine), make special requests for this and include a place on your forms for them, since once a toxicity is expected, it often goes unremarked in the record, particularly if it is not considered dangerous by the physician caring for the patient.

Another important instruction that must be included in this section is what to do if there is severe toxicity (see Chapter 13 also). Expected but unusually severe toxicity and, particularly, *unexpected* severe toxicity should be reported promptly by the investigator to the drug sponsor and the Food and Drug Administration (FDA). If the drug is already on the market, then the investigator should report unexpected severe toxicity to the drug company as well as directly to the FDA. An example of an unhappy surprise with a drug which has been used by the medical community for a while occurred when BCNU (bischloroethyl nitrosourea), a drug that had been given intravenously to many patients with brain tumors, was given intraarterially in an investigational setting. In the first few patients the drug was found to cause blindness if injected into the carotid artery proximal to the takeoff of the ophthalmic artery (6). Blindness had never before been reported with this drug and the oncologic community needed to be rapidly alerted to this problem. Central reporting serves as an early warning system to all investigators using a particular agent or protocol. The National Cancer Institute's *Investigator's Handbook* (7) describes the method for this sort of notification.

REQUIRED LABORATORY AND CLINICAL DATA

The list of required studies should be as short as possible while still including all the information needed to evaluate the extent of disease and the toxicity of the treatment. It is usually necessary to require some tests that are consistent with good medical practice and which, in the long run, may not be used for evaluation of the therapy. An example might be some tests to determine the risks of urate nephropathy in patients with acute leukemia or lymphoma at the time of presentation. The more tests required, however, the more expensive and more difficult it will be for the patients and the harder it will be to have evaluable patients on study. The intervals at which tests are required should also be carefully considered. If liver functions need only be assessed every 4 weeks, before each dose of medicine, they should not be required on a weekly basis just out of curiosity. More evaluations for toxicity will be necessary when agents or combinations about which little is known are being studied. Review the work of others and make this section as efficient and "lean" as possible. Remember that no matter how interested you might be in studying a new technique such as magnetic resonance imaging in the evaluation of a tumor, the proper facilities may not be available in every institution participating in your study and you may decrease patient accrual if you require such a study for each entry. Discuss these with your colleagues before you write your final protocol draft.

CRITERIA FOR EVALUATING THE EFFECT OF TREATMENT

These must also be extremely specific. The definition of what constitutes complete response, partial response, and progressive disease should be spelled out including which tests are to be used to define each one (see Chapter 2). Defining disease response in terms of the measurement of individual lesions may not be sufficient. If a previously packed bone marrow of a patient with leukemia becomes aplastic, is this a complete response, or do you insist that normal marrow cellularity, cell composition, and peripheral counts be established before the patient is considered to have responded? Is second-look surgery required before a patient is considered to have been completely evaluated? Which tests specifically need to be repeated? Just the ones that were abnormal when therapy began or all the initial tests? Are there new tests that should be added? For example, a patient who originally had disease grossly visible on chest X-ray and who now has a normal chest X-ray might be required to have, in addition, a CT scan of the chest to define complete remission.

CRITERIA FOR REMOVING A PATIENT FROM STUDY

The criteria for removing a patient from study should be just as precise as those for patient eligibility. If toxicity will be a cause for removal then state what grade; if patients will be removed from study if they fail to respond or show progressive disease, then these terms must be defined as well as the number of treatments to be given before this decision is made.

STATISTICAL CONSIDERATIONS

The statistical considerations vary from one type of trial to the next (see Chapters 3–6). An appropriate general description of the methods to be used should be given. The section in the protocol must explain what the anticipated minimal and maximal patient accrual will be to meet the needs of the study and how rapidly it is expected that this goal will be met. Some sort of stopping rule should be described so that if one arm turns out to be more toxic or significantly less effective than anticipated, patients will not be entered indefinitely on such therapy. A description should be given as to how often and by whom the data will be evaluated to determine whether the study should continue, and what techniques will be used to achieve this.

REFERENCES

These do not need to be exhaustive but they should be complete enough to allow readers to evaluate for themselves the statements made in the background section and should serve as the basis for the discussion section in the eventual report of the study. If the protocol is aimed at clarifying a debated issue, references supporting both points of view should be included.

FORMS

Data management is a very important part of the conduct of a clinical trial, particularly for multiinstitutional studies. Obtaining reliable data requires the same planning and professional expertise as the other aspects of the study. You cannot expect that your co-workers will spontaneously note items about a patient that might be of interest to you unless you include those items on the forms and specifically request them. For example, if you wish to have the patient weighed on a regular basis, you must provide a place on the form where weight can be recorded and then review those forms from time to time to see whether those boxes are being filled out, and encourage people to do so if they are not.

Every question on your forms should require an answer even if the answer is "not done" or "not examined" (8). Too often it is assumed that a test was done and was normal if there is no notation. In addition, forms should be designed so that the answers given on them can be easily coded for entry into a computer. That means that nonnumerical information should be reduced to numerical codes, for example, for a Hodgkin's disease study under histology:

1 = Nodular sclerosing
2 = Mixed cellularity
3 = Lymphocyte predominant
4 = Lymphocyte depleted
8 = Other ___(describe)___

Every question on your forms should require an answer and you should think through all possible answers. An entry such as:

Liver scan   1. normal   2. metastases

is not as helpful as:

Liver scan   1—normal   2—metastases   9—not done.

An even more helpful question could be:

Liver scan: 1—normal;   2—metastases;
        8—other abnormality (describe);   9—not done.

As with required tests, required observations should be kept to the minimum that is consistent with the information needed. Forms should be arranged with sufficient space for all the necessary information.

The question of whether information should be directly entered into a computer, if the capability exists, should also be considered. The advantage of computer flow sheets is that the material is available in a form that permits easy analysis without reentry, and therefore with one less possibility for error in transferring. The disadvantages are that, if you are going to deal with your information principally on paper, the printouts are bulkier and harder to follow than a flow sheet that has been filled in by hand, and the marginal comments which may summarize or explain an observation are often lost.

On-Study Forms

Some sort of initial synopsis or summary of the patient status at the time of entry on study must be made. Generally it should include diagnosis, how it was established, and staging with details of what examinations were performed and what the results were, including relevant negative studies. What other demographic information do you want about the patient? Does it matter if the patient has siblings and is therefore a potential allogeneic marrow transplant candidate? What items in the prior history do you want to know? Are the patient's smoking or drinking habits relevant? Do not waste your time collecting information you are never going to use. How will you record the prior treatment (if any)? If this is a randomized study, be sure to indicate which arm of treatment the patient was randomized to receive, since you will need this information later to check on whether they actually got what they were supposed to get.

Flow Sheets

The next set of forms you require may be the flow sheets for follow-up information about the patients. Make sure that you have sufficient room on the flow sheets to record the information you need. Remember that there are certain critical items that need to appear on all sheets. The date must be noted, including *year*, which is often not entered by the investigator and should be checked by the principal investigator when reviewing the sheets. Sheets should be numbered, but that is often forgotten too and if you have neither year nor the number it may be very difficult to reconstitute the patients' course in a long study if you get the sheets out of order.

What medications were given and in what dose? Make sure that the dose recorded is clearly marked as the dose given or the dose/m^2 or dose/kg. For some medications a total lifetime dose should be recorded as well. Radiation therapy should be noted with daily dose as well as total dose. Record surgery and the findings; operations required by protocol will probably require a separate set of forms. Should other medications that are given, such as antibiotics, transfusions, and antiemetics, be recorded? The collection and analysis of these data entail hours of work, and should perhaps be omitted if they are not necessary for the interpretation of the study.

The physical status of the patient, including performance status and certain critical historical items and physical findings need to be recorded. These latter will vary by which disease you are following. For patients on a leukemia study, adenopathy, hepatosplenomegaly, and testicular size are crucial items. For patients with a brain tumor, these items could be omitted but certain features of a minimal neurologic exam should be recorded. See Table 11.3 for examples of how widely the physical examination portion of flow sheets may differ in different diseases.

The item that is usually least well recorded is tumor size. Index lesions should be measured at each visit and the size recorded. If this cannot be done, the reason should be noted. These measurements should be reviewed by the study chairman with sufficient frequency, that if the measurements are not being recorded, this can be called to the attention of the primary physician who is supposed to be doing it. Measurements should be recorded while the patient is present, particularly if one is seeing several patients in one day, for these measurements are difficult to remember precisely, let alone determine precisely.

TABLE 11.3. *Physical examination portion of brain tumor and hematology flow sheets*[a]

Brain Tumor Flow Sheet

					Comments
Date		___	___	___	
General Neuro. Exam					
24. Conscious state		___	___	___	
25. Headache		___	___	___	
26. Nausea/vomiting		___	___	___	
27. Seizures		___	___	___	
28. Abnormal gait		___	___	___	
29. Double vision		___	___	___	
30. Blurred vision		___	___	___	
31. Muscle strength		___	___	___	
32. Babinski		___	___	___	
33. Papilledema		___	___	___	
34. Reflexes: Biceps		___	___	___	
35. Triceps		___	___	___	
36. Patellar		___	___	___	
37. Ankle		___	___	___	
Infratentorial					
38. Romberg's sign		___	___	___	
39. Nystagmus H/V		___	___	___	
40. Finger/nose		___	___	___	
41. Heel/shin		___	___	___	
42. Posit. sense (toe)		___	___	___	
43. EOM function		___	___	___	
44. Bladder/bowel function		___	___	___	
Supratentorial					
45. Time/place		___	___	___	
46. Calculation		___	___	___	
47. Object recognition		___	___	___	
48. Extinction		___	___	___	
49. Hemianopsia		___	___	___	
50. Aphasia		___	___	___	
Response					
51. Performance status		___	___	___	
52. Objective tumor size		___	___	___	
53. Subjective		___	___	___	
54. Same/better/worse		___	___	___	

Hematology Flow Sheet

				Comments
Date	___	___	___	
Physical Exam				
41. Temp.	___	___	___	
42. Wt. (kg) Ht. (cm)	___	___	___	
43. Liver (cm)	___	___	___	
44. Spleen (cm)	___	___	___	
45. Max. node (cm) Cerv.	___	___	___	
46. Ax.	___	___	___	
47. Ing.	___	___	___	
48. Left testis (cm)	___	___	___	
49. Right testis (cm)	___	___	___	
50. Infection	___	___	___	
51. Performance	___	___	___	

[a]All observations are numbered for computer compatibility.

NOTE: The portion of the brain tumor flow sheet which deals with the physical examination is markedly different from that for leukemia. The blank space at the side remains open for remarks.

In addition, laboratory data will have to be recorded: hematology, chemistry, tumor marker data. There will have to be a place to record studies done such as X-rays, bone scans, lumbar punctures. Any instruction necessary for filling out the forms should be included on the form, for example, if you are asking your co-workers to note the grade of a particular toxicity, then make sure the definitions of those grades are present on the back of the form, or the task will be done inaccurately. There is often not sufficient room to record both the actual data and the grade of a toxicity and leave the flow sheet only one page long. It is always preferable to have the actual data and then grade the toxicity yourself as you review the flow sheet. Any flow sheet should have space for freehand comments since there has to be some place where the physician can indicate important items such as why a medication dose was held or reduced. These cannot all be anticipated and coded in advance. For example, one of the authors held medicine on some patients because of a hurricane which made it impossible for them to get to clinic on a particular day. Remember, if you are keeping computerized flow sheets there has to be some mechanism developed for making sure that all information, including any marginal freehand comments are entered in the computer memory.

Off-Study Forms

The next form that might be needed is an off-study form if the patient should relapse, or show progressive disease or intolerable toxicity. Here again, the items that need to be recorded should be carefully considered as the form is drawn up. Describe the reason for a patient coming off study. Note tumor progression, tumor response, toxicity (describe), and death. Is the treatment complete as called for in the protocol? Other? The form must provide adequate space for this information.

If the patient remains in continuous complete remission on the protocol, there will be a need for regular follow-up and check on the patients' status. There may also be a need for a study of late effects of treatment. These forms are often developed after an original protocol when some appreciation has developed of what possible late effects there might be.

Notification of Death

Even if the patient has been off study for some time when this occurs, it is often necessary to have this information so that survival analyses can be performed.

Evaluation Forms for the Study Coordinator

Separate forms should be developed, if the study is large enough to warrant them, that the study coordinator can use to summarize all the patients' data. These should also be compatible for computer entry. They will presumably not be necessary for a Phase II trial which entered only 15 patients in whom no response was seen, but will be necessary for a large, multiinstitutional Phase III study and should be drafted together with the statistical office personnel.

Informed Consent

This topic is covered in the next chapter. A protocol cannot be activated without a formal consent form, which must be reviewed and approved by the appropriate committees within and outside your institution. This form is explained to each individual who enters the study and signed by them before they are registered as participants.

The writing of the protocol is only one step in the development of a study. Once the protocol has been written, it must be reviewed by colleagues within the institution and often outside as well. A good protocol is the foundation of a good experiment and the time invested in making it an excellent scientific document will not be wasted.

REFERENCES

1. Webster's Ninth New Collegiate Dictionary, (1983). Merriam Webster, Inc. Springfield, Massachusetts.
2. Sullivan, M. P., Fuller, L. M., Chen, T., et al. (1982): Intergroup Hodgkin's disease in children, study of Stages I and II: A preliminary report. *Cancer Treat. Rep.*, 66:937–947.
3. Simon, R. M. (1982): Design and conduct of clinical trials. In: *Cancer: Principles and Practice of Oncology*, edited by V. T. DeVita, Jr., S. Hellman, and S. A. Rosenberg, pp. 198–225, 1st ed. Lippincott, Philadelphia.
4. Zimm, S., Ettinger, L. J., Holcenberg, J. S., et al. (1985): Phase I and clinical pharmacological study of mercaptopurine administered as a prolonged intravenous infusion. *Cancer Res.*, 45:1869–1873.
5. Yates, J., Glidewell, O., Wiernik, P., et al. (1982): Cytosine arabinoside with daunorubicin or adriamycin for therapy of acute myelocytic leukemia: A CALGB study. *Blood*, 60:454–462.
6. Greenberg, H. S., Ensminger, W. D., Chandler, W. F., et al. (1984): Intraarterial BCNU chemotherapy for treatment of malignant gliomas of the central nervous system. *J. Neurosurg.*, 61:423–429.
7. *Investigator's Handbook* (1986): Cancer Therapy Evaluation Program, Division of Cancer Treatment, National Cancer Institute.
8. DePauw, M., and Buyse, M. (1984): Design of forms for cancer clinical trials. In: *Cancer Clinical Trials: Methods and Practice*, edited by M. E. Buyse, M. J. Staquet, and R. J. Sylvester, pp. 64–82. Oxford University Press, Oxford.

CHAPTER 12

Protection of Human Subjects

Research involving human beings differs in many obvious ways from the scientific study of laboratory animals, cells, or cell-free systems. The dual role of research physician and care giver is sometimes an uneasy one, and ethical dilemmas of one sort or another intrude quite commonly in the design and conduct of human experimentation. As the process has matured over the years, society has evolved certain rules that serve as procedural and ethical guidelines. These rules have not evolved in a vacuum, of course; to the contrary, they have resulted in part from some terrible experiences that occurred in settings that either lacked adequate societal oversight or were altogether devoid of normal ethical standards. In this chapter we shall examine briefly how current notions of informed consent and the protection of human subjects in research arose. We shall also outline the current standards in the U.S. for the protection of human subjects. Protection is assured chiefly by two processes: (a) the institutional review of studies involving human subjects; (b) the informed consent process.

BACKGROUND

Although the procedures necessary to assure protection of human subjects is both time consuming and sometimes frustrating, the process is essential. The large-scale coopting of the German medical profession by the Nazis and the participation of many physicians in the torture of prisoners under the guise of ''scientific research'' illustrate starkly what can happen when the process of research goes mad along with the society in which it is embedded.

In 1947, the Nuremberg code was drafted as a set of standards for judging physicians and scientists who had conducted biomedical experiments on concentration camp prisoners. This code became the prototype of many later codes including the Helsinki Declaration of 1964, intended to assure that research involving human subjects would be carried out in an ethical manner (1).

Unfortunately, unethical research is not confined to wartime settings or rabidly racist societies. In an interesting review, Beecher (2) examined 100 consecutive human studies published in 1964 in an excellent journal. He judged 12 of them to be unethical. He includes examples of 22 studies which represent various categories of experimentation. The categories include research on patient volunteers and normal subjects; therapeutic research; and experimentation on a patient not for his benefit but for that, at least in theory, of patients in general. Two examples are reproduced here:

Example 1

In a study of the effect of thymectomy on the survival of skin homografts, 18 children, age 3 months to 18 years of age, about to undergo surgery for congenital heart disease, were selected. Eleven were to have total thymectomy as part of the operation, and 7 were to serve as controls. As part of the experimentation, full thickness skin homografts from an unrelated adult donor were sutured to the chest wall in each case. Total thymectomy is occasionally, although not usually part of the primary cardiovascular surgery involved, and whereas it may not greatly add to the hazards of the necessary operation, its eventual effects in children are not known. This work was proposed as part of a long-range study of the "growth and development of these children over the years." No difference in the survival of the skin homograft was observed in the 2 groups.

Regardless of the specific ethical dilemmas this work is an example of badly flawed experimental design. Even with highly inbred mice the difference in survival time of skin grafts is small enough that large numbers of animals are required for reliable detection of differences. In the clinical trial described above a three- to fourfold difference in survival times of the grafts would have been required to approach a statistically significant result with this small number of patients.

Example 2

Melanoma was transplanted from a daughter to her volunteering and "informed" mother, "in the hope of gaining a little better understanding of cancer immunity and in the hope that the production of tumor antibodies might be helpful in the treatment of the cancer patient." Since the daughter died on the day after the transplantation of the tumor into her mother, the hope expressed seems to have been more theoretical than practical, and the daughter's condition was described as "terminal" at the time her mother volunteered to be a recipient. The primary implant was widely excised on the twenty-fourth day after it had been placed in the mother. She died from metastatic melanoma on the 451st day after transplantation. The evidence that this patient died of diffuse melanoma that metastasized from a small piece of transplanted tumor was considered conclusive.

The death of the mother in this case adds to the horror of the story, but even without it, this study was badly flawed, since it was performed in a patient far too ill to benefit.

It is clear from these examples that certain experiments conducted by individuals ostensibly in the mainstream of academic medicine should never have been performed. The need of the medical profession to monitor itself according to ethical standards is obvious. As we note later, ethical dilemmas may well diminish if clinical trials are designed with attention to reasonable scientific principles.

INSTITUTIONAL REVIEW

In response to the growing concern with the protection of human subjects, the concept arose that all research projects must be reviewed by an Institutional Review

Board (IRB) which would include as members other scientists, individuals from nonscientific disciplines, and lay people. In other words, the researcher himself is no longer considered an adequate sole judge of the ethics of his research. Each IRB is a local organization serving the institution within which it operates. If the institution is receiving federal support for research, then the IRB must operate within the scope of broad federal guidelines. These, however, are procedural rather than substantive, and federal regulation recognizes the primacy of the local IRB in determining what may or may not proceed within its institution (3).

In a typical large research institution, most often associated with a major university, research involving human subjects is carried out under an "assurance of compliance." This is a formal agreement with the federal government and includes descriptions of the administration of the institution and the process by which protocols involving human subjects (except for a few specifically exempt categories, such as some noninvasive behavioral research) will be forwarded to an IRB for review and approval. Members of the IRB are required to possess expertise in the scientific disciplines most closely related to the research to be reviewed. Additionally, there must be at least one nonscientist member of the board and at least one member of the board who is in no other way affiliated with the institution. In addition to this general assurance, each specific protocol submitted to a federal agency for funding must be accompanied by certification of IRB review and approval. Each active protocol must be reviewed at least annually by the IRB. All of these procedures must not only be completed but documented by the individual investigator as well as by the institution. The investigator should realize that his compliance with the appropriate regulations reflects on his entire institution.

INFORMED CONSENT

The earliest medical consent lawsuits arose when surgery was done without consent, and the courts found the surgeons liable for battery. If consent is obtained, even if it is later judged that insufficient information was given to the patient, the courts have held that the consent will protect from liability for battery. It is "informed consent," however, that protects from liability for negligence (4). Courts have developed two standards for determining the adequacy of disclosure. The "reasonable physician" standard holds that the disclosure should be that which a reasonable medical practitioner would make under the same or similar circumstances. The "reasonable patient" standard provides that the duty to disclose is determined by the informational needs of the patient, not by professional practice. Research activities generally adhere to the "reasonable patient" standard; and the patient should be provided with the amount and quality of information any reasonable individual would need to make a decision under the circumstances.

In its broadest sense, informed consent refers to the entire complex process by which the patient is made to understand the treatment that is being proposed. Thus, the informed consent process may include a series of interactions involving many physicians and may extend over hours, days, or months. Informed consent does not start when the study is proposed, nor does it stop once the patient has agreed to participate in a trial. It should rather be viewed as an ongoing educational effort, one that requires patience and reinforcement.

In a narrow sense, however, informed consent is often used to denote the process surrounding the signing of a specific document that outlines certain relevant details about the particular study and acknowledges the patient's willingness to participate in it. For studies supported by federal funds, the consent form must include certain elements deemed essential by federal regulation (5) (see Table 12.1). Federal regulation does not prescribe how the consent form is to be worded; it merely stipulates that the consent form must address in adequate and understandable fashion certain generic issues common to all research protocols. The precise wording of the consent form is a local matter and is under the jurisdiction of the local IRB, which is responsible for reviewing and approving the consent form before it is used. If the protocol involves administration of investigational agents, the sponsor of the research (e.g., the National Cancer Institute or a pharmaceutical firm) must also review the form for the presence of the essential elements and for adequacy of disclosure.

ELEMENTS OF INFORMED CONSENT

All of the elements listed in Table 12.1 must appear in the form in understandable lay language (5). These include a description of the patient's diagnosis and condition, a description of the proposed study with an explanation of its purpose, and

TABLE 12.1. *Elements of informed consent*

A. Basic elements
    1. State that it is research
        a. Give purposes
        b. Describe planned treatment
        c. Specify which procedures are experimental
    2. Describe risks
    3. Describe benefits
    4. Describe alternatives to participation
    5. Describe confidentiality
    6. Explain compensation or treatment for injury
    7. State whom to contact for answers in regard to:
        a. Research
        b. Subjects' rights
        c. Injury
    8. Explain right to refuse and withdraw
B. Additional elements required when appropriate
    1. Currently unforseeable risks
    2. Why an investigator might withdraw a subject
    3. Additional costs to subject
    4. Consequences of subjects' withdrawal
    5. Informing patient of new findings
    6. Number of patients
C. Assent form may be required from a minor

Adapted from Ref. 5.

a clear statement as to which elements of the treatment are experimental. The treatment must be described in general including what studies and procedures will be required, and how long the treatment will last. It must be clear how the treatment the patient is to receive is selected. If the trial is randomized, consent must be secured before randomization, so the patient must agree to any of the proposed arms, as well as to the process of randomization itself. The patient must be informed about the known risks of the treatment and the possibility of unknown risks. The possible benefits should be described. It must be made clear that the patient's participation is voluntary and the patient must also be told what would be considered standard therapy for this condition, if such exists, or at any rate whether any alternative therapies exist that are worthy of mention, including, perhaps, no active therapy at all.

Patients must understand that if they refuse randomization, they *cannot* choose to receive experimental therapy. The patient should not get the impression that he is being offered a choice of A, X, *or* a randomization between the two. Truly experimental therapy should be offered only in the setting where knowledge about efficacy will be gathered and this can only be in the context of a clinical trial.

There must be some discussion of the effect the patient's decision will have on the care at a particular institution. If the institution does only experimental therapy, may the patient stay if he does not agree to be on study? If the experimental drug would be free, will a patient have to pay if he or she wishes to have standard therapy? In addition, the responsibilities that the institution or sponsoring drug company is willing or not willing to assume in the event of possible injury should be carefully spelled out. The patient must also be informed of the extent to which individuals outside of the immediate medical staff will have access to his or her medical record. Sponsors of experimental therapy or representatives of the Food and Drug Administration, for example, may require access for various reasons, and patient consent for this should be part of the informed consent process.

For randomized trials, there should be some sort of assurance that if it should turn out that Arm A is clearly better than Arm B, the patients will be informed and given a chance for the more effective treatment if medically appropriate. In one notorious case, prisoners in Tuskegee, Alabama, were randomized to receive or not receive penicillin for syphilis. Years later, when it had clearly been proven that antibiotic therapy was beneficial, the control group was not contacted and notified that they should be treated (6). The scandal which surrounded the discovery of this oversight was one of the stimuli to the development of the current regulations.

In a cancer treatment study, where the endpoint is disease recurrence or death, it is often not practical to consider switching the patient to the other arm of the study. If the trial involves an untreated control group, and it appears that the treatment is effective in delaying appearance of metastatic disease, it might be reasonable to state, as part of the protocol that the patient will receive the treatment should disease recur. In a recent multiinstitutional study of osteosarcoma (7), for example, all patients with disease recurrence on the untreated control arm had metastatic disease resected where possible, and were started on chemotherapy. Here the only safeguard is to assure the patient that the data will be closely supervised and that the randomization will be discontinued as soon as the investigators are convinced that there is a real difference between the two arms of the study.

A copy of the form should be given to the patient for later reference. In addition, the form must include the name and telephone number of someone whom that patient can call if they have questions or problems. Most institutions will have outlines and sample forms that meet their individual requirements.

Despite the time and effort it takes to construct a consent form and the number of individuals who will end up reviewing it, the most important communication with the patient is not the form, but rather the ongoing interaction with the patient and the physician's direct explanation of the study. Most patients and families are distracted and concerned with the clinical problem at the time the informed consent document is presented. Thus they are sometimes not able to concentrate on a form and absorb the information on it. They will rely most heavily on what the physician tells them, and, in fact, many may have decided to sign the form before they have read it. One must be certain, therefore, to explain the treatment adequately, with repetitions as often as needed. In addition, the patient and family should be given as much time as possible to consider the decision, even if it is only a day or so, before they are asked formally to sign the document.

SPECIAL CONSIDERATIONS REGARDING CHILDREN

There are special procedures for research relating to pregnant women, fetuses, and children (5). In general, since most anticancer agents given in therapeutic doses may be teratogenic or lead to the death of a fetus, pregnant women with cancer are not included in trials of experimental agents. The only exception might be a trial for an agent to treat a pregnancy-associated tumor such as choriocarcinoma. Children with cancer, on the other hand, are regularly involved as subjects in clinical trials. A child is defined as a person who has not attained the legal age for consent in the jurisdiction in which the research will be conducted. In most states this will be age 17 or 18 or younger if they are "emancipated," i.e., living independently without parental control or support. Federal regulations state that research involving more than minimal risk can be conducted in children only if the procedures hold out the prospect of direct benefit to the individual. Research may also be carried out if the risk is more than minimal but is about the same as conventional medical management and likely to yield generalizable knowledge about the subject's disorder.

Subjects over the age of 7 may also be required to sign an "assent" form even if the parents are the ones giving formal consent. The determination of whether children are capable of assenting is within the jurisdiction of the local IRB. In making this determination the IRB takes into account the ages of maturity and psychological state of the children involved. This judgment can be made for all children involved in research on a particular protocol or for each child as the IRB deems appropriate. Thus, the formal requirement for an "assent" procedure varies from one institution to another.

ASSESSMENT OF PATIENTS' REACTIONS

It seems clear where the sense of urgency to develop proper consent forms arose. As we have mentioned, the form itself is only part of the process, and the explanation is really the critical factor. However, a major ethical and legal question is, "Is there really any such thing as informed consent?" (8). The reason for this question is twofold: (a) The concept of consent, freely given, would seem to be jeopardized if a subtle form of coercion is involved, as, for example, in the consent of a prisoner, or the consent of a less knowledgeable person to one he perceives as more knowledgeable; (b) the patient may still not be truly "informed" even if he has been told everything appropriate for him to be told. Regarding the second point, a study at Montefiore Hospital in 1977 (9) demonstrated that a majority of surgical patients denied after surgery that they had been told about all the possible undesirable outcomes prior to the surgery, even though discussion of possible undesirable outcomes ran for an hour and a half prior to the surgery and was tape recorded. As Herbert (8) says:

> If the brain does not record, store, or recall the information supplied to it, or even suppresses that information, has there been informed consent? Is the concept of informed consent really a legalistic rather than an ethical one, with the legalisms being used instead of ethics rather than in support of ethics? In other words, if the consent form is given to the patient to sign, but the information is not registered, is it merely being used as a device to protect the physician?

Despite intense interest in these issues, things seem not to have changed much from the patients' point of view over the past 10 years. Penman et al. (10) interviewed 144 patients and 68 physicians at three cancer centers for their perceptions of the consent procedure in which they participated 1 to 3 weeks earlier. The primary reasons that the patients gave for accepting the treatment were the belief the treatment would help, trust in the physician, and fear that the disease (viewed as highly serious) would get worse without it. Nearly a fourth did not recall the information that the treatment was investigational. The consent form played no role in decision making for 69%. All patients remembered that toxicity had been discussed, but when asked to recall specific toxicities, they most commonly recalled those that related to unpleasant physical symptoms such as nausea, vomiting, or hair loss, rather than potentially more dangerous side effects such as decreased white count and infection. The physicians in general felt that therapeutic benefits would exceed potential problems for most patients, and they viewed many of the patients as not eager for discussion of details and as passive in decision making. In general, the patients felt the physicians wanted them to participate in the study and that, although they had made their own decision, they had done so principally because they had faith in their physician and the physician's institution and feared their disease. The information provided to them had little influence on their decision. The investigators concluded that the perceptual set of both parties placed inadvertent constraint on patient's autonomy in decision making.

The role of the individual who obtains consent as both the informer and the protector of the patient seems clear. However, Curran (11) writes that:

> . . . many researchers do not understand their protective duty to patients. They have heard so much about the requirement for informed consent that they assume it purifies every research design. It does not. Entry into the research study at all must be essentially reasonable for the patients. They rarely can be subjected to nonbeneficial choices not in their best interests.

ASSESSMENT OF PHYSICIANS' REACTIONS

Informed consent also poses difficulties for the physician. A certain number of physicians hesitate to offer randomized choices to patients, because they fear that doing so will compromise their relationship with the patient.

In 1974, the National Surgical Adjuvant Breast Project (NSABP) completed a randomized surgical trial demonstrating that total mastectomy, with or without radiation, was as effective as radical mastectomy in the primary treatment of cancer of the female breast. Within 38 months, 34 of the 75 NSABP institutions entered a total of 1765 patients in this controlled trial. A follow-up study was initiated to compare outcome for one of three treatments which were randomly assigned: segmental mastectomy (''lumpectomy'') without radiation, segmental mastectomy with radiation, or total mastectomy. It was projected that the accrual rate for the second trial would be equal to or higher than that in the first trial with a projected accrual of 75 patients per month. After 44 months, only 519 patients had been enrolled, an actual accrual rate of approximately 12 patients per month, or 16% of the expected rate. Thus, nonaccrual was threatening the successful completion of the trial.

A questionnaire was mailed to the 94 investigators to find out why patients were not being accrued to the new study (12). All but 2 responded; 32 (35%) had entered none, 34 (38%) some, and 25 (27%) had entered all of their eligible patients. The 66 physicians who did not enter all eligible patients on study offered the following explanations:

1. Concern that the doctor–patient relationship would be affected by a randomized clinical trial (73%). By this they meant that participation in a clinical trial, with the indecision which needed to be discussed with the patient, potentially compromised the authority of the physician.

2. Difficulty with informed consent format itself (38%).

3. Dislike of open discussions involving uncertainty (22%).

4. Perceived conflict between the roles of scientist and clinician (18%).

5. Practical difficulties in following procedures, e.g., the increased time required to obtain consent (9%).

6. Feelings of personal responsibility of the treatments were found to be unequal (8%) (12).

Most of these reasons can be summarized by saying that the surgeons participating in the trial had difficulty describing to patients their indecision about what was the best surgical procedure, and felt their traditional role as an expert with individualized decision-making power on behalf of their patients was threatened by the need to obtain consent for a randomized procedure. A major question, which was apparently not addressed by the questionnaire, was why these investigators who had entered patients on a previous trial of radical versus simple mastectomy had such difficulty with the current trial of mastectomy versus lumpectomy. One must presume that the same problems would have applied in the previous study. Angell (13) postulates that, although the treatments being compared were not known to differ in terms of their efficacy, they did differ in terms of their impact on the patients' lives and the physicians knew this. In other words, the difference to a patient between a radical and a simple mastectomy is not as great as the difference between simple mastectomy and lumpectomy. As she says: ''It is not enough for the physician to have no reason to prefer one treatment over the other; in addition, there must be no reason for the patient to prefer one treatment.''

The NSABP attempted to solve its dilemma by allowing the investigators to perform prerandomization as proposed by Zelen (14). In this design a patient is randomized without his knowledge to receive either best standard (control) treatment or experimental treatment. Zelen argued that since the control patients were receiving standard treatment, it would not be necessary to obtain informed consent from this group. Only patients who were prerandomized to the experimental therapy arm would learn that they were participating in a study and would be required to give their informed consent to participate. After much heated discussion of the ethics of this procedure, it was subsequently modified to a ''double consent randomized design'' in which patients on both study arms provided informed consent (15). Using this latter method, accrual increased sixfold to the NSABP study, which was then completed.

There are practical concerns with this type of prerandomization (16). Because the patients are randomly assigned to treatment before giving consent, there will be some proportion of randomized patients on each arm who refuse the assigned treatment. This will complicate the analysis and mean that more total patients are required to complete the trial. In addition, there are ethical problems with pre-randomization. Notably, the manner in which patients are informed about the study may be affected by the treatment assignment. Knowledge by the physician of the assigned treatment allows conscious or subconscious tailoring of the study presentation to predispose the patient to accept the assigned therapy. If the patient has been assigned to standard therapy, the physician may stress the experimental nature of the new therapy, its potential risks, and the possibility that the new therapy may be worse than the standard one. If the patient has been assigned to the experimental therapy, the physician may stress the unsatisfactory track record of the standard therapy and the promising earlier studies that indicated that the experimental therapy may be an improvement. The physician may gloss over or even omit the information that treatment has been chosen by a random mechanism and imply to the patient that the assigned therapy has been individually selected for them. One must question whether patients receiving such presentations are being completely and honestly informed about the nature and objectives of the study.

The lesson to be learned from this experience is that there are often great practical difficulties in offering patients choices that are so widely disparate (e.g., mastectomy versus lumpectomy) that the physicians themselves feel uncomfortable explaining to the patient their own uncertainty about the relative efficacy of the treatments.

ETHICS OF CLINICAL TRIALS

The idea that somehow there may be an adversary relationship between patient and physician in the course of the performance of a randomized clinical trial as opposed to the "supportive" relationship which exists between patient and physician when the latter "chooses the best treatment" for the patient in our minds is not a rational one. A physician is obligated to do the best he can for his patient within the limits of his knowledge. If he does not know, he can make an educated guess. Why should guessing what is best for an individual patient under the guise of personalized treatment be more ethical than performing a well-designed clinical trial that will have the added benefit of providing data that will render guessing no longer necessary? As Roy (17) points out, the concept of "physician versus clinical investigator" as a polarized relationship is antithetical to the conduct of reasonable ethical discourse on the subject of clinical trials.

A properly designed clinical trial should offer reasonable therapy to all groups of patients and should be closely monitored. The legal requirements (18) are that the risk–benefit ratio be reasonable, that the investigator obtain outside review before doing the research, and that informed consent be obtained. The scientific requirements are that the trial be designed in such a way that there will be accrual of valid and reliable data that lead to useful knowledge while patient welfare is adequately safeguarded. If one is to obtain true informed consent from the patient one must be properly informed oneself about the background and rationale for the trial and about the adequacy of the trial design. This will obviate some of the problems in obtaining consent because one will be comfortable that there is, in fact, a dilemma, a decision that needs to be made about this clinical situation and that the necessary knowledge does not already exist. Some of the difficulty in saying "I don't know" to a patient arises when one feels if one only had done one's homework one would know. But if the answer is really not known, then saying "I do not know" becomes very easy indeed.

REFERENCES

1. The National Commission for the Protection of Human Subjects of Biomedical and Behavioral Research: The Belmont Report: Ethical principles and guidelines for the protection of human subjects of research (1978): DHEW Publ. No. 78-0012. Washington, D.C.
2. Beecher, H. K. (1966): Ethics and clinical research. *N. Engl. J. Med.*, 274:1354–1360.

3. McCarthy, C. (1983): Experience with boards and commissions concerned with research ethics in the United States. In: *Research Ethics*, pp. 111–122. Alan R. Liss, New York.
4. Miller, R. D. (1986): *Problems in Hospital Law*, Chap. 13, pp. 255–286, 5th ed. Aspen, Rockville, Maryland.
5. Code of Federal Regulations. Title 45, Part 46. Protection of Human Subjects.
6. U.S. Public Health Service (1973): Final report of the Tuskegee Syphilis Study Ad Hoc Advisory Panel. U.S. Government Printing Office. Washington, D.C.
7. Link, M. P., Goorin, A. M., Miser, A. W., et al. (1986): The effect of adjuvant chemotherapy on relapse free survival in patients with osteosarcoma of the extremity. *N. Engl. J. Med.*, 314:1600–1606.
8. Herbert, V. (1977): Acquiring new information while retaining old ethics. *Science*, 198:690–692.
9. Robinson, G., and Merav, A. (1977): Informed consent: Recall by patients tested postoperatively. *Ann. Thorac. Surg.*, 22:209–212.
10. Penman, D. T., Holland, J. C., Bahna, G. F., et al. (1984): Informed consent for investigational chemotherapy: Patients' and physicians' perception. *J. Clin. Oncol.*, 2:849–855.
11. Curran, W. J. (1979): Reasonableness and randomization in clinical trials: Fundamental law and governmental regulation. *N. Engl. J. Med.*, 300:1273–1275.
12. Taylor, K. M., Margolese, R. G., and Soskolne, C. L. (1984): Physicians' reasons for not entering eligible patients in a randomized clinical trial of surgery for breast cancer. *N. Engl. J. Med.*, 310:1363–1367.
13. Angell, M. (1984): Patients' preferences in randomized clinical trials. *N. Engl. J. Med.*, 310:1385–1387.
14. Zelen, M. (1979): A new design for randomized clinical trials. *N. Engl. J. Med.*, 300:1242–1245.
15. Zelen, M. (1982): Strategy and alternate randomized designs in cancer clinical trials. *Cancer Treat. Rep.*, 66:1095–1100.
16. Ellenberg, S. (1984): Randomization designs in comparative clinical trials. *N. Engl. J. Med.*, 310:1404–1408.
17. Roy, D. J. (1986): Controlled clinical trials: An ethical imperative. *J. Chronic Dis.*, 39:159–162.
18. Robertson, J. A. (1981): Legal considerations in clinical cancer research. *Semin. Oncol.*, 8:442–445.

CHAPTER 13

Quality Control

A clinical trial is a complex experiment that may require years of effort from many people. Once the scientific question is specifically formulated, it then remains to do the experiment as carefully as possible. The terms "quality control" or "quality assurance" are used to denote in aggregate the procedures that insure reliability of the data.

Quality control is important at an individual institutional level. Unless the procedures for entering patients on study and making measurements are rigorously defined, the data may lack internal consistency; it will then be impossible to know exactly how to interpret results of the study. The potential for certain kinds of variability may, of course, be much less for single institution studies than for group trials; a small and cohesive group of surgeons, for example, are probably more likely to perform the "same" modified radical mastectomy than a much larger group spread all over the country. Nevertheless, the potential problems are there all the same. Quality control procedures have been most rigorously developed and widely disseminated for multiinstitutional group studies to assure reliability and comparability of data across all participating institutions. These procedures are the ones that will be considered here.

Consider the complexity of this task for a moment. A typical comparative study in one of the clinical cooperative groups may involve hundreds of patients at one-to three-dozen institutions, at each of which physicians, nurses, pharmacists and data managers participate actively. Data from institutions get funneled into the statistical center where they are coded, processed, and analyzed collaboratively with the principal investigator(s). Some basic questions that arise are as follows: Were all required baseline, follow-up, and off-study tests performed at the appropriate times? Was the treatment given as specified in the protocol? Have the clinical data been recorded accurately? Do the data in the research record (the flow sheets and/or the computerized data base at the statistical center) accurately reflect the data in the patient's chart or the hospital's service laboratories, or the pharmacist's or nurses' records of administered drug dose?

We shall discuss several steps in this process. First, how does one assure oneself that the participants (the institutions and investigators) are adequately qualified? Next, how are procedures for data gathering properly established both at the institutional level and at the central office? Third, how might properly collected data in therapeutic trials be analyzed? Finally, we shall review briefly the process of external auditing and some of the regulatory aspects of using investigational drugs.

QUALIFICATION OF THE PARTICIPANTS IN A CLINICAL TRIAL

Initial Screening of Institutions

Before it can participate in any cooperative group trial, an institution must demonstrate to the group that it has the proper personnel and facilities. Each cooperative group has its own requirements for eligibility. For multimodal trials each subspecialty must contribute qualified physicians. The effort also requires diverse support personnel such as nurses, pharmacists, and data managers. These individuals must attest to their commitment to the group activities by agreeing to participate in protocol activities, by attending group meetings regularly, by participating in verbal and written communication about protocol design and compliance, and by submitting required records in a timely fashion. In addition, the institution must demonstrate access to sufficient patients for the appropriate studies and a commitment to enter these patients on study. In recent years the National Cancer Institute (NCI) has also required that each cooperative group in its clinical trials network establish written policies and procedures for its affiliate (or satellite) institutions in the community, so that the data from these institutions are also controlled.

Specific facilities may also be reviewed. For radiotherapy the Quality Assurance Review Center (QARC) (1), in addition to reviewing the responsible staff, visits each institution to assess the adequacy of the equipment; the calibration of the instruments is checked by the Radiological Physics Center.

Education of the Participating Investigators

An ongoing intensive educational program is crucial for assuring data quality. Discussions and updates of results on each protocol occur at the twice yearly or more frequent group meetings. In connection with specific trials that involve complex procedures, educational sessions held before the start of the trial and during its course are invaluable in assuring protocol compliance and standardization of protocol procedures. For example, an ongoing National Surgical Adjuvant Breast Project (NSABP) protocol studying the effectiveness of colon cancer adjuvant chemotherapy given via the portal vein was preceded by sessions for the surgical membership in which audiovisual aids were used to demonstrate the proper technique for regional drug administration.

Quality Control in Diagnosis

Many of the cooperative groups now have panels of pathologists who undertake central pathology review of clinical material. An example of the necessity for such reviews is the demonstration of disagreement 15–20% of the time among pathologists as to the subcategory of lung cancer to which a specimen belongs (2,3). For other tumors that are more difficult to classify (e.g., non-Hodgkin's lymphoma), disagreement may reach even higher rates (2). In addition to central pathology review for solid tumors, central reference laboratories have been established (e.g., by the Pediatric Oncology Group) to which leukemia cells are sent for classification with newer diagnostic techniques that might be outside the scope of many of the individual participating institutions.

The advantage to such a review, in addition to standardization, is that it gives an opportunity for pathology research. Analysis of the size of the tumor, histologic pattern of the neoplasm, number of lymph nodes involved, and other features has uncovered valuable information about the prognosis and indications for adjuvant therapy in patients with breast carcinoma in the NSABP (4). In the Wilms' tumor study, new pathologic subtypes of anaplastic and sarcomatous variants of Wilms' tumor were discovered to be prognostically important (5). This type of analysis could not be performed without access to larger quantities of material than is usually available from a single institution. The results are often disseminated back to the individual institutions as valuable teaching material. Admittedly these reviews are often quite time consuming, and therefore cannot often be used prospectively as a stratification factor.

DATA COLLECTION AND SUBMISSION AT THE INSTITUTIONAL LEVEL

Each protocol has specific requirements for patient eligibility, and for the monitoring of treatment and toxicity. Most of them have special forms and flow sheets that must be completed. The overall responsibility for this activity rests with the physician, but much of the record keeping may be done by a data manager.

A description of the data management procedures in one cooperative group, the Eastern Cooperative Oncology Group (ECOG) has recently been published (6). In this group each data manager is specially trained, there are numerous workshops held for data managers at all levels, and an extensive Data Managers' Manual describes the group's policies and procedures in this area. The completion of necessary forms and flow sheets is the responsibility of the data manager and the physician. Before any material is sent to the central office, certain protocol items must be reviewed by the institutional data managers. These include patient eligibility; checks on treatment administration; a review of the records to be kept, especially specific forms for specific diseases; and a table of parameters to be followed. The importance of properly trained and motivated data managers in scheduling the required procedures and treatments, as well as in proper record keeping cannot be overstated. The data manager may also be responsible for the retrieval of the specific records from all departments within the hospital. This can be particularly important when the reports come from departments other than those of the principal investigator.

The data manager makes sure that the appropriate data have been submitted to the central office. For the QARC, this will include the documents that allow the central office to assess the irradiated volume as well as the treatment dosimetry (7). Simulator films, port films, and some of the initial diagnostic clinical films as well as a photocopy of the patient's radiotherapy treatment chart are submitted, tailored to the needs of each protocol. Although the amount of material required for submission is considerable, with practice good compliance can be achieved. The QARC found that within 5 years of the introduction of their monitoring system, the percent of complete data submission rose from 20 to > 90% (1).

DATA MANAGEMENT AT THE CENTRAL OFFICE

Once submitted to the central office the data are reviewed by statistical office data managers, the biostatistical staff, and the principal investigator of the study. Data managers at the statistical center are generally assigned to individual studies. They check submitted forms for completeness, consistency, and accuracy. For some radiotherapy protocols, treatment is reviewed at a different central office (QARC) (1). Protocols are filed with this Center and their requirements entered into a computer. Comparisons can then be made as to whether the treated volume and the dose rate and amount were given as called for by the protocol (7). In this case the reviewers include a radiotherapist and a medical physicist.

Either the protocol chairman or the statistical office or both can generate, if necessary, query letters to the institutions. Both the data manager and the computer check compliance on drug doses, monitor blood counts, and evaluate toxicity as reports come in. Other specific reviews may be required as appropriate. For example, a study that calls for the assessment of drug levels may require another level of review. Computer checks can be performed to assure that data are complete, that each data element not falling within a reasonable range is flagged, and that data are internally consistent. For example, a height of 36 cm is very unlikely for any one not on a pediatric study and is certainly not consistent with a weight of 140 kg. Other checks can be incorporated into the system as appropriate. For a pediatric study lasting several years, one might want to reassess body size and m^2 at least yearly.

Of major importance to the quality of the data is timeliness. The Statistical Center produces regular requests for outstanding data as well as reports of institutional performance in timeliness of data submission. Although data on extremely active studies may be requested every 3 months, most are requested every 6 months, to correspond with the preparation of reports for group meetings; a few may be requested at even less frequent intervals. For certain types of data and interventions, it is possible to detect mistakes as the trial is ongoing and provide rapid feedback to the investigator so that the mistake can be corrected. During the delivery of radiotherapy, for example, port or simulation films can be assessed centrally and errors called to the attention of the treating radiotherapist before a significant fraction of the total dose has been given (7). In the QARC program this kind of real-time notification of infraction has been worthwhile. As investigators were notified of their failure to comply with specific protocols, the incidence of major deviations fell from 35% to 5% (1).

Even if certain types of errors cannot be corrected by ongoing surveillance techniques in real time, it is important to characterize the extent to which they occurred in a protocol, so that these deviations from the planned protocol can form part of the assessment of the overall therapeutic strategy. What were the extent and types of major and minor violations in the execution of the study? How many patients were inevaluable for the major endpoints? One cannot evaluate the scientific validity of the study without such information.

DATA ANALYSIS

Assessing the Amount of Therapy Administered

It must be emphasized that these issues are of much more than regulatory interest. Consider the question of administered dose: Was the patient in fact given the prescribed dose at the prescribed time and via the prescribed route? If these data have been adequately collected, then it should be possible to calculate what *proportion* of the proposed medication was given. For example, if the protocol called for 4 weekly doses of 1.5 mg/m^2 of vincristine, and the patient, because he developed ileus, had one dose delayed 1 week and was then given a half dose, the 4-week dose would be only 3.75 mg/m^2 instead of the required 6 mg/m^2, or the total induction dose (assuming that the final dose of vincristine was eventually given) would be 5.25 mg/m^2 as opposed to 6 mg/m^2. It is important to report the fraction of each drug administered, and how this fraction was calculated. One might choose to report the above data by saying that the patient received $5.25/6 = (88\%)$ of the prescribed total dose of vincristine. This summary of the administered dose will help in comparing the results of one trial with another or even in comparing the amounts of therapy administered to different patient groups. One method of comparing the amount of drug administered to different groups of patients is to construct a comparison of dose per unit time for different schedules of the same drugs (8).

Patient Compliance

Variations in compliance can cause variable results in a clinical trial. The extent of compliance cannot even be evaluated if data are not properly collected. Compliance means following both the intervention regimen and trial procedures (e.g., clinic visits, laboratory procedures, taking prescribed medications, and filling out forms) (9). Any clinical trial is likely to have less than 100% compliance. People tend to forget, they develop side effects, and they change their minds regarding participation. Compliance can be improved by educating the subject and the family about the nature and importance of the trial and by making the trial as simple as possible.

One of the most difficult areas to assess properly is what oral medication the patient has taken at home. This is partly because the information is often not well recorded in the flow sheets and partly because the patient, once he leaves the hospital, often does not take the suggested medication. A check on whether or not the patient has taken his medication can be made via pill count or patient diary, though the reliability of these techniques is questionable. Compliance can also be measured by looking at the blood levels of the appropriate medication. Smith et al. (10) measured urine 17-ketogenic steroids in patients who were supposed to be taking prednisone. They found that 33% of patients who by protocol and instruction were supposed to be receiving prednisone were not complying. Separate analysis of adolescents revealed an even more alarming 59% noncompliance rate. It is not surprising that compliance may vary within patient groups in the same study, and this factor may need to be taken into account when subset analysis is performed. Measurement of drug levels can also be useful to determine whether patients are taking drug who should *not* be taking it. In a study of aspirin versus placebo for prevention of myocardial infarction, urine salicylate levels were measured both in the group randomized to receive aspirin (around 87% positive) and in the group randomized to placebo (around 4% positive) (9).

Another important reason for measuring patient compliance is that patient behavior may, in and of itself, represent a prognostic factor without any obvious pharmacologic explanation. The study by the coronary Drug Project Research Group (11), in which patients who took their placebo faithfully had a lower incidence of heart attacks compared with those who did not, has already been discussed.

SYSTEMATIC VARIABILITY IN INSTITUTIONAL PERFORMANCE

Once data have been collected at the central office one can assess whether or not there are significant deviations in results from one institution to another. Any such differences might be due to differences in the prevalence of key prognostic factors; for example, if one institution sees only patients on referral, then it might see only patients well enough to survive the trip or, on the other hand, only patients sick enough to make their physicians willing to refer them.

On the other hand, one might also find that systematic variations in the percentage of drug administered by different institutions occur because of differences in institutional philosophy. Buyse (12) analyzed a multicenter Phase III trial in which all institutions were to give cyclophosphamide, methotrexate, and 5-fluorouracil at the same doses. He found that four institutions varied from one in which no patient received < 50% of the projected full dose of methotrexate to another in which nearly half the patients received < 50% of the projected dose. The dosage of other drugs was also similarly less in the latter institution. The exact factors which led to this variation were not immediately obvious, but they were consistent from one institution to the next and they were not related to patient prognostic factors. This is the type of systematic variation that quality control procedures are designed to detect and help explain.

Toxicity reporting may also vary from institution to institution. Figure 13.1 (12) shows the proportion of patients for whom side effects or toxicities to a new chemotherapeutic agent were reported in a multicenter Phase II study involving 15 European institutions. Institution A systematically reports fewer cases with toxicity than all the other institutions; perhaps surprisingly, this is true of both hematologic and nonhematologic toxicities. Conversely, in institution B, there is a relative over-reporting of cases with toxicity. Note that institutions A and B entered, respectively, 28 and 31 patients in the study (out of a total of 111 patients) and were the two major participants, hence the wide differences in percentages are not just due to small denominators. Multivariate analyses showed that these differences were not attributable to apparent variations in the patient population (age, extent of disease, etc.) or in the treatment administration. It seems likely, therefore, that these differences actually reflect differences in reporting rather than differences in true toxicity. One feature that may have contributed to some of the variability is that the most frequent toxicities of this particular drug were gastrointestinal and therefore difficult to quantitate. It is important that there be a minimal subjective component in assigning a grade to a toxicity.

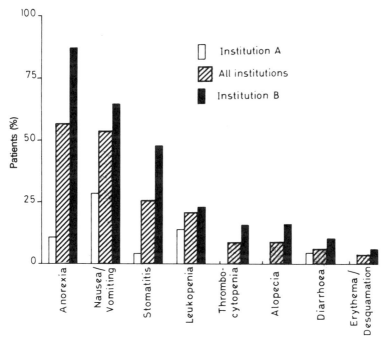

FIG. 13.1. Percentages of patients with various toxicities in two institutions, A and B, compared with all institutions participating in a multicenter trial (12).

WHAT CONSTITUTES A DEVIATION?

Just as it is important to define the level of difference from normal function that will be called "toxicity," an investigator must decide, in advance, what level of departure from the prescribed course of treatment will be called "deviation." For a number of studies, more than 10% variation between the dose of chemotherapy prescribed by protocol and the dose administered is considered a major deviation (13). For the QARC studies a minor deviation was defined as ± 5% and major as ± 10% beyond the radiation dose required in the protocol (1). As with other measurements, one must be sure that the amount of variance that is considered a deviation is indeed detectable. For example, if patients were taking one-half a scored tablet daily, a 10% variation in dose would be impossible to detect without weighing the pieces.

Methods of Educating Investigators

No monitoring program will be effective if the data cannot be translated into something that changes an investigator's behavior. We have already noted that informing investigators that their normal practices or reports are inadequate has a marked impact on behavior. Martin et al. (14) attempted to reduce the ordering of laboratory and radiology tests by medical residents in their first postgraduate year. They divided the residents into three groups and compared the effects of concurrent chart review and discussion in one group with the effect of a moderate financial incentive for limited ordering of tests in a second group. The third group of residents served as a concurrent control. Chart review produced the most dramatic (47%) and sustained reduction. The financial incentive seemed to be of no value when the testing pattern of this group was compared with that of the control group. Thus, perhaps the "stick" of being embarrassed before your colleagues if you don't do things properly is more important than the "carrot" of modest reimbursement.

REGULATORY ASPECTS

Federal Regulations and Definition of Terms

The Kefauver Amendment (1962) to the Food, Drug and Cosmetic Act of 1938 states that a drug may not be introduced into interstate commerce until it has been proven to be safe and effective for its intended use (15). The determination of whether a drug has proven to be safe and effective rests with the Food and Drug Administration (FDA). Before this has been established, the drug is considered investigational. Any organization or individual seeking to sponsor clinical trials with such drugs must first apply to the FDA for permission.

The FDA grants this permission by issuing a Notice of Clinical Exemption for an Investigational New Drug, often referred to as an IND. The sponsor can then conduct trials with the new agent or authorize others to conduct trials on its behalf. The sponsor, however, must see to it that all trials performed under its aegis are done in accordance with FDA regulation. The sponsor also has overall responsibility for formulating and executing the development plans for the new agent.

Although INDs are sometimes held by individuals, it is much more common for sponsors to be large organizations, such as pharmaceutical firms or the NCI. If you wish to perform clinical trials with an investigational agent, you must submit your request to the sponsor. Each sponsor has its own procedures for reviewing and approving such requests. Current NCI policies and procedures are summarized in its *Investigators Handbook* (16). When the submitted protocol has been approved, the sponsor supplies its investigator with a clinical brochure, which contains information about the preclinical and clinical characteristics of the new agent.

Once a sponsor considers that all the requirements to demonstrate safety and efficacy of an agent in a particular tumor type have been met, it may submit all the data to the FDA in the form of a new drug application (NDA). In the case of a biological product, this document is called a Product Licensing Application (PLA). Approval by the FDA means that the new agent may be sold commercially and advertised for the approved indications.

On-site Monitoring

As part of its responsibility to insure the integrity of its clinical trials, the sponsor conducts site visits at participating institutions. This aspect of quality assurance, though expensive and time consuming for all concerned, is an essential part of the process of data verification. Although the site visit programs of various sponsors differ in detail, all of them have the same general goals, which we shall outline below. The frequency of these site visits depends somewhat on the type of study. For trials that will be pivotal in a pharmaceutical company's NDA or PLA, however, a frequency of one visit per institution every 6–8 weeks is not unusual.

The NCIs monitoring program for the cooperative groups began in the late 1970s as certain events, including one widely publicized instance of data falsification, gave investigators, the NCI, and the FDA much cause for concern. This episode led the ECOG to set up a site-visit monitoring program of its own. The NCI then broadened the requirement for site-visit monitoring to include the entire cooperative group program. In the 1977 recommendations, the FDA also mandated site visits by all sponsors of INDs (15).

In the case of the cooperative groups, the NCI has delegated the responsibility for organizing and conducting these site visits to the groups themselves. Visits are conducted by teams of peers selected from the group membership on a rotating basis. Representatives from the NCI attend about 10–20% of the site visits (13). All cooperative group members are audited at least once every 3 years on a random basis.

The purposes of the on-site audit are several. First, they verify data by comparing the research record with the hospital chart and other primary sources. Unfortunately, in 1982 during routine audits of affiliate institutions, two separate cooperative groups found that two affiliates had submitted falsified data. A total of 56 patient cases was misrepresented (13). The groups immediately dropped the affiliates and expunged all data submitted by them. These occurrences highlighted the need for periodic checks to assure that the data submitted to the statistical offices of the groups has a basis in reality. The auditors also check research data, such as patient eligibility data and tumor response data, to assure that the assessment of the auditors agrees with that of the investigators in the primary institution.

Another element of the on-site audit is to look into institutional practices regarding human subjects' protection. Is there evidence that the execution of the study was accompanied by the necessary steps to insure full protection of the study participants, as mandated by federal and local regulations? Was the protocol approved by the Institutional Review Board? Was informed consent obtained appropriately before the patient was enrolled on study? In the course of the monitoring program (1982–1984) the percentage of institutions having $> 30\%$ of protocols not submitted to their review boards fell from 20 to 6 (13).

Compliance with the sponsor's drug accountability system is also examined at the site visit. Since the sponsor is legally responsible for the uses to which experimental agents distributed under its aegis are put, most sponsors have implemented a drug accountability system to assure that experimental drugs have been given only to patients on the protocols for which the agents are authorized. This is an area in which documentation is harder to cite, but it appears that about 15% of major institutions had some difficulty in this area during recent audits.

The NCI has recently assessed the initial experience with site-visit monitoring in the cooperative groups (13). Overall, about 10–15% of major institutions have had severe enough infractions that repeated site visits were required, and about another 5% were placed on probation or dropped. Of affiliate institutions in the first year, around 20% required a second site visit and another 20% were suspended or dropped. By the third year there had been an improvement in the performance of affiliate institutions with no suspensions or probations. This may have been the result of either increased educational efforts by the groups or the voluntary dropping of many affiliates that were poor performers.

Perhaps the most important function of the site-visit monitoring program is an educational one. The individuals who are doing the monitoring at every level, including study chairmen and site visit auditors, are themselves group members. As they become involved in supervising others, they become more familiar both with regulatory requirements and with many of the potential pitfalls in clinical trials methodology. In addition, once a realistic assessment of the sources of error in the implementation of a particular protocol has been made, this information can be used to assist the investigator in writing better, more standardized, unambiguous, internally consistent protocols that can be adhered to more easily.

Quality assurance efforts can have more specific benefits relative to scientific and medical issues as well. The monitoring program of one cooperative group, for example, found that assessment of response of lung cancer patients by audited investigators varried significantly from that of the audit teams. This led to a general reevaluation of the criteria for these studies within the group (13).

Analysis of the infractions may lead to useful information about how to improve patient treatment. In one QARC analysis of a protocol (CALGB 7611) in which some patients were to receive cranial radiation as "prophylaxis" against central nervous system (CNS) leukemia, it was discovered that the majority of infractions were related to treating the patient with the head facing sideways, rather than face up as was required by the protocol. The usual error consisted of excessive blocking of radiation doses to the orbit. Identification of this systematic error, which occurred in about half the cases, highlighted the changes required for better treatment in future protocols (17).

Another QARC review of radiotherapy for limited small cell carcinoma of the lung found a variation in doses administered to different patients because of differences in shielding techniques. When 3500–3800 cGy were given, 8/10 cases had an in-field recurrence; at 3800–4000 cGy, 15/32 cases failed in the chest. At 4100–4400 cGy, 10/32 patients failed locally. Of the 14 cases who received 4400 cGy, no in-field failures occurred. A dose–response curve for small cell carcinoma of the lung has been derived from these data and incorporated into the next study (18).

Unacceptable Levels of Performance

Most clinical trials groups set limits for acceptability of data below which group participation will not be permitted until the situation is remedied. In the ECOG (6), failure to reply to more than 20% of the biennial requests for delinquent data lead to suspension of randomization privileges for that institution. Once this measure was put into place, the percentage of outstanding forms fell from 36 to 3%.

Noncompliance with group requirements for data quality that are not responsive to educational measures can lead to suspension of an institution's privileges to enter patients on group studies. Lack of attention to the rules regarding human subjects' protection may also jeopardize a member's standing in a group and lead to an investigation by the Office for Protection from Research Risks (OPRR) of the National Institutes of Health (NIH). Improper use of investigational agents can result in the suspension or revocation of an investigator's FD 1573, the form establishing that the investigator is legally authorized to administer experimental agents. An investigator found to have submitted fraudulent data to an NIH sponsored study is liable to disbarment from funding by Department of Health and Human Services.

The site-visit monitoring program has found that these kinds of serious offenses against good clinical trials practice and federal regulation are very uncommon indeed. As noted previously (13), however, evidence of less than meticulous clinical trials practice is not uncommon. Early indications are that the educational efforts of the entire quality assurance effort are resulting in a measurable improvement in clinical trials data.

Reporting of Adverse Events

An important responsibility of sponsors is the qualitative and quantitative assessment of the toxicities of a new agent. What kinds of toxicities can a new agent produce? What is the incidence of the various toxic manifestations of a new drug? In addition, when new and unexpected toxicities are observed, the sponsor must disseminate the information as quickly as possible to its investigators, in order to insure the safety of patients on clinical trials. These goals are obviously impossible to fulfill without accurate and timely reporting of adverse events by the investigators to the sponsor.

NCI's requirements for the reporting of adverse reactions to investigational agents under its sponsorship are outlined in Table 13.1. Special forms are provided from the NCI for this type of reporting. These reports do not languish unexamined in some anonymous government file cabinet. They are looked at carefully with the intent of establishing whether the relationship between drug administration and the

TABLE 13.1. *Requirements for reporting adverse reactions to agents in trials sponsored by the Division of Cancer Treatment, NCI[a]*

Phase I Studies

a. All life-threatening events (Grade 4) which may be due to drug administration.	Report by phone to IDB within 24 hr. Written report to follow within 10 working days.[b]
All fatal events while on study.	
b. First occurrence of any toxicity (regardless of grade).	Report by phone to IDB drug monitor within 24 hr. A written report may be required.

Phase II and III Studies

Unknown reaction		Known reaction	
Grades 2–3	Grades 4 and 5	Grades 1–3	Grades 4 and 5
Written report to IDB within 10 working days.[b]	Report by phone to IDB within 24 hr. Written report to follow within 10 working days.	Not to be reported as ADRs. These toxicities should be submitted as part of study summary.	Written report to IDB within 10 working days. (Grade 4 myelosuppression not to be reported.) Aplasia in leukemia patients.

[a]Adapted from official form. Special form to report ADRs with DCT sponsored agents.
[b]Report to: Investigational Drug Branch, P.O. Box 30012, Bethesda, Maryland, 20814. 24-hr telephone number: 301-496-7957.
ADR, adverse reaction; DCT, Division of Cancer Treatment; IDB, Investigational Drug Branch.

adverse reaction is highly likely, probable, possible, or unlikely. These data become a part of the total experience with an agent and may figure importantly in the execution of an agent's development plan. Commercial sponsors will have similar requirements.

Examples of new toxicities that appeared unexpectedly in "repeat Phase I trials" at high doses of old drugs have been given in Chapter 3. Other toxicities may come as the result of the simultaneous or sequential administration of several medications. The increase in CNS toxicity of chemotherapy, particularly with methotrexate (MTX), when given to individuals who have already had cranial radiation, is well known. A recent surprising life-threatening toxicity was reported when MTX and the non-steroidal antiinflammatory, ketoprofen, was given (19). Four cycles of MTX administration were characterized by severe toxicity which was fatal in 3 cases. Simultaneous administration of ketoprofen was found to be associated with prolonged and striking enhancement of serum MTX levels. This association, once noted, was rapidly published and disseminated by the NCI to all investigators working with high-dose MTX. It is this ability for rapid dispersal of the knowledge about toxicity to all involved individuals (because they are listed as investigators) which makes the centralized reporting of this sort of data so important even if the drug being studied is commercially available.

APPLICATION TO SINGLE INSTITUTIONS

The impressive and effective series of quality assurance measures in place in the cooperative groups has only fragmentary and occasional representation within single centers for nongroup studies. Admittedly, institutions differ widely in the attention they pay, as institutions, to setting up the kinds of centralized, shared resources necessary to exert a positive effect on data quality. In recent years, a few centers have set up centralized patient registration procedures, centralized data management, and an institutional protocol office. This healthy trend ought to expand in the next few years, so that assurances of the quality of data from single center trials will be at least as strong as those of the cooperative groups.

CONCLUSIONS

Quality assurance or quality control programs have been instituted since the 1970s to assure that study participants are qualified, that data are properly collected and consistent from one investigator or institution to the next, and that errors, when they occur, can be detected and analyzed so that something is learned from them. Data are monitored at three levels—the individual institution, the central reference office for the appropriate modality or group, and through on-site audits at the individual institutions. Both major (rare) and minor (relatively common) infractions have been detected, but in general, as investigators become more conscious of the issues involved, their performance is improving. In fact, one report recently described a "learning curve" for clinical investigators showing gradual improvement in compliance with repeated use of a protocol (20).

REFERENCES

1. Glicksman, A. S., Reinstein, L. E., McShan, D., and Laurie, F. (1981): Radiotherapy quality assurance program in a cooperative group. *Int. J. Radiat. Oncol. Biol. Phys.*, 7:1561–1568.
2. Kempson, R. L. (1985): Pathology quality control in the cooperative clinical cancer trial programs. *Cancer Treat. Rep.*, 69:1207–1210.
3. Feinstein, A. R., Gelfman, N. A., and Yesner, R. (1970): Observer variability in the histopathologic diagnosis of lung cancer. *Am. Rev. Respir. Dis.*, 101:671–684.
4. Fisher, E. R., Fisher, B., Sass, R., and Wickerham, L. (1984): Pathologic findings from the National Surgical Adjuvant Breast Project (Protocol No. 4), XI. Bilateral breast cancer. *Cancer*, 54:3002–3011.
5. Beckwith, J. B. (1983): Wilms' tumor and other renal tumors of childhood. A selective review from the National Wilms' Tumor Study Pathology Center. *Hum. Pathol.*, 14:481–492.
6. Wolter, J. M. (1985): Quality assurance in a cooperative group. *Cancer Treat. Rep.*, 69:1189–1193.
7. Reinstein, L. E., McShan, D., and Glicksman, A. S. (1982): A dosimetry review system for cooperative group research. *Med. Phys.*, 9:240–249.
8. Hryniuk, W., and Bush, H. (1984): The importance of dose intensity in chemotherapy of metastatic breast cancer. *J. Clin. Oncol.*, 2:1281–1288.
9. Friedman, L. M., Furberg, C. D., and DeMets, D. L. (1982): *Fundamentals of Clinical Trials.* John Wright, PSG, Boston.
10. Smith, S. D., Rosen, D., Trueworthy, R. C., and Lowman, J. T. (1979): A reliable method for evaluating drug compliance in children with cancer. *Cancer*, 43:169–173.
11. The Coronary Drug Project Research Group (1980): Influence of adherence to treatment and response of cholesterol on mortality in the coronary drug project. *N. Engl. J. Med.*, 303:1038–1041.
12. Buyse, M. E. (1984): Quality control in multi-centre cancer clinical trials. In: *Cancer Clinical Trials: Methods and Practice*, edited by M. E. Buyse, M. J. Staquet, and R. J. Sylvester, pp. 102–123. Oxford University Press, Oxford.
13. Mauer, J. K., Hoth, D. F., Macfarlane, D. K., et al. (1985): Site visit monitoring program of the clinical cooperative groups: Results of the first 3 years. *Cancer Treat. Rep.*, 69:1177–1187.
14. Martin, A. R., Wolf, M. A., Thibodeau, L. A., et al. (1980): A trial of two strategies to modify test ordering behavior of medical residents. *N. Engl. J. Med.*, 303:1330–1336.
15. A Brief Legislative History of the Food, Drug, and Cosmetic Act (1974): U.S. Government Printing Office 26-062, Washington, D.C.
16. Investigators' Handbook (1986): Cancer Therapy Evaluation Program, Division of Cancer Treatment, National Cancer Institute, Bethesda, Maryland.
17. Reinstein, L. E., Maddock, P., Landmann, C., et al. (1982): The effect of patient position on radiotherapy protocol deviations in the treatment of acute lymphocytic leukemia. *Am. J. Clin. Oncol.*, 5:303–306.
18. Glicksman, A. S., Reinstein, L. E., and Laurie, F. (1985): Quality assurance of radiotherapy in clinical trials. *Cancer Treat. Rep.*, 69:1199–1206.
19. Thyss, A., Milano, G., Kubar, J., et al. (1986): Clinical and pharmacokinetic evidence of a life-threatening interaction between methotrexate and ketoprofen. *Lancet*, i:256–258.
20. Michelson, S., and Glicksman, S. A. (*submitted*): Provider adherence and learning: Issues in a study design, performance, and analysis.

CHAPTER 14

Reporting a Trial

In this chapter we consider some of the issues that arise when one is preparing either to report a completed trial or to evaluate an already published report. A number of journals have published formal guidelines for prospective authors concerning reports of clinical trials (1,2). The guidelines of Simon and Wittes (1) are given as Table 14.1. These were originally adopted by the editorial board of *Cancer Treatment Reports* where they first appeared. They have subsequently been adopted by the *Journal of Clinical Oncology*, *Cancer*, and the *American Journal of Clinical Oncology* as well as several journals published abroad.

Many of these guidelines relate to matters of trial design, so that mistakes, if made early on, cannot be rectified by improving the final report. An analysis of clinical trials reported in four journals (3) and a separate analysis of a series of randomized controlled clinical trials of breast cancer published before July, 1984 (4) found many deficiencies. The most frequent included the description of patient eligibility or the patient population which was adequate less than half the time. Loss to follow-up and withdrawals were discussed in the majority of papers, but only 41% of the breast cancer studies included all patients in the analyses. The report of side effects was adequate in only 64% and 52% of the series. Statistical methods were often poorly described. The description of the randomization process was adequate in only 19% of the reports; only 16% of the breast cancer studies in reporting major endpoints gave both the *p* values and the statistics from which they had been calculated so that the reader could make an independent check. Formal discussion of the power of completed studies was rare. It appeared that the involvement of a biostatistician in the research team was positively associated with the improvement of the internal validity (i.e., the quality of design and execution of the study), but not of the external validity (defined as the presentation of the information required to determine the generalizability of the study). The general lesson of such methodological surveys of the literature is that there is ample room for improvement.

The customary format of a paper that presents new results consists of a Summary, Introduction, Materials and Methods, Results, and Discussion, usually in that order. These divisions are useful because they structure the presentation and facilitate the reader's efforts to locate information quickly. Papers published in abbreviated "Brief Report" formats contain the same kind of information but often telescoped into combined categories (e.g., "Results and Discussion").

TABLE 14.1. *Methodologic guidelines for reports of clinical trials*

---

1. Patients studied should be adequately described. Applicability of conclusions to other patients should be dealt with carefully. Claims of subset-specific treatment differences must be carefully documented statistically as more than the random results of multiple-subset analyses.
2. All patients registered on study should be accounted for. The report should specify for each treatment the number of patients who were not eligible, who died or withdrew before treatment began. The distribution of follow-up times should be described for each treatment, and the number of patients lost to follow-up should be given.
3. Authors should discuss briefly the quality control methods used to ensure that the data are complete and accurate. A reliable procedure should be cited for ensuring that all patients entered on study are actually reported on. If no such procedures are in place, their absence should be noted. Any procedures employed to ensure that assessment of major endpoints is reliable should be mentioned (e.g., second-party review of responses) or their absence noted.
4. The study should not have an inevaluability rate for major endpoints of > 15%. Not more than 15% of eligible patients should be lost to follow-up or considered inevaluable for response due to early death, protocol violation, missing information, etc.
5. In randomized studies, the report should include a comparison of survival and/or other major endpoints for all eligible patients as randomized, that is, with no exclusions other than those not meeting eligibility criteria.
6. The sample size should be sufficient to either establish or conclusively rule out the existence of effects of clinically meaningful magnitude. For "negative" results in therapeutic comparisons, the adequacy of sample size should be demonstrated by either presenting confidence limits for true treatment differences or calculating statistical power for detecting differences. For uncontrolled Phase II studies, a procedure should be in place to prevent the accrual of an inappropriately large number of patients, when the study has shown the agent to be inactive.
7. Authors should state whether there was an initial target sample size and, if so, what it was. They should specify how frequently interim analyses were performed and how the decisions to stop accrual and report results were arrived at.
8. All claims of therapeutic efficacy should be based on explicit comparisons with a specific control group, except in special circumstances where each patient is his own control. If nonrandomized controls are used, the characteristics of the patients should be presented in detail and compared with those of the experimental group. Potential sources of bias should be adequately discussed. Comparison of survival between responders and nonresponders does not establish efficacy and should not generally be included. Reports of Phase II trials that draw conclusions about antitumor activity but not therapeutic efficacy generally do not require a control group.
9. The methods of statistical analysis should be described in detail sufficient that a knowledgeable reader could reproduce the analysis if the data were available.

From Ref. 1.

When actually setting about to write a paper, however, many authors find it easiest to start with the Materials and Methods section and describe how the study was conducted. The Results section then presents the data and the statistical analysis. The observations should be organized in a way that illuminates the points to be considered later in the Discussion. The Summary and the Introduction will then be relatively easy to write, once the author is thoroughly familiar not only with what the data show but also with what he or she wishes to emphasize about the data.

MATERIALS AND METHODS

The materials and methods of the study must be described in sufficient detail that the reader could reproduce the study. In essence, this section tells the reader how the experiment was done. Without a clear and complete description, the results will be uninterpretable.

Materials and Methods sections of clinical trials reports must describe the nature of the disease studied, the criteria employed for diagnosis, whether or not there was central review of the pathology, the criteria used for staging and patient eligibility, and the population base from which the patients were selected. As we have stated before, without this information it will be impossible to decide how generalizable the results might be, and no single reader will be able to decide whether the results as reported are likely to be applicable to his or her own patients. Important characteristics of the patient population, such as demographic features, the amount of prior therapy, and extent of disease, should be included as part of the description.

The reporting of the protocol treatment plan should be outlined in sufficient detail that the therapy can be duplicated by another physician. If the written protocol provided for a deescalation or escalation of dose(s) as a function of toxicity, details of the dose modification criteria should be given (2). The study design should be outlined and a schema is often helpful to the reader.

The definition of the endpoints used in the study must be clear. Response criteria should always be either precisely defined in the text or reference made to standard previously published criteria. Any procedures employed to ensure that assessment of major endpoints is reliable should be mentioned (e.g., second-party review of responses) or their absence noted (1).

The methods for selecting treatments must be well described. If the patients were randomized, then the technique of randomization should be detailed. As we have noted elsewhere in this text, there are acceptable and unacceptable ways to "randomize" patients, and the reader deserves to know exactly how treatment allocation was made.

The methods used to analyze the data must also be described or referenced in such a way that a knowledgeable reader could reproduce the analysis.

Authors should also state whether there was an initial target sample size and, if so, what it was. They should specify how frequently interim analyses were performed and how the decisions to stop accrual and report results were arrived at (1).

RESULTS

The distinction between Materials and Methods and Results is often somewhat arbitrary. In general, Materials and Methods describe what you planned to do; Results describes what happened when you did the experiment.

The patient sets and subsets studied are usually described under Materials and Methods. If, however, a particular subset analysis is going to be undertaken, then the subsets to be analyzed should be described under results. It should be reemphasized that retrospective subset analysis based on response (e.g., the comparison of survival between responders and nonresponders) should not be performed as a way of demonstrating efficacy of treatment (5). If there is more than one important subset of patients, for example, if more than one diagnosis is included in the trial, then response must be reported for each subset. It is most frustrating to be told, "Eleven patients with brain tumors were treated, 9 with glioma and 2 with ependymoma. There were 3 responders," when one is trying to estimate response rates for either glioma or ependymoma separately.

In describing the results of treatment, the description of the therapy actually received by patients must be given. We have discussed at some length in Chapter 13 the fact that the doses as written in the protocol may not always be given to patients. Summary measures such as average relative intensity, average dose per course, proportion of patients receiving incomplete courses, proportion of patients receiving full doses, and average number of courses should be provided (2). It should also be made clear whether the doses were changed according to the toxicity criteria spelled out in the protocol (which have been described under Materials and Methods) or whether unanticipated factors arose which required dosage modification, such as patient refusal to take doses for symptoms that would not have been deemed dangerous by the physicians designing the trial.

The endpoints have already been described in Materials and Methods. In Results the endpoints are compared, and the follow-up period for the patients should be given separately for each treatment. Although claims for activity may be made from an uncontrolled Phase II trial, all claims of therapeutic efficacy should be based on explicit comparisons with a specific control group. Analysis should include data from all patients assigned to each treatment group, not just those who received the treatment. An additional analysis may of course be made by patient group according to the treatment received, separate from the analysis of response by treatment assigned. In a well-designed, well-conducted trial there should be no major differences between these two, since the shifting of significant numbers of patients to groups other than the ones to which they were originally assigned implies some systematic flaw in the trial.

Trials in which the endpoints are survival and disease-free survival may have many censored patients for the usual variety of reasons: patient has not experienced an adverse event (relapse or death), death from other causes, irretrievable losses to follow-up. All of these reasons for censoring and the impact of this censoring on the analysis should be described.

As we have noted elsewhere, the sample size should be sufficient to establish or conclusively rule out the existence of effects of clinically meaningful magnitude. For "negative" results in therapeutic comparisons, the adequacy of sample size should be demonstrated either by presenting confidence limits for true treatment differences or by calculating statistical power for detecting differences. One of the most common errors in performing clinical trials is a sample size so small that a "negative" result is really "indeterminate" (6). In addition, the likelihood of a false positive increases with the number of analyses performed (2).

DISCUSSION

This section is comprised of a summary, defense, and discussion of the conclusions drawn from the data presented in Results. The earlier review of the relevant literature, performed when writing the initial background section of the protocol, should be updated and reanalyzed here and presented in the order of the points that you wish to make from your own trial. Here you begin to analyze critically the data presented elsewhere in the literature in light of your own findings. How do the patients studied in other trials compare to yours? Was the toxicity in your study comparable to what has been seen in other trials? If there were differences in either response or toxicity, how can you account for them? Be careful to try to find the most complete and recent report of any trial that you discuss here. Trials reported with ''initial promising results'' in abstract form may no longer show any difference between treatments by the time the formal, final analysis is performed.

You may be able to check the statistical analysis in other papers for yourself or you may need assistance from a biostatistical colleague. In an analysis of statistical techniques used in oncology journals, Hokanson et al. (7) found that 27% of the papers did not contain any description of statistical methods at all.

In the majority of cases, the statistics presented in journal articles have not been reviewed by a statistician other than the statistical coauthor. George (8) surveyed the editors of 98 medical journals and concluded that many editors rely solely on subject matter reviewers to spot problems. He points out that in a survey of one journal (9), over one-third of all papers seen only by a subject matter referee could be rejected on statistical grounds. He also argues that those articles most in need of a statistical review are those in which there are actually very few statistical methods used. Improper application of simple t-tests or chi-square tests is a common flaw in medical papers. Articles requiring or using sophisticated statistical designs or analyses call attention to themselves simply by this use and are more likely to receive a statistical review than articles that use little or no statistical methods. His message to editors is that each paper should receive a statistical review. It is his message to the reader, however, that is most germane to this chapter: If a paper is critical for your understanding of a problem and you don't understand the statistics yourself, get someone who does understand it to go over it with you.

REVIEWING THE LITERATURE

To write a good discussion, one should perform a thorough review of the literature. Since none of us is ever as up to date as we would like to be, this should involve a formal search of the current literature, aided by the several computerized data bases that index the literature. A good description of how to use the library and how to set up one of your own is given by Sackett et al. (10).

We should emphasize here, however, that it is most important to read the articles critically which you are citing. Examples of errors that may occur if this is not done, particularly if the data are from small samples, can include (a) data recycling, in which the same data are included twice or more; and (b) data misreading, in which mistakes frequently occur in quoting the small numbers involved. Hillcoat (11) reviewed and analyzed the reports of the treatment of ovarian cancer with etoposide. All the series were small. He notes one report of 1/6 patients responding. This report originally appeared in two different journals in different languages in 1975. One of the reports was included in a pooled report published in 1979 and then added again to a pooled report published in 1982. The original author performed a review in 1982 as well, in which he added his second report to the previous pooled data, so that the one response he had observed had now been multiplied to 4 (Fig. 14.1). Other data were recycled as well in the final summary report. Although the correct ratio of 8/101 responses is similar to the final one of 18/161, the similarity is fortuitous, as it depends on a similar response rate in the recycled data compared with the true rate (see Fig. 14.1). In this article, Hillcoat also gives several examples of data misreading, such as quoting 1/7 responders instead of 1/6 and citing inaccurate references.

In addition to the problems of inaccurate pooling of data, one must be sure that there has not been inaccurate splitting, such as reporting only a portion of a study with misleading results. Data from a single institution which has participated in a multiinstitutional trial, for example, should never be reported separately as though it were itself a controlled, randomized trial. Aside from the questionable ethics of such an action, the protections against bias conferred by the structure of a concurrent randomized trial are not applicable here, and it is misleading to imply otherwise (12).

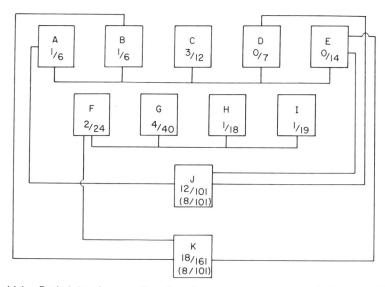

FIG. 14.1. Pooled data from small studies of ovarian carcinoma treated with etoposide. Recycling of data is apparent (11).

Beyond the factors that may lead to confusion in the analysis of literature, the results themselves may simply be confusing. Bailar (13) has written an editorial accompanying two papers published back-to-back in the *New England Journal of Medicine*, each of which appears quite sound in itself, that come to conclusions which are diametrically opposed to one another. He analyzes the possible reasons why this might happen but finally concludes that he "simply cannot tell from present evidence whether (the use of hormonal therapy in the postmenopausal patient) added to the risk of various cardiovascular diseases, diminished the risk, or left it unchanged." Thus, even after a sophisticated review, one may not be able to conclude exactly what the role of a treatment is in the management of a particular disorder from a small number of reports.

One factor contributing to this confusion is the relative unwillingness of editors to publish confirmatory studies, because they are considered unoriginal. One can readily imagine that an article citing a result that contradicts current clinical thinking might have an easier time getting published than one that states facts all clinicians think they already know. Nevertheless, confirmatory clinical reports are important. It is probably also true that positive results have an easier time in the journal peer-review process than negative results, and the investigator himself is more likely to want to describe and submit positive results for publication. Thus, in surveying the literature one should remember that positive responses, or responses that run counter to the general trend of prior observations, are more likely to be published than those that merely confirm the nature and degree of previous responses. This may help explain some confusion, but still will not eliminate it all.

In addition to relying on the analysis of the data presented in an article, Sackett suggests (10) that one should take the track record of the author into account when evaluating the validity of a paper. Perhaps, in the field of oncology, it is equally valid to suggest that the track record of the investigative group should be considered in evaluating a paper.

REFERENCES

1. Simon, R., and Wittes, R. E. (1985): Methodologic guidelines for reports of clinical trials. *Cancer Treat. Rep.*, 69:1–3.
2. Zelen, M. (1983): Guidelines for publishing papers on cancer clinical trials: Responsibilities of editors and authors. *J. Clin. Oncol.*, 1:164–169.
3. DeSimonian, R., Charette, L. J., McPeek, B., and Mosteller, F. (1982): Reporting on methods in clinical trials. *N. Engl. J. Med.*, 306:1332–1336.
4. Liberati, A., Himel, H. N., and Chalmers, T. C. (1986): A quality assessment of randomized control trials of primary treatment of breast cancer. *J. Clin. Oncol.*, 4:942–951.
5. Bertino, J. R. (1986): Guidelines for reporting clinical trials (Editorial). *J. Clin. Oncol.*, 4:1.
6. Frieman, J. A., Chalmers, T. C., Smith, H., Jr., and Keubler, R. R. (1978): The importance of beta, the type II error and sample size in the design and interpretation of the randomized control trial: Survey of 71 "negative" trials. *N. Engl. J. Med.*, 299:690–694.
7. Hokanson, J. A., Luttman, D. J., and Weiss, G. B. (1986): Frequency and diversity of use of statistical techniques in oncology journals. *Cancer Treat. Rep.*, 70:589–594.
8. George, S. L. (1985): Statistics in medical journals: A survey of current policies and proposals for editors. *Med. Pediatr. Oncol.*, 13:109–112.

9. Gardner, M. J., Altman, D. G., Jones, D. R., and Machin, D. (1983): Is the statistical assessment of papers submitted to the *British Medical Journal* effective? *Br. Med. J.*, 286:1485–1488.

10. Sackett, D. L., Haynes, R. B., and Tugwell, P. (1985): *Clinical Epidemiology: A Basic Science for Clinical Medicine*. Little, Brown, Boston.

11. Hillcoat, B. L. (1984): Data recycling and misreading: Two potential errors in pooled data from small studies. *J. Clin. Oncol.*, 2:1047–1049.

12. Green, S. B., Byar, D. P., Strike, T. A., and Walker, M. D. (1981): Proper analysis of clinical trials for malignant glioma. *Cancer Treat. Rep.*, 65:920–922.

13. Bailar, J. C., III. (1985): When research results are in conflict. *N. Engl. J. Med.*, 313:1080–1081.

Subject Index